Springer Optimization and Its Applications

Volume 189

Aims and Scope

Optimization has continued to expand in all directions at an astonishing rate. New algorithmic and theoretical techniques are continually developing and the diffusion into other disciplines is proceeding at a rapid pace, with a spot light on machine learning, artificial intelligence, and quantum computing. Our knowledge of all aspects of the field has grown even more profound. At the same time, one of the most striking trends in optimization is the constantly increasing emphasis on the interdisciplinary nature of the field. Optimization has been a basic tool in areas not limited to applied mathematics, engineering, medicine, economics, computer science, operations research, and other sciences.

The series **Springer Optimization and Its Applications (SOIA)** aims to publish state-of-the-art expository works (monographs, contributed volumes, textbooks, handbooks) that focus on theory, methods, and applications of optimization. Topics covered include, but are not limited to, nonlinear optimization, combinatorial optimization, continuous optimization, stochastic optimization, Bayesian optimization, optimal control, discrete optimization, multi-objective optimization, and more. New to the series portfolio include Works at the intersection of optimization and machine learning, artificial intelligence, and quantum computing.

Volumes from this series are indexed by Web of Science, zbMATH, Mathematical Reviews, and SCOPUS.

More information about this series at https://link.springer.com/bookseries/7393

Antonios Fytopoulos • Rohit Ramachandran
Panos M. Pardalos

Editors

Optimization of Pharmaceutical Processes

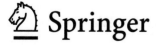 Springer

Editors
Antonios Fytopoulos
Department of Chemical
Engineering, KU Leuven
Leuven, Belgium

School of Chemical Engineering
NTUA, Athens, Greece

Rohit Ramachandran
Department of Chemical and Biochemical
Engineering
Rutgers University
Piscataway, NJ, USA

Panos M. Pardalos (iD)
Department of Industrial and Systems
Engineering
University of Florida
Gainesville, FL, USA

ISSN 1931-6828   ISSN 1931-6836   (electronic)
Springer Optimization and Its Applications
ISBN 978-3-030-90926-0   ISBN 978-3-030-90924-6   (eBook)
https://doi.org/10.1007/978-3-030-90924-6

Mathematics Subject Classification: 49M99, 93A10

This Springer imprint is published by the registered company Springer Nature Switzerland AG
The registered company address is: Gewerbestrasse 11, 6330 Cham, Switzerland

Preface

Although manufacturing industries have made huge achievements in many sectors, in the pharmaceutical sector the need of a more structured approach and better control and optimization of pharmaceutical processes is still the main goal of industry and academia. The demand for better quality, higher yield, more efficient-optimized and green pharmaceutical processes indicates that optimal conditions for production should be applied. Optimization and control methods are very powerful tools and can pave the way towards this direction. However, the application of such methods is not trivial in the pharmaceutical industry, as in a process, many unwanted phenomena can take place compromising total control. Thus, experimental values given in real time and modelling provide the required framework for better under-standing and control of the processes. In this volume, world leading researchers summarize a number of practical applications and methodologies that can help pharmaceutical and chemical engineers apply modelling, optimization and control methodologies in several aspects of pharmaceutical manufacturing.

The book starts with chapter "Process Control and Intensification of Solution Crystallization" that summarizes the design and optimization of solution crystalliza-tion process. In this chapter, topics such as the application of intensification methods and optimization of seeding are discussed among others. In chapter "Method of Characteristics for the Efficient Simulation of Population Balance Models", the method of characteristics (MOCH) is presented as a methodology able to reduce the computational cost of Population Balance Models. Numerical examples that demonstrate the accuracy and efficiency of this method are mentioned.

Chapter "Linearized Parameter Estimation Methods for Modeled Crystallization Phenomena Using In-Line Measurements and Their Application to Optimization of Partially Seeded Crystallization in Pharmaceutical Processes" focusses on the linearized parameter estimation methods coupled with in-line measurements using Process Analytical Technologies. Optimal operating conditions are applied to the case study of partially seeded crystallization of L-arginine. Chapter "Mathematical Modeling of Different Breakage PBE Kernels Using Monte Carlo Simulation Results" covers the modelling of breakage processes. The authors discuss the development of different breakage kernels that can be used in PBMs and their ability to describe different breakage types, such as linear–nonlinear breakage and sonofragmentation.

The book continues with chapter "Optimization of Tablet Coating", where the significance of coating is discussed and different optimization techniques are presented. Chapter "Continuous Twin-Screw Granulation Processing" places the focus on continuous twin screw granulation processing. In this chapter, the advantages of TSG are mentioned and examples of granule optimization achieved by the implementation of QbD approach and PAT monitoring are included.

Chapter "Continuous Powder Feeding: Equipment Design and Material Considerations" covers the continuous feeding of raw materials and highlights its effect on the designing of robust and efficient manufacturing of solid dosage forms, while chapter "Ultrasound for Improved Encapsulation and Crystallization with Focus on Pharmaceutical Applications" gives an overview of the application of ultrasounds as a tool for improved encapsulation and crystallization.

In chapter "Nonsmooth Modeling for Simulation and Optimization of Continuous Pharmaceutical Manufacturing Processes", non-smooth formulation approach is demonstrated for dynamic simulation and optimization of continuous pharmaceutical manufacturing. This powerful method optimizes the overall campaign performance in terms of productivity and yield. Chapter "Integrated Synthesis, Crystallization, Filtration, and Drying of Active Pharmaceutical Ingredients: A Model-Based Digital Design Framework for Process Optimization and Control " is on integrated synthesis, crystallization, filtration and drying of APIs. In this chapter, the authors demonstrate a structured approach for process analysis and optimization of the aforementioned processes based on mathematical models.

Chapter "Fast Model Predictive Control of Modular Systems for Continuous Manufacturing of Pharmaceuticals" introduces methodologies that can be used for the plant-wide optimization and control of nonlinear modular systems. In this chapter, dynamic optimization is used as a tool to determine optimal trajectories for quadratic dynamic matrix control in order to control the plant. In chapter "Dynamic Modeling and Control of a Continuous Biopharmaceutical Manufacturing Plant", a dynamic modelling is used for a continuous biopharmaceutical manufacturing plant. Effectiveness and control are achieved and the method is applied to the case study of lovastatin.

Chapter "Overview of Scheduling Methods for Pharmaceutical Production" reviews the most important scheduling methods for pharmaceutical production. General concepts and challenges are discussed and mathematical programming models are applied to several case studies. Chapter "Model-Based Risk Assessment of mAb Developability" discusses the model-based risk assessment of mAb developability. Optimality in terms of time needed for manufacturing is presented.

Chapter "Design Framework and Tools for Solid Drug Product Manufacturing Processes" describes a design framework for solid drug product production. Simulation-oriented analysis is conducted leading to a more efficient and rational process design. Finally, in chapter "Challenges and Solutions in Drug Product Process Development from a Material Science Perspective" the impact of material attributes on drug production is discussed. Optimal product quality and robustness is proved to be correlated with material science.

We wish to thank all invited contributors and their groups who made this work possible. The editors want also to express their gratitude to the editors of Springer for their guidance and support through the entire project.

Leuven, Belgium   Antonios Fytopoulos
Piscataway, NJ, USA   Rohit Ramachandran
Gainesville, FL, USA   Panos M. Pardalos

Contents

Contributors

Sara Badr Department of Chemical System Engineering, The University of Tokyo, Tokyo, Japan

Massimiliano Barolo CAPE-Lab—Computer-Aided Process Engineering Laboratory, University of Padova, Padova, Italy

Paul I. Barton Process Systems Engineering Laboratory, Massachusetts Institute of Technology, Cambridge, MA, USA

Mohammad Amin Boojari Biotechnology Group, Faculty of Chemical Engineering, Tarbiat Modares University, Tehran, Iran

Richard D. Braatz Department of Chemical Engineering, Massachusetts Institute of Technology, Cambridge, MA, USA

Daniel Casas-Orozco Davidson School of Chemical Engineering, Purdue University, West Lafayette, IN, USA

Pierre-François Chavez UCB Pharma, Braine l'Alleud, Belgium

Giorgio Colombo Process and Systems Engineering Centre (PROSYS), Department of Chemical and Biochemical Engineering, Technical University of Denmark, Kgs. Lyngby, Denmark

Abina M. Crean University College Cork, Cork, Ireland

Ashok Das Department of Mathematics, Indian Institute of Technology Kharagpur, Kharagpur, West Bengal, India

Francesco Destro CAPE-Lab—Computer-Aided Process Engineering Laboratory, University of Padova, Padova, Italy

Tumpa Dey Faculty of Engineering and Science, School of Science, University of Greenwich, Kent, UK
CIPER—Centre for Innovation and Process Engineering Research, Kent, UK

Dennis Douroumis Faculty of Engineering and Science, School of Science, University of Greenwich, Kent, UK
CIPER–Centre for Innovation and Process Engineering Research, Kent, UK

Julie Fahier UCB Pharma, Braine l'Alleud, Belgium

Mohammad Fakroleslam Process Engineering Department, Faculty of Chemical Engineering, Tarbiat Modares University, Tehran, Iran

Zhenguo Gao Tianjin University, Tianjin, China

Krist V. Gernaey Process and Systems Engineering Centre (PROSYS), Department of Chemical and Biochemical Engineering, Technical University of Denmark, Kgs. Lyngby, Denmark

J. Glassey School of Engineering, Newcastle University, Newcastle upon Tyne, UK

Parag Gogate Chemical Engineering Department, Institute of Chemical Technology, Mumbai, India

Junbo Gong Tianjin University, Tianjin, China

Matteo Grossi Process and Systems Engineering Centre (PROSYS), Department of Chemical and Biochemical Engineering, Technical University of Denmark, Kgs. Lyngby, Denmark

Izumi Hirasawa Department of Applied Chemistry, Waseda University, Tokyo, Japan

Yashraj Jagtap Chemical Engineering Department, Institute of Chemical Technology, Mumbai, India

Mark Nicholas Jones Process and Systems Engineering Centre (PROSYS), Department of Chemical and Biochemical Engineering, Technical University of Denmark, Kgs. Lyngby, Denmark

M. Karlberg School of Engineering, Newcastle University, Newcastle upon Tyne, UK

Brian M. Kerins University College Cork, Cork, Ireland

A. Kizhedath School of Engineering, Newcastle University, Newcastle upon Tyne, UK

Jitendra Kumar Department of Mathematics, Indian Institute of Technology Kharagpur, Kharagpur, West Bengal, India

Daniel J. Laky Davidson School of Chemical Engineering, Purdue University, West Lafayette, IN, USA

Corentin Larcy UCB Pharma, Braine l'Alleud, Belgium

Seyed Soheil Mansouri Process and Systems Engineering Centre (PROSYS), Department of Chemical and Biochemical Engineering, Technical University of Denmark, Kgs. Lyngby, Denmark

Christos T. Maravelias Andlinger Center for Energy and the Environment and Department of Chemical and Biological Engineering, Princeton University, Princeton, NJ, USA

Ikuma Masaki Department of Applied Chemistry, Waseda University, Tokyo, Japan

Kensaku Matsunami Department of Chemical System Engineering, The University of Tokyo, Tokyo, Japan

Shamik Misra Department of Chemical and Biological Engineering, University of Wisconsin, Madison, WI, USA

Zoltan K. Nagy Davidson School of Chemical Engineering, Purdue University, West Lafayette, IN, USA

Uttom Nandi Faculty of Engineering and Science, School of Science, University of Greenwich, Kent, UK
CIPER—Centre for Innovation and Process Engineering Research, Kent, UK

Morteza Nikkhah Nasab Process Systems Engineering Laboratory, Department of Chemical Engineering, AmirKabir University of Technology (Tehran Polytechnic), Tehran, Iran

Anastasia Nikolakopoulou Massachusetts Institute of Technology, Cambridge, MA, USA

Mehrdad Pasha UCB Pharma, Braine l'Alleud, Belgium

Mayur M. Patel Department of Pharmaceutics, Institute of Pharmacy, Nirma University, Ahmedabad, India

Michael Patrascu Department of Chemical Engineering, Technion-Israel Institute of Technology, Haifa, Israel

Simone Perra Process and Systems Engineering Centre (PROSYS), Department of Chemical and Biochemical Engineering, Technical University of Denmark, Kgs. Lyngby, Denmark

Gabrielle Pilcer UCB Pharma, Braine l'Alleud, Belgium

Gintaras V. Reklaitis Davidson School of Chemical Engineering, Purdue University, West Lafayette, IN, USA

Ali M. Sahlodin Process Systems Engineering Laboratory, Department of Chemical Engineering, AmirKabir University of Technology (Tehran Polytechnic), Tehran, Iran

Chinmayee Sarode Chemical Engineering Department, Institute of Chemical Technology, Mumbai, India

Seyed Abbas Shojaosadati Biotechnology Group, Faculty of Chemical Engineering, Tarbiat Modares University, Tehran, Iran

Fanny Stauffer UCB Pharma, Braine l'Alleud, Belgium

Hirokazu Sugiyama Department of Chemical System Engineering, The University of Tokyo, Tokyo, Japan

Isuru Udugama Process and Systems Engineering Centre (PROSYS), Department of Chemical and Biochemical Engineering, Technical University of Denmark, Kgs. Lyngby, Denmark

Joi Unno Department of Applied Chemistry, Waseda University, Tokyo, Japan

Preksha Vinchhi Department of Pharmaceutics, Institute of Pharmacy, Nirma University, Ahmedabad, India

Matthias von Andrian Massachusetts Institute of Technology, Cambridge, MA, USA

Lifang Zhou Department of Chemical Engineering, Massachusetts Institute of Technology, Cambridge, MA, USA

Xiaoxiang Zhu Department of Chemical Engineering, Massachusetts Institute of Technology, Cambridge, MA, USA

Process Control and Intensification of Solution Crystallization

Junbo Gong and Zhenguo Gao

Solution crystallization attracts more and more attention in the pharmaceutical industries because of the functions of separation and the tuning ability of solid-state properties at the molecular level. Generally, the research of solution crystallization includes crystal engineering and crystallization process design and control. The crystallization process design and control have achieved great progress in the past decade, in which process analytical technology (PAT) has come to the real manufacturing practice and the conversion from batch to continuous is becoming a clear tendency. In this chapter, the design and optimization of the crystallization process are summarized that covers process control, seeding technique, intensification by external fields, and the solution crystallization in continuous manufacturing.

1 Solution Crystallization Process Control

1.1 Introduction of Solution Crystallization Process Control

As a unit operation for separating and purifying solid products, crystallization is widely used in the fields of medicine, food, microelectronics, and fine chemicals. The crystallization process determines the purity, morphology, polymorph, particle size, and particle size distribution of the solid product and many other characteristics, which have a significant impact on the performance of the drug and the efficiency of the post-processing process [1]. Therefore, the precise control of the crystallization process is of great significance to the production process and the quality of products.

J. Gong (✉) · Z. Gao
Tianjin University, Tianjin, China
e-mail: junbo_gong@tju.edu.cn

© The Author(s), under exclusive license to Springer Nature Switzerland AG 2022
A. Fytopoulos et al. (eds.), *Optimization of Pharmaceutical Processes*, Springer
Optimization and Its Applications 189, https://doi.org/10.1007/978-3-030-90924-6_1

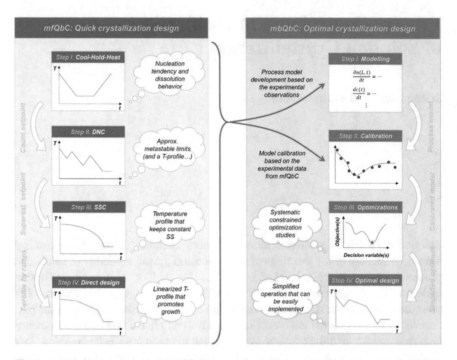

Fig. 1 A high-level overview of the efficient combination of model-free and model-based QbC approaches for rapid (model-free) and optimal (model-based) crystallization process design. (Caption and figure reprinted with permission from Ref. [5]

The actual purpose of crystallization control is to govern the crystal nucleation and growth. Based on modeling and experimental methods, there are a lot of researches on the control of polymorph, shape, and size [2–4]. The control of the crystallization process usually aims to control the crystallization path in a safe operation zone that ensures a robust manufacturing process. The crystallization control strategies can be divided into two major categories: model-free and model-based control approaches. Model-free techniques are based on feedback control algorithms relying on in situ PAT measurements that provide the critical quality attributes of the product, including size distribution, crystal shape, fewer impurities, and target crystal form. Model-based control involves using a mathematical model and numerical simulation to design the process by solving process optimization problems. Nagy [5] proposed a general framework for the optimal design of crystallization processes, which combined the application of two QbC methods: model-free (mfQbC) and model-based (mbQbC). In addition to its robust operating procedures, mfQbC also automatically generates model parameters and experimental data required by the mbQbC. As shown in Fig. 1, the derived model can be used for optimal crystallization process design.

For a classical cooling crystallization process, the mfQbC includes the following main steps: first, cooling-holding-heating experiments under different heating rates and cooling rates, these experiments provide the nucleation rate and solubility kinetics. In the second step, the direct nucleation control (DNC) experiment obtains the width of the metastable zone of primary nucleation and secondary nucleation. The third step is to guide the supersaturation control (SSC) experiment according to the crystal phase diagram obtained from the DNC experiment to obtain the temperature control curve. Finally, to be easily implemented in an industrial distributed control system, the temperature curve generated by the SSC is approximated by a linear ramp to obtain the given temperature curve designed by mfQbC. The process control technology plays an increasingly important role in the controlling of product polymorph, purity, shape, particle size, and particle size distribution.

1.2 Polymorphic Control

Drug polymorphism refers to two or more molecular assembly modes when the drug molecules crystallize from solution to solid state [6]. Polymorphism is a common phenomenon in the crystallization process. Since the different crystal forms of the drug may seriously affect the stability, bioavailability, therapeutic effect, and product quality, so ensuring the consistency of the crystal form is crucial to the drug production process. There are challenges in polymorphic control, for example, the transformation of the crystal form will lead to difficult control of the polymorphism in which the purity of the crystal form is hard to control during the production process.

In response to the challenge of polymorphic control, feedback control strategies provide a pathway for solving the difficulties in the control process. The control of polymorphs in the crystallization process mainly controls the nucleation of nontarget crystals and promotes the growth of target crystals. For polycrystalline materials, different ways to produce supersaturation may result in different crystal forms. Supersaturation is the driving force of the crystallization process, and many researchers have shown that an optimal supersaturation exists for a crystallization process, and various methods for supersaturation measurement and implementation of constant SSC strategy have been investigated. The SSC control strategy is based on the understanding that the crystallization process needs to be operated in the metastable region in the phase diagram, as shown in Fig. 2a. This method can specify an arbitrary concentration target curve in the phase diagram, which is particularly useful for the control of the polymorphic crystallization process. In the polymorphic crystallization process, a complex operation trajectory is designed to selectively control a specific crystal form [7]. Besides, setting the operation trajectory in the crystallization phase diagram can greatly reduce the sensitivity of the crystal size distribution to process disturbances and can prevent the crystallization process crossing the metastable zone and causing undesired explosion nucleation. The advantage of this method is that by specifying the operation trajectory in the crystalline phase diagram, the best operation trajectory in the time domain (such as

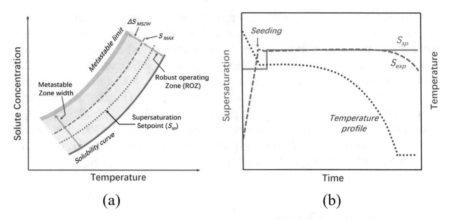

Fig. 2 Crystallization phase diagram (**a**); supersaturation and corresponding temperature profiles obtained during the SSC process (**b**)

the cooling curve) is automatically determined, and it can be implemented on an industrial scale through a standard tracking control system.

By using traditional open-loop control approaches to implement the cooling profile, such as simple linear cooling, it is hard to maintain the concentration operating curve along with an expected trajectory. The SSC is a higher-level control approach through controlling the crystallization operating trajectory in the phase diagram than controlling the process by just following the timely determined temperature profile (or solvent/anti-solvent ratio). The main advantage of this approach over uncontrolled crystallization is that the operating curve can be directly maintained within a "robust operating zone," which can represent the nucleation metastable zone or the targeted polymorph nucleation/growth region. In this way, SSC can avoid undesired nucleation and polymorph transformation and achieve optimal crystallization performance without a large number of experiments for investigating the influence mechanism of process conditions [8–10]. The schematic representation of the SSC approach is shown in Fig. 2b.

The SSC strategy can directly control the crystallization process on the phase diagram, which is a relatively intuitive control method. However, when the crystallization phase diagram is greatly affected by disturbances or the nucleation rate is high, the robustness of this method will be greatly reduced [11]. In addition, the concentration feedback control strategy cannot directly control the properties of solids, which means that even if the supersaturation levels of the two batches are the same in the batch process, the product properties may still be quite different due to process disturbances.

The temperature cycle during the crystallization process is beneficial to dissolve the metastable crystal form produced during the crystallization process. Pataki et al. [12] used Raman to detect nontarget crystal forms in the crystallization process and trigger automatic heating to dissolve and eliminate metastable crystal forms. Tacsi et al. [13] adopted polymorph concentration control to separately refine two crystal forms of carvedilol. During the crystallization process, Raman detected a nontarget crystal form to trigger temperature-rising dissolution, and the products obtained were all target crystal forms. Active polymorphic feedback control realizes the refining of the stable crystal form of OABA in the case of impure seed crystal form. Raman detects that the metastable crystal form triggers heating and dissolution, and then the system performed supersaturation control to prepare stable crystals [14].

In the past 20 years, in situ monitoring of polymorphism in the crystallization process has developed rapidly, including online Raman, in situ XRD, in situ laser backscattering, and in situ process image microscopy. Although none of these technologies can be applied to all solute-solvent systems for online monitoring of polymorphs, for most systems, at least one sensor technology can be used to monitor the conversion between different crystal forms [15]. In recent years, process detection and online analysis methods have been widely used in polymorphic selective crystallization processes. Based on this, the development of polymorphic feedback control (or closed-loop control) strategies has also made continuous progress.

1.3 CSD and Morphology Control

In industrial crystallization process, crystal morphology, crystal size, and crystal size distribution (CSD) are important properties of crystals, because these properties play a vital role in determining the quality of the final product and the efficiency of downstream processes. Also, a poor particle size distribution may lead to solvent entrainment, and then leading to impurity problems, resulting in a reduced purity. The process control technology is playing an increasingly important role in improving yield and purity, ensuring the consistency of crystal products in terms of particle size and crystal morphology, and avoiding particle coalescence and solvent encapsulation.

Generally, the explosion nucleation process will promote the crystallization process to produce fine particles, and the dissolution process will be the dissolution of fine particles. Therefore, the heating-cooling cycle can eliminate fine crystals and prepare larger crystals. The DNC strategy is based on the idea that the smaller the system particles, the larger the product particle size and the temperature cycle is beneficial to eliminate fine crystals. The DNC strategy shows good consistency in the crystallization process, because this method does not need to know the crystallization process model, kinetics, and the width of the metastable zone in advance, and these parameters change due to the hydrodynamic properties during the amplification process. Changes often occur, so it is a robust feedback control strategy. When the number of monitored crystal count changes, DNC automatically adjusts the operating conditions, which can well overcome the adverse effects of process disturbances. The most significant feature of the DNC strategy is the ability to directly monitor and control the crystal properties, which can be achieved through a controllable growth and dissolution cycle (cooling/heating cycle or anti-

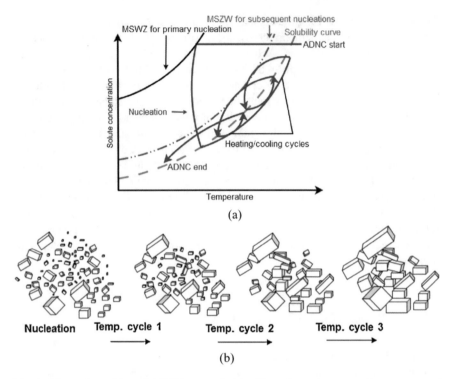

(a)

(b)

Fig. 3 Schematic working of ADNC approach (**a**); effect of temperature cycling on a crystal suspension (**b**) (Caption and figure reprinted with permission from Ref. [19]

solvent/solvent addition cycle). The advantage of DNC is that it can produce crystal products with a more regular particle size in line with expectations [16], reduce particle coalescence and solvent occlusion [17], and improve the purity of crystal [18]. This is because the direct nucleation control can inhibit the adsorption of impurities on the crystal surface by repeatedly dissolving the growth cycle, and the fine particles and impurities on the crystal surface will dissolve continuously during the heating process. Thus, in the subsequent cooling process, crystal growth is promoted, and the crystal with a larger particle size has a smaller specific surface area, which reduces the adsorption of impurities on the surface, as shown in Fig. 3.

The DNC nucleation strategy is also suitable for anti-solvent crystallization. Nagy et al. [20] used the DNC strategy to control the CSD of glycine by controlling the flow of solvent and anti-solvent. Most of the crystallization process indirectly affects CSD through real-time temperature control or anti-solvent to follow the supersaturation set in the phase diagram. Using the SSC strategy during the crystallization process can keep the supersaturation constant at the set value, and reduce or avoid secondary nucleation during the entire crystallization process to promote crystal growth. And the image analysis-based direct nucleation control method based on image processing has a very significant effect on the control of particle size and particle shape [21]. The smaller the number of crystals at the crystallization endpoint, the larger the crystal size. Griffin et al. [22] used mass-count graphs for feedback control to optimize the CSD of paracetamol.

Model-based closed-loop optimization and control strategies for improving the crystal morphology of products obtained from the crystallization process have been considered a challenging topic, mainly due to the limitations of existing monitoring technology and modeling capabilities. In recent years, monitoring technology and modeling capabilities have continuously improved, and certain progress has also been made in crystal morphology control. Comprehensive simulation and experimental studies applied to the feedback control approach for the evolution of particle shape have also been reported [23–26]. The precise control of the crystallization process can tailor the solid properties such as polymorph, crystal morphology, particle size, and particle size distribution, which has a significant effect on the overall efficiency of the solid production process and the quality of the final product.

2 Seeding in the Solution Crystallization

2.1 Targets of Seeding in the Solution Crystallization

In the pharmaceutical solution crystallization, the strategy of seeding is widely used, and it is an effective technique to optimize the product quality and improve the process efficiency. In some crystallization processes, seeding is essential because the seeds can effectively avoid uncontrollable primary nucleation and have a profound impact on secondary nucleation and crystal growth. Before the seed strategy was utilized, one should fully understand what specific targets the seed strategy can achieve. In general, the purposes of seeding can be divided into crystal quality-oriented (e.g., purity, particle and particle size distribution, morphology, polymorph) seeding strategies and process-oriented (e.g., oiling out, process reproducibility, process efficiency) seeding strategies. The design and implementation of the seeding strategies vary according to the specific targets to be achieved. Besides, not only the characteristics of the seeds itself but also the process operating conditions should be considered. Common targets in solution crystallization, seed characteristics, and process operating conditions are summarized in Table 1. In this section, three targets in pharmaceutical crystallization are mainly highlighted.

Particle Size and Particle Size Distribution (PSD). **PSD** is one of the key indicators of the quality of drug crystal products. It will directly affect the dissolution rate, flowability, tableting performance, anticaking property, and so on. The core of particle size and particle size distribution control is to inhibit the occurrence of secondary nucleation as far as possible so that the supersaturation of the solution system is consumed in the crystal growth of seeds added. There are usually two scenes. The first scene is that the crystals obtained by spontaneous

Table 1 The specific targets, seed characteristics, and operating conditions to be considered in the design and implementation of the seeding strategy

Targets	Seed characteristics	Operating conditions
Products quality-oriented: • Purity • Particle Size and Particle Size Distribution (PSD) • Morphology • Polymorph **Process-oriented:** • Process efficiency • Process repeatability • Process scale-up	• Purity • Loading amount • Size and size distribution • Morphology • Polymorph • Surface Roughness	• Supersaturation • Supersaturation generation rate • Temperature • Mixing quality • Timing of seed addition • Holding time after seeding

nucleation are too tiny, and crystals with larger size and a narrow PSD are desired. An effective solution is to add enough seeds to provide enough growth surfaces while keeping the system at a low supersaturation and using mild stirring. Gentle mixing and low supersaturation level can effectively inhibit secondary nucleation which may cause bimodal particle size distribution of crystal products. Another scene is that the size of crystals obtained by spontaneous nucleation and subsequent growth is too large; the crystals with smaller size and a narrower PSD are preferred. In the second situation, compared with the first scene, a greater number of seeds with smaller crystal sizes are expected to be added to ensure that the supersaturation of the system can be highly dispersed on more seeds. Overall, based on the specific optimization objectives, the factors that may affect the secondary nucleation and seed growth should be considered, such as seed loading amount, seed size, seed surface property, supersaturation control, and so on.

Polymorphism. The polymorphism phenomenon determines many important properties of pharmaceutical crystals, such as solubility, dissolution rate, bioavailability, and long-term stability, and these properties may even influence therapeutic efficacy. Therefore, precise control over polymorph is of vital importance in solution crystallization. Usually, the seeds act as heterogeneous nuclei to ensure that the solute molecules crystallize isomorphically with the seed crystals. According to Ostwald's rule, the conventional polymorph systems tend to crystallize into the metastable form first, and then the metastable form transforms into the stable one through solvent-mediated transformation. However, some special systems do not follow Ostwald's rule, that is, they crystallize directly into the stable form in the solution, so that it is difficult to obtain metastable form whose properties (such as solubility, dissolution rate, morphology, etc.) may be more preferred in production and market. In addition, the transformation rate from the metastable form to the stable form may be too slow in some polymorphic system, resulting in the failure to obtain the stable crystal form or the appearance of the mixed crystal forms. Remarkably, the seed with a specific crystal form can not only be added before the

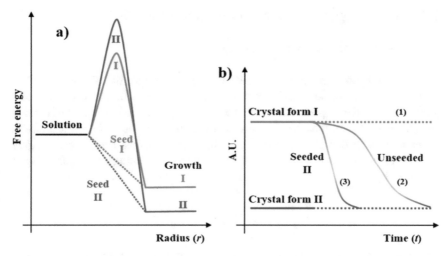

Fig. 4 Schematic of seeding for polymorphic control: (**a**) energy level representation of nucleation, growth, and the role of seeding for two polymorphs and (**b**) polymorphic transformation with and without seeding optimization

spontaneous nucleation of the solution system to induce the preferential nucleation of the desired crystal form but also play a role in the polymorphic transformation process to promote the transformation from the metastable form to the stable form (see Fig. 4).

Process Robustness. The process robustness is the key to ensure the reproducibility of the crystallization procedure as well as the consistency of crystals' quality between different batches. In the solution crystallization without seed addition, due to the stochastic nature of the primary nucleation, the number and size distributions of the first crystal population have little reproducibility between different batches, resulting in the fluctuation of product quality. Besides, primary nucleation often occurs at high supersaturation, and a massive number of nuclei are generated in a short time, resulting in crystal agglomeration, solvent entrapment, and crystallizer encrustment. Oiling out, also called liquid-liquid phase separation (LLPS), may also take place. All of these would greatly reduce the efficiency of the crystallization process. It is worth mentioning that seeding is an effective approach to avoid uncontrollable primary nucleation and prevent the liquid phase from entering the metastable liquid-liquid phase region. Besides, for a specific crystallization process, such as tubular continuous crystallization, a constant seed flow can achieve steady-state operation and improve the process robustness.

2.2   Seeds Properties and Seeding Techniques

Seed Loading Amount and Seed Size

The loading amount and size of the seeds represent the quantity of crystal surface areas that the seeds can provide for the supersaturated solution, which are key parameters for the implementation of seed strategy. It's obvious that the loading amount of seeds and their particle size will determine the size of crystal products obtained by a seeded crystallization. A simple mass-balance Eq. (1) can roughly estimate the size of products harvested according to the loading amount and size of the seeds added:

$$\left(\frac{d_{seed}}{d_{product}}\right)^3 = \frac{m_{seed}}{m_{seed} + m_{product}} \tag{1}$$

where d_{seed} and $d_{product}$ are the average size of the seeds and final products, respectively, while m_{seed} represents the mass of the seeds added and $m_{product}$ represents the mass of the products that can be obtained theoretically in the crystallization process without seed. Besides, based on different optimization targets in solution crystallization, there are four levels of seed loading amount: trace addition (~0.1 wt%), small addition (~1 wt%), large addition (~10 wt%), and massive addition (>10 wt%). In general, a trace or small addition amount can avoid uncontrolled nucleation or oiling out, and also start a nucleation event at a specific point. In contrast, when the optimization goal is to control the particle size and particle size distribution of the crystal products, a large or massive addition is adopted, combined with a low supersaturation and a mild mixing. It can ensure that the supersaturation of the system is consumed on the seed growth to the maximum extent so that the crystals with a narrow particle size distribution can be harvested. On the other hand, the size of the seed determines the effective surface area that can facilitate the growth of crystals. Usually, seeds with a larger surface area are preferred, and sufficient surface area of seeds is favorable to suppress secondary nucleation at lower supersaturation. Porte et al. [27] investigated the effect of seeded surface area on particle size distribution in the cooling crystallization of glycine and found that only when the seed surface area reaches a critical value can the PSD be controlled effectively. However, the larger surface area means a smaller size. These small particles with a large surface area have a greater tendency to agglomerate, thus affecting the quality of the final product.

Seed Surface Roughness

Whether the target of seed strategy is to control the particle size distribution, crystal form, or the process robustness, the surface properties of seeds require high attention. This is because the occurrence of secondary nucleation and the crystal growth rate of seeds are closely related to the seed surface roughness. Roughness can be caused by pores, specific topological structure, and a fractured or smooth surface on the crystals, all of which can affect seeding performance through the confinement effect and angular matching between the surface features and the growing lattice [28]. In practice, one can increase the roughness of the seeds by milling, ultrasonic, and high-speed stirring. A rougher surface leads to a larger seed surface area with more active nucleation sites. It may induce faster secondary nucleation kinetics and a higher crystal growth rate. It is found that the dislocation or roughness of seeds surface has a more profound impact on crystal growth than secondary nucleation because the fast growth of the crystals generates imperfections in the crystal surface.

Seed Polymorphism

For the seed strategy aiming to control the polymorphic outcome, it is easy to understand how to select the seeds. That is, if we want to harvest the crystal products of a specific crystal form, just add the seeds of the corresponding crystal form. However, the success ratio of the crystallization process with metastable crystal form as a target crystal form is much lower than that with stable form. This is due to the risk of the polymorphic transformation of the metastable form. Therefore, additional efforts need to be made to reduce the transformation kinetics of metastable form. Beckmann [29] reviewed the seeding techniques for the desired polymorph during crystallization from solutions based on the theoretical and practical considerations.

Timing of Seed Addition

The choice of seeding time is critical to the success of the seeding strategy. The seed crystal should be added in the metastable zone of the crystallization system. If it is added too early, the seed crystal will be partially or completely dissolved, which will greatly reduce the surface area provided by the seeds. On the contrary, if the seeds are added too late, that is, the system exceeds beyond the metastable zone, spontaneous nucleation will occur, resulting in the precipitation of a large number of crystal nuclei. However, the most difficult problem is how to determine the appropriate addition location of seed within the metastable region. Solubility curve and metastable zone width (MSZW) of the crystallization system are the basic data for judging the addition time. A common rule of thumb suggests that the addition point should be in the region between the solubility curve and 1/4–1/2 unit of metastable zone width beyond the solubility curve [30].

2.3 Seed Preparation

In practice, seed usually comes from the crystal products of previous crystallization. However, in order to meet the requirements of specific optimization objectives on seed characteristics, such as particle size, particle size distribution, surface roughness, etc., the seed often needs further processing, such as milling and sieving. The key to preparing seed is to obtain seeds with a narrow particle size distribution and a good dispersion. Dry milling and wet milling are the commonly used processing methods to obtain desired small seeds with a narrow particle size distribution. Although dry milling is very convenient in operation, it has some obvious disadvantages, such as milling-induced polymorphic transformation, severe seed agglomeration, as well as poor dispersion of seeds when added into the solution. The advantage of wet milling compared is that it is easier to achieve scale-up and the continuous operation of crystallization [31]. In addition, due to the presence of solvents, the former can also stabilize specific crystal form and prevent the desolvation of solvates. An alternative way to prepare the seeds is to suspend them in the same solvent as used in the crystallizer. During the suspension process, very tiny crystals may be dissolved; amorphized surfaces may recrystallize. Besides, it is convenient to apply ultrasonic intensification to the suspension process, which can further improve the dispersion of the seeds.

3 Intensification of Solution Crystallization

3.1 The Role of Intensification for Product and Process Robustness and Efficiency

For pharmaceuticals, numerous studies devoted to optimizing the crystallization process parameters and control recipes to improve product quality and process robustness [32–34]. To optimize a pharmaceutical process, the process intensification is needed for product production, which could be divided into two methods, including the physical field technology and equipment enhancement. Considering the best economic impact, such as the product specifications and further downstream processing, these intensification technologies have achieved more attention. The physical field technology is widely applied in the nucleation process for pharmaceutical manufacturing, control of the crystal size distribution [35], preparation of uniform crystals [36], and obtaining the specific crystal polymorph [37]. The equipment enhancement can shorten the processing time, obtain higher heat and mass transfer efficiency, achieve higher yield purities, and better process efficiency and reliability [38].

3.2 Physical Field Technology-Assisted Intensification

In the early twenty-first century, the effects of electric field on solution crystallization process have been widely studied, which is a relatively new research field. The role of the electric field in the crystallization experiments could be divided into two configurations: (1) The internal electric field, immersing the electrodes in the solution, releases small voltage and current to limit the faradic reaction. (2) The external electric field is another way to influence the solution crystallization process that the electrodes do not contact the solution [39]. Alexander et al. [39] summarized the researches of the influence of the electric field on the solution crystallization process, showing that the protein crystallization process is the most common system that can be affected by the electric field. The electric field could reduce the induction time, increase the product yield, improve the crystal quality, optimize the crystal size, control the crystal growth orientation, and affect crystal polymorph outcome [40–45].

Taleb et al. [39] studied the crystallization kinetics of lysozyme in the presence of an electric field. The equilibrium time was shortened in the electric field, which was essential to the aging of the protein crystals and influencing the crystal quality. Li et al. [46] measured the induction time and nucleation rate of the lysozyme crystals. Depending on the electrode shape and surface area, the enhancement or inhibition of protein crystallization could be controlled. Parks et al. [42] modeled the paracetamol crystallization kinetics with electric field vector, obtaining a new paracetamol polymorph and controlling the crystal morphology. It is the molecule conformation and packing pattern that determine the crystal polymorph and material property. The electric field could change the molecule spatial orientation, and maximize the alignment between the electric dipole and the applied electric field vector, resulting in a new polymorph.

Laser-induced crystallization is widely studied in the field of crystallization of amino acids and proteins [47–49]. There are two common crystallization mechanisms influenced by laser. Nakamura et al. verified by using the experimental setup as shown in Fig. 5 [50]. When the intense femtosecond laser is irradiated into the supersaturated solution, the nonlinear phenomenon is generated, such as shockwaves, cavitation bubbles, and jet flow [50]. The bubbles generated by the intense femtosecond could act as a preferential field for enhancing the crystallization process. Another mechanism is thought to be the influence of the optical Kerr effect. The optical Kerr effect could induce the partial alignment of the organic molecules, in which anisotropically polarizable molecules began to generate torsion making the polarizable axis being parallel to the polarization direction of the incident light [38, 51]. The laser field could induce the alignment of solute molecules to generate a prenucleation cluster, which can intensify the nucleation process. Tsuri et al. [52] prepared the aspirin form II in the presence of laser, for the reason that the cavitation bubbles induced by laser lower the interface energy and finally reduce the nucleation barrier. Except for the promotion of nucleation and control polymorph, the laser field could also be used to control the morphology to prepare the single

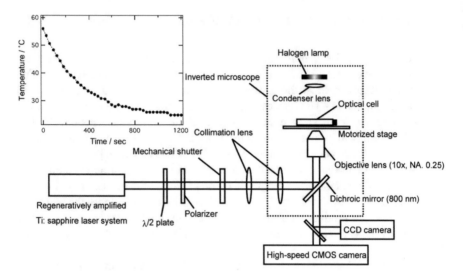

Fig. 5 Experimental setup femtosecond laser-induced crystallization. The inset indicates the temporal profile of the temperature of the sample solution on the microscope. (Reprinted with permission from Ref. [50]. Copyright 2007 ACS)

crystal. Liu et al. [47] studied the repetition rate, pulse energy, and focal position dependencies, finding that the frequency of the cavitation bubble generated by laser could significantly affect the crystal morphology. Finally, the single crystal was prepared by optimizing the laser parameters, such as the power and shot number.

The ultrasound devices with frequencies ranged from 20 kHz up to several gigahertz could form acoustic cavitation in liquid, resulting in the initiation and enhancement of crystallization in a supersaturated solution [53, 54]. In 1927, it was the first time to introduce the ultrasound to the solution crystallization. The application of ultrasound in a crystallization process, also known as sonocrystallization, could modify the crystal morphology [55, 56], change the crystal size and CSD [57, 58], control polymorph formation [59, 60], affect crystal agglomeration [61], enhance process robustness [62], and accelerate the solvent-mediated polymorph transformation process. The cavitation phenomenon, which is the formation, growth, and collapse of cavitation bubbles, is the main factor for influencing the nucleation process [53, 63, 64]. The collapse of cavitation bubbles could generate high pressure and high temperature by the rapid adiabatic compression of gas in the bubbles. At the same time, the shockwaves, microjets, and microturbulences are created, improving the mixing effect, intensifying the mass transfer process, and finally promoting the nucleation process in the solution. The ultrasonic equipment commonly used in the studies could be divided into three types: ultrasonic horn, ultrasonic bath, and multiple-frequency flow cell [65]. But there are also some defects existing in the above ultrasonic equipment. For example, in the case of the ultrasonic horn, the horn is always exposed to the liquid medium, which may corrode the transducer surface and contaminate the pharmaceutical solution. For another example, it is inconvenient to control the crystallizer temperature in the ultrasonic bath. Thus, making improvement to the ultrasonic equipment is necessary for the technological requirement. To adapt for various solution crystallization conditions, the aim of reconstructing ultrasonic equipment is to obtain a uniform distribution of cavitation activity and maximal cavitation yield.

The metastable zone widths (MSZWs) and induction time are widely studied in the ultrasound-assisted crystallization process, and the nucleation kinetic parameter is also calculated for evaluating the nucleation process. Mastan et al. [66] calculated the nucleation parameters by MSZW data, using four different nucleation models to state the effect of ultrasound on the nucleation process respectively. To evaluate the product quality and prepare for the downstream process, the morphology and crystal size distribution should be investigated for better control. In the ultrasound-assisted crystallization of mefenamic acid, Iyer et al. [56] improved the yield of mefenamic acid product, decreased crystal size distribution, and obtained plate-shaped morphology which was different from the needle-shaped morphology without ultrasound.

The magnetic field is usually applied in protein crystallization and inorganic crystal crystallization [67–72]. The magnetic field could narrow the crystal size distribution, broaden the metastable zone width, influence the ratio of the crystal polymorphs, and improve crystal quality [67, 73]. In this section, the solution crystallization process is especially emphasized, and the protein crystallization acts as a model compound to explain the effect of magnetic field on the solution crystallization. Huang et al. [70] proposed a new method to realize the high-throughput protein crystallization. The author designed a crystallization setup with capillaries as containers for holding crystallization solution, and put all of these capillaries in the same magnetic field conditions, resolving the uncertainties in the protein crystallization screening. Yin et al. [69] combined the magnetic field with levitated containerless droplets, expecting to produce high-quality protein crystals.

To obtain favorable crystal quality, it is essential to investigate the influential factors which could control the nucleation process and crystallization kinetic. The physical field mentioned above could influence the product quality directly, while the scale-up of the solution crystallization system that assisted by the physical field is hard. The crystallizers are usually made of metal, which could have safety concerns with high voltage in the electric field. The ultrasound irradiation is usually accompanied by a loud noise, which will increase noise pollution for the environment. Besides, for industrial applications, the increased investment could also be the problem needed to be solved. To deepen the comprehending of the effect of physical fields on the crystallization process, more attention should be paid to the combination of various crystal preparation methods with physical fields. The final target is the realization of continuously producing high-quality crystals with the assistance of physical fields.

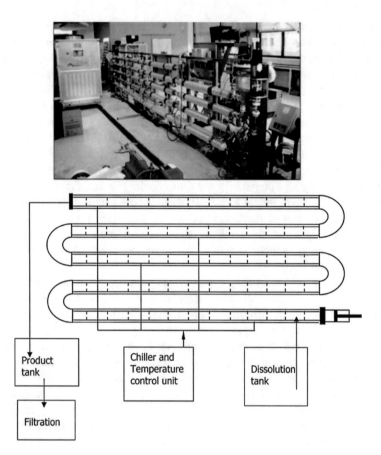

Fig. 6 Continuous oscillatory baffled crystallizer (Reprinted with permission from Ref. [74]. Copyright 2009 ACS)

3.3 Equipment Enhancement in the Solution Crystallization Process

The continuous oscillatory baffled crystallizers (COBC), as shown in Fig. 6 [74], is a series of baffles in long tubes that own the high length-to-diameter ratio. The appearance of COBC is similar to the plug flow crystallizer with baffles. When the flow stream in the COBC interacts with baffles, the production and disappearance of vortices intensify the mixing, which is thus decoupled from net flow-driven turbulence. As the vortex circulates, strong radial motion is generated, so that each baffle area has uniform mixing and plug flow conditions accumulated along the column length, which would otherwise lead to a laminar-flow state [75]. The COBC have shown their advantages in shortening the processing time, increasing the operating scaling, and improving the transfer efficiency [74]. Compared with the stirred tank reactors, the COBC has the linear scale-up capability, which could provide a better understanding of the connection between laboratory scale and industrial operation [76].

Concerning the solution crystallization of pharmaceutical production, there are many studies relating to designing a better crystallization process with COBC or promoting the understanding of magnifying the laboratory-scale production [77–80]. Callahan et al. [78] studied the nucleation mechanism in the cooling crystallization of sodium chlorate. The author stated that solution situations and structure conditions in the COBC favored seed-dissimilar secondary nucleation, such as the scraping between the outer edge of the baffle and the inner surface of the column wall, the evaporating supersaturated solution caused by the oscillatory motion, and the variational mixing condition closed to the seed [78]. According to changing these solution situations and structure conditions, seed-dissimilar crystals could be promoted or avoided, and the secondary nucleation could be predominant in the continuous crystallization process. Peña et al. [79] realized a continuous preparation of the spherical agglomerates of benzoic acid in an oscillatory flow baffled crystallizer. This spherical crystallization technique separated the nucleation, growth, and agglomeration process, which could control each section better and intensified the crystallization process ultimately.

The Couette-Taylor (CT) crystallizer consists of two annular cylinders, the inner and the outer cylinder, as shown in Fig. 7a [81]. As shown in Fig. 7b [81], the Taylor vortex fluid motion is generated between the gap of the two cylinders, in which the inner cylinder is rotated to generate the Taylor vortex fluid and the outer cylinder remains stationary. The Taylor vortex crystallizer has been widely used in various crystallization processes to improve desired crystal properties, such as product purity, crystal shape, crystal size distribution, polymorphic crystallization, and production efficiency [82–85]. Kim's group developed the crystallization in a CT crystallizer and demonstrated that the Taylor vortex flow is highly effective for promoting heat and mass transfer [85].

A coiled flow inverter (CFI) is a helical tube with ninety degree bends at constant intervals along the length of the tube [86]. The bends change the direction of the centrifugal force, and the Dean vortices are produced and parallel to the cross section of the tube. Dean vortices promote the radial mixing of fluid elements and finally narrow the residence time distribution [86]. Many studies explored the role of CFI crystallizer in improving the pharmaceutical process and controlling the crystal property [87–89]. Hohmann et al. studied the L-alanine crystallization in a self-designed CFI crystallizer, and the metastable zone width and mean residence time were studied to characterize the nucleation property [87]. The author also stated that the scale-up from lab to the production scale could be promoted by the accurate design guidelines, but retaining the flow property. Two years later, the author studied the crystal size distribution property in the CFI crystallizer with L-alanine/water system and proved that the CFI crystallizer could solve the difficulties of product quality from the batch operation to the continuous operation [88].

The continuous plug flow crystallizer (CPFC) is a commonly used continuous crystallizer. The supersaturation ratio is usually generated by the cooling operation

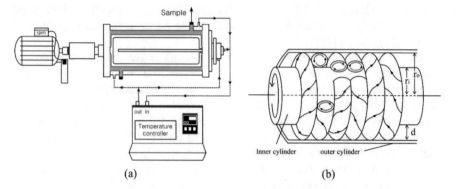

Fig. 7 Experimental system crystallization process: (**a**) Couette-Taylor (CT) crystallizer, (**b**) schematic drawing of Taylor vortex flow (Reprinted with permission from Ref. [81]. Copyright 2015 ACS)

or anti-solvent addition [90, 91]. The radial direction of the CFPC could provide perfect mixing, but the axial direction does not make any contribution to the mixing. Besenhard et al. [92] realized three crystallization processes in the CPFC, including the removal of fine crystals, the tuning of crystal shapes, and the transition between polymorphic forms. The crystallization process in a CPFC could also be intensified to increase the process yield and narrow the particle size distribution [93, 94]. Besides, the development of continuous crystallizer can also improve the process of safety and controllability and reduces the equipment cost and operating cost [95].

4 Solution Crystallization in Continuous Pharmaceutical Manufacturing

4.1 From Batch to Continuous Manufacturing

Traditionally, for simplification of crystallization equipment and manual operation, chemical enterprises tend to adopt the method of batch crystallization [96]. However, the existence of dead-flow zones in the crystallizer leads to concentration gradients in both space and time, eventually resulting in a decline of the product quality. And other circumstances, such as inevitable batch-to-batch variations, would make the batch process worse. Hence the pharmaceutical industry has begun to show much more interest in continuous manufacturing (CM), since it has advantages in product quality and process efficiency [97]. Continuous processes have also many benefits over batch mode such as a shorter development period to reach pilot-scale and/or commercial production; lower facility cost and space requirements; fewer product quality fluctuations; and better amplification and intelligent process

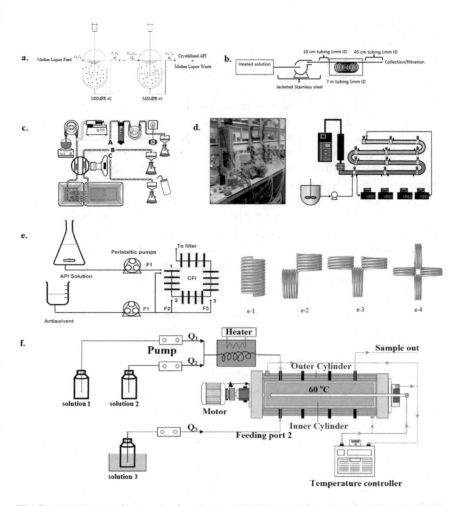

Fig. 8 (**a**) A diagram of a cascade of continuous MSMPR crystallizers. Reprinted from Ref. [98]. Copyright 2018 American Chemical Society. (**b**). A diagram of a laminar-flow tubular crystallizer. Reprinted from Ref. [99]. Copyright 2018 American Chemical Society. (**c**) Schematic draft of a crystallization process design based on gas-liquid continuous segmented flow. Reprinted from Ref. [100]. Copyright 2017 American Chemical Society. (**d**) A continuous oscillatory baffled crystallizer setup (left) with a schematic (right). Reprinted from Ref. [101]. Copyright 2017 American Chemical Society. (**e**) A diagram of the coiled flow inverter anti-solvent crystallizer, different geometries of the crystallizers shown from e-1 to e-4. Reprinted from Ref. [102]. Copyright 2019 American Chemical Society. (**f**) Schematic diagram of the continuous Couette-Taylor crystallizer. Reprinted from Ref. [103]. Copyright 2018 Elsevier B.V. All rights reserved

control. A few commonly used continuous crystallizers are graphically presented in Fig. 8.

As mentioned above, though the batch operation is still the main approach for the crystallization in pharmaceutical production, a lot of researchers have devoted to the shift from traditional batch production toward continuous manufacturing (CM) [104, 105]. Actually, the realization of continuous solution crystallization relies on the process data, which can be experimentally obtained from batch operations, including but not limited to thermodynamic equilibrium data, MSZW, nucleation, and growth kinetics parameters. Besides, seed crystals and feed suspensions suitable for continuous crystallization need to be prepared by the batch operation [106–108].

A study of shifting from batch process to continuous process was done by Siddique et al. [109], where a continuous crystallization was presented combined with an advanced control strategy. The entire transformation was divided into three consecutive steps. Firstly, fundamental thermodynamic data and solvent screening were accomplished in a batch stirred tank crystallizer. Secondly, the kinetic data including MSZW, growth kinetics, dissolution kinetics, and seed loading were determined within an oscillatory baffled crystallizer, which ensures a similar geometry to mimic mixing and heat transfer. Based on the two steps, a complete set of basic kinetic and thermodynamic data consistent with the continuous operation were established for lactose crystallization using FBRM and mid-IR. In the last step, a new systematic approach was proven to develop a continuous sonocrystallization process using the inline PAT and direct control approach, in which the crystal habit, crystal size distribution (CSD), yield, and polymorph purity could be controlled. The comparison between continuous operation and batch operation has never been restricted by the type of crystallizer, the way of supersaturation accumulation, and the diversity of compound, and the focus of comparison is product quality including CSD, mean size, polymorphic form, and final yield [95, 110].

Controlling particle size and CSD are the basic requirements for pharmaceutical manufacturing companies to produce APIs. Because a fair amount of drugs are poorly soluble, which leads to poor bioavailability and biocompatibility, thus there is a demand to produce small size crystals to enhance the dissolution rate. Neugebauer and Khinast [111] compared a continuous cooling crystallization of lysozyme in a multi-segmented tubular crystallizer with a slug flow to a batch crystallizer. The smaller mean size was obtained by tubular crystallizer than the batch because the nucleation zone was separated from the growth zone by the use of multiple water baths resulting in a well-controlled supersaturation along the main flow direction. Different from cooling crystallization, both anti-solvent crystallization and reactive crystallization require the introduction of two or more streams (reactant or anti-solvent) to generate supersaturation, so the quality control of the final product is considered more difficult. Anti-solvent continuous crystallization of benzoic acid in a plug flow crystallizer (PFC) was investigated by Ferguson et al. [112] A premixing segment was realized by the use of a Roughton mixer before nucleation in the tube. Experiment results showed that much narrower CSD, more crystal counts, and smaller crystals in the PFC were obtained compared to the fed-batch one. Smaller crystals were also produced by a continuous reactive crystallization system. Stihl et al. [113] pointed out the shorter residence times and proper mixing design of the inlet flows are the main reasons of the narrower CSD and smaller crystals.

4.2   Coupled Configuration of Solution Crystallization Process

Although in some cases the design of a continuous crystallization process including only one crystallizer can achieve effective control of product properties, productivity, and yield, a relatively low production efficiency caused by high residence time and the high energy consumption will severely restrict the further application of the continuous design. Coupled configuration of continuous devices is to use the advantages of different continuous units, providing the possibility for precisely solid-liquid separation or the refining of crystalline product. In this section, we discussed the experimental work that has been reported.

Polymorphism control is considered one of the most challenging problems in the pharmaceutical industry. In the batch crystallization process, the polymorph can be precisely produced by controlling the appropriate temperature profile or seeding point to avoid uneven mass and heat transfer. However, since the steady-state condition is difficult to achieve and maintain in continuous crystallization, precise control of specific crystal forms remains challenges. According to the study by Myerson's research group [114], the polymorph of L-glutamic acid crystals could be effectively controlled by varying the residence time and temperature in single-stage MSMPR crystallization. To obtain the desired crystal form at a steady state while optimizing other control variables, Lai et al. [115] tried to use an MSMPR cascade to increase throughput and improve product quality. The researchers obtained the desired enantiotropic p-aminobenzoic acid polymorph and the desired yield simultaneously by using an MSMPR cascade at different temperatures. The two-stage MSMPR crystallizer separated the nucleation and growth stages of the crystallization process and facilitated the nucleation of the α-form during the first stage. The first-stage suspension was then transferred into the second stage, which provided a large number of growth sites for secondary nucleation and growth of the desired form. This strategy could also improve the situation of apparent inconsistency between crystal polymorph selectivity and yield. As a part of the Novartis-MIT Center for Continuous Manufacturing project, Quon et al. [116] described a two-stage MSMPR continuous reactive crystallization. Since the reaction rate, solubility, and production efficiency were all affected by temperature, the researchers controlled the yield and purity of the product using a reasonable selection of the temperature of the two-stage MSMPR cascade, and accordingly, the mathematical modeling of the continuous crystallization process was established. Powell et al. [117, 118] contrived a novel periodic MSMPR crystallizer cascade to select a desired polymorphic form of urea-barbituric acid (UBA) cocrystals. The system consisted of a three-stage MSMPR crystallizer cascade that was characterized by periodic transfer of slurry with high velocities of addition and withdrawal. This new crystallizer could not only precisely harvest the target cocrystal but also ensured the state-state of the continuous operation. In addition, the authors used an integrated process analysis tool to detect and optimize crystallization processes for improvement of UBA purity.

Enantiomers are stereoisomers that are mirror images of each other. In the synthetic production of materials with specific optical properties, it is hard to prevent the appearance of enantiomer from spontaneously accompanying the targeted product. Chaaban et al. [119] achieved a continuous preferential crystallization of DL-asparagine monohydrate in an aqueous solution using a two-stage MSMPR crystallizer with an exchange of their clear liquid phases. By seeding the two types of pure enantiomers in the two MSMPR crystallizers separately, they were able to improve the yield of each crystallizer. The D and L types had purities of 100% and 92%, respectively. The authors attributed the relatively low purity of the L enantiomer to surface nucleation of the enantiomer on the surface structure of the seeds. Köllges and Vetter [82] presented a difference between preferential crystallization and Viedma ripening. The results of process model calculations and experimental verification showed that although the use of a multiple-crystallizer cascade could increase the crystallization yield, the preferred crystallization process still had superior enantiomeric purity. Some researchers have coupled three crystallization devices to separate racemic mixtures. A dissolver vessel was applied to circulate the liquid phase containing a suspension of a racemic mixture, which was successfully applied at the laboratory and industrial scales [120].

Some scholars have also paid attention to the continuous combination of tubular crystallizers and MSMPR systems to meet the requirements of polymorph and particle size distribution control. Agnew et al. [101] combined COBC and MSMPR systems to produce paracetamol form II with enhanced dissolving ability and compressibility. They monitored the large-scale production of the desired form with inline PAT, which showed the system to have better efficiency than individual MSMPR or COBC crystallizers. Sulttan and Rohani [121] developed a continuous-seeding MSMPR-helical tubular crystallizer. In their work, a computational fluid dynamics simulation coupled with a population balance equation model was established to describe the CSD. The reliability of precise control of a crystalline polymorph by the crystallization apparatus was verified by Gao et al. [122] through consideration of the initial concentration, nucleation temperature, stirring impact, and residence time distribution. They successfully harvested the desired α-form of L-glutamic acid with a narrow size distribution.

Wet mills are also usually coupled within continuous crystallization to realize particle size distribution control of the crystalline product. Yang et al. [123] integrated the rotor-stator wet mill and continuous mixed-suspension mixed-product removal (MSMPR) crystallizer to optimize the crystallization process. The wet mill is applied in two different configurations: one is in the downstream recycle loop to continuously reduce particle size via controlled secondary nucleation and breakage; and the other is in the upstream as a high shear nucleator to continuously generate seed crystals. It was observed that smaller crystals (55 μm) with uniform distribution were obtained when the wet milling was used in the downstream processing. While, when the wet mill was used in the upstream stage, small crystals were obtained when the tip speed was high, whereas large crystals can be produced when the tip speed was low. This is because the high tip speed of the wet mill results in a high primary nucleation rate and a large amount of small seed crystals, and therefore only a small amount of supersaturation is available for crystals to grow in the MSMPR.

Despite these successes, many practical issues indeed remain in scaling up to industrial-scale continuous crystallization operation. On the lab scale, the supersaturation is almost uniformly distributed. However, on larger scales, problems due to scale-up can appear. For example, mixing issues such as particle suspension, particle attrition, etc. [124] should be considered in the crystallizers. At present, industrial-scale continuous crystallization is still limited in the production of inorganic salts (e.g., sodium chloride, lithium carbonate). For the pharmaceuticals, it has higher requirements on the continuous crystallization development because, in addition to the purity and yield, the crystal shape and CSD need to be optimized to ensure the downstream filtration efficiency, granulation, tableting, etc.

4.3 Continuous Flow for on-Demand Pharmaceutical Manufacturing

Continuous manufacturing has been recognized as a method for process intensification in the specialty and commodity chemical industry. The whole continuous manufacturing (end-to-end) of a targeting API has been considered to integrate unit operations including upstream synthesis and downstream filtration, drying, granulation, lubrication, etc. [125] As shown in Fig. 9a, Polster et al. realized a pilot-scale integration of continuous synthesis and crystallization of an API, which showed a good-quality control ability compared with the batch process. The most significant attributes are the consistency of crystal products and the scalability of the industrial process. The fouling occurred in the plug flow reactor and also the tubular crystallizer, which raised a higher requirement of the continuous process. Besides, compared with batch process, the continuous manufacturing process has great advantages in project footprint and investment. Domokos et al. reported an end-to-end process from chemical synthesis to the tableting process of acetylsalicylic acid, as shown in Fig. 9b. The 100 mg dose strength tablets have obtained that start from the raw materials. Based on the researches of continuous synthesis, crystallization, drying, etc., the integration of the individual technological steps has become the tendency to develop the end-to-end system, in which the realization of the continuous flow from the synthesis of APIs to the graduation and formulation process is difficult and, what's more, the in situ monitoring such as the purity of the synthesis product, the crystal polymorph and CSD in the crystallization process, the blending performance, etc. needs to be implemented in the whole manufacturing process to meet the quality by design strategy.

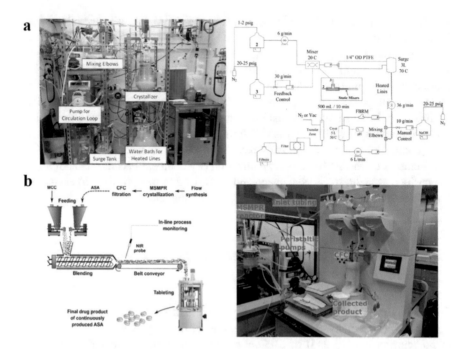

Fig. 9 (**a**) Photograph (left) and schematic (right) of pilot-scale continuous equipment to realize amide formation and reactive crystallization (left). Reprinted from Ref. [125]. Copyright 2014 American Chemical Society. (**b**) Experimental setup of the continuous blending and tableting (left), and integrated continuous crystallization and filtration (right). Reprinted from Ref. [97]. Copyright 2020 Elsevier B.V. All rights reserved

References

1. Nagy, Z. K.; Fevotte, G.; Kramer, H.; Simon, L. L., Recent advances in the monitoring, modeling and control of crystallization systems. *Chemical Engineering Research & Design* **2013,** 91, (10), 1903–1922.
2. Pena, R.; Nagy, Z. K., Process Intensification through Continuous Spherical Crystallization Using a Two-Stage Mixed Suspension Mixed Product Removal (MSMPR) System. *Crystal Growth & Design* **2015,** 15, (9), 4225–4236.
3. Liu, W.; Wei, H.; Zhao, J.; Black, S.; Sun, C., Investigation into the Cooling Crystallization and Transformations of Carbamazepine Using in Situ FBRM and PVM. *Organic Process Research & Development* **2013,** 17, (11), 1406–1412.
4. Luo, Y.-H.; Tu, Y.-R.; Ge, J.-L.; Sun, B.-W., Monitoring the Crystallization Process of Methylprednisolone Hemisuccinate (MPHS) from Ethanol Solution by Combined ATR-FTIR- FBRM- PVM. *Separation Science and Technology* **2013,** 48, (12), 1881–1890.
5. Szilagyi, B.; Eren, A.; Quon, J. L.; Papageorgiou, C. D.; Nagy, Z. K., Application of Model-Free and Model-Based Quality-by-Control (QbC) for the Efficient Design of Pharmaceutical Crystallization Processes. *Crystal Growth & Design* **2020,** 20, (6), 3979–3996.
6. Cruz-Cabeza, A. J.; Reutzel-Edens, S. M.; Bernstein, J., Facts and fictions about polymorphism. *Chemical Society Reviews* **2015,** 44, (23), 8619–8635.

7. Kee, N. C. S.; Tan, R. B. H.; Braatz, R. D., Selective Crystallization of the Metastable alpha-Form of L-Glutamic Acid using Concentration Feedback Control. *Crystal Growth & Design* **2009**, 9, (7), 3044–3051.

8. Liotta, V.; Sabesan, V., Monitoring and feedback control of supersaturation using ATR-FTIR to produce an active pharmaceutical ingredient of a desired crystal size. *Organic Process Research & Development* **2004**, 8, (3), 488–494.

9. Nonoyama, N.; Hanaki, K.; Yabuki, Y., Constant supersaturation control of antisolvent-addition batch crystallization. *Organic Process Research & Development* **2006**, 10, (4), 727–732.

10. Hermanto, M. W.; Braatz, R. D.; Chiu, M.-S., Integrated Batch-to-Batch and Nonlinear Model Predictive Control for Polymorphic Transformation in Pharmaceutical Crystallization. *Aiche Journal* **2011**, 57, (4), 1008–1019.

11. Nagy, Z. K.; Chew, J. W.; Fujiwara, M.; Braatz, R. D., Comparative performance of concentration and temperature controlled batch crystallizations. *Journal of Process Control* **2008**, 18, (3–4), 399–407.

12. Pataki, H.; Csontos, I.; Nagy, Z. K.; Vajna, B.; Molnar, M.; Katona, L.; Marosi, G., Implementation of Raman Signal Feedback to Perform Controlled Crystallization of Carvedilol. *Organic Process Research & Development* **2013**, 17, (3), 493–499.

13. Tacsi, K.; Gyurkes, M.; Csontos, I.; Farkas, A.; Borbas, E.; Nagy, Z. K.; Marosi, G.; Pataki, H., Polymorphic Concentration Control for Crystallization Using Raman and Attenuated Total Reflectance Ultraviolet Visible Spectroscopy. *Crystal Growth & Design* **2020**, 20, (1), 73–86.

14. Simone, E.; Saleemi, A. N.; Tonnon, N.; Nagy, Z. K., Active Polymorphic Feedback Control of Crystallization Processes Using a Combined Raman and ATR-UV/Vis Spectroscopy Approach. *Crystal Growth & Design* **2014**, 14, (4), 1839–1850.

15. Howard, K. S.; Nagy, Z. K.; Saha, B.; Robertson, A. L.; Steele, G.; Martin, D., A Process Analytical Technology Based Investigation of the Polymorphic Transformations during the Antisolvent Crystallization of Sodium Benzoate from IPA/Water Mixture. *Crystal Growth & Design* **2009**, 9, (9), 3964–3975.

16. Saleemi, A. N.; Rielly, C. D.; Nagy, Z. K., Comparative Investigation of Supersaturation and Automated Direct Nucleation Control of Crystal Size Distributions using ATR-UV/vis Spectroscopy and FBRM. *Crystal Growth & Design* **2012**, 12, (4), 1792–1807.

17. Simone, E.; Nagy, Z. K., A link between the ATR-UV/Vis and Raman spectra of zwitterionic solutions and the polymorphic outcome in cooling crystallization. *Crystengcomm* **2015**, 17, (34), 6538–6547.

18. Simone, E.; Zhang, W.; Nagy, Z. K., Application of Process Analytical Technology-Based Feedback Control Strategies To Improve Purity and Size Distribution in Biopharmaceutical Crystallization. *Crystal Growth & Design* **2015**, 15, (6), 2908–2919.

19. Saleemi, A. N.; Steele, G.; Pedge, N. I.; Freeman, A.; Nagy, Z. K., Enhancing crystalline properties of a cardiovascular active pharmaceutical ingredient using a process analytical technology based crystallization feedback control strategy. *International Journal of Pharmaceutics* **2012**, 430, (1–2), 56–64.

20. Abu Bakar, M. R.; Nagy, Z. K.; Saleemi, A. N.; Rielly, C. D., The Impact of Direct Nucleation Control on Crystal Size Distribution in Pharmaceutical Crystallization Processes. *Crystal Growth & Design* **2009**, 9, (3), 1378–1384.

21. Borsos, A.; Szilagyi, B.; Agachi, P. S.; Nagy, Z. K., Real-Time Image Processing Based Online Feedback Control System for Cooling Batch Crystallization. *Organic Process Research & Development* **2017**, 21, (4), 511–519.

22. Griffin, D. J.; Kawajiri, Y.; Rousseau, R. W.; Grover, M. A., Using MC plots for control of paracetamol crystallization. *Chemical Engineering Science* **2017**, 164, 344–360.

23. Botschi, S.; Rajagopalan, A. K.; Morari, M.; Mazzotti, M., Feedback Control for the Size and Shape Evolution of Needle-like Crystals in Suspension. IV. Modeling and Control of Dissolution. *Crystal Growth & Design* **2019**, 19, (7), 4029–4043.

24. Rajagopalan, A. K.; Botschi, S.; Morari, M.; Mazzotti, M., Feedback Control for the Size and Shape Evolution of Needle-like Crystals in Suspension. III. Wet Milling. *Crystal Growth & Design* **2019**, 19, (5), 2845–2861.

25. Rajagopalan, A. K.; Botschi, S.; Morari, M.; Mazzotti, M., Feedback Control for the Size and Shape Evolution of Needle-like Crystals in Suspension. II. Cooling Crystallization Experiments. *Crystal Growth & Design* **2018**, 18, (10), 6185–6196.

26. Boetschi, S.; Rajagopalan, A. K.; Morari, M.; Mazzotti, M., Feedback Control for the Size and Shape Evolution of Needle-like Crystals in Suspension. I. Concepts and Simulation Studies. *Crystal Growth & Design* **2018**, 18, (8), 4470–4483.

27. Lung-Somarriba, B. L. M.; Moscosa-Santillan, M.; Porte, C.; Delacroix, A., Effect of seeded surface area on crystal size distribution in glycine batch cooling crystallization: a seeding methodology. *Journal of Crystal Growth* **2004**, 270, (3–4), 624–632.

28. Artusio, F.; Pisano, R., Surface-induced crystallization of pharmaceuticals and biopharmaceuticals: A review. *International Journal of Pharmaceutics* **2018**, 547, (1–2), 190–208.

29. Beckmann, W., Seeding the desired polymorph: Background, possibilities, limitations, and case studies. *Organic Process Research & Development* **2000**, 4, (5), 372–383.

30. Lafferrere, L.; Hoff, C.; Veesler, S., In situ monitoring of the impact of liquid-liquid phase separation on drug crystallization by seeding. *Crystal Growth & Design* **2004**, 4, (6), 1175–1180.

31. Li, Y.; O'Shea, S.; Yin, Q.; Vetter, T., Polymorph Selection by Continuous Crystallization in the Presence of Wet Milling. *Crystal Growth & Design* **2019**, 19, (4), 2259–2271.

32. Xu, A.-W.; Dong, W.-F.; Antonietti, M.; Coelfen, H., Polymorph switching of calcium carbonate crystals by polymer-controlled crystallization. *Advanced Functional Materials* **2008**, 18, (8), 1307–1313.

33. Garg, R. K.; Sarkar, D., Polymorphism control of p-aminobenzoic acid by isothermal anti-solvent crystallization. *Journal of Crystal Growth* **2016**, 454, 180–185.

34. Parambil, J. V.; Poornachary, S. K.; Tan, R. B. H.; Heng, J. Y. Y., Template-induced polymorphic selectivity: the effects of surface chemistry and solute concentration on carbamazepine crystallisation. *Crystengcomm* **2014**, 16, (23), 4927–4930.

35. Maghsoodi, M., Role of Solvents in Improvement of Dissolution Rate of Drugs: Crystal Habit and Crystal Agglomeration. *Advanced Pharmaceutical Bulletin* **2015**, 5, (1), 13–18.

36. Ferrari, E. S.; Davey, R. J.; Cross, W. I.; Gillon, A. L.; Towler, C. S., Crystallization in polymorphic systems: The solution-mediated transformation beta to alpha glycine. *Crystal Growth & Design* **2003**, 3, (1), 53–60.

37. Maghsoodi, M., How spherical crystallization improves direct tableting properties: a review. *Advanced pharmaceutical bulletin* **2012**, 2, (2), 253–7.

38. Zaccaro, J.; Matic, J.; Myerson, A. S.; Garetz, B. A., Nonphotochemical, laser-induced nucleation of supersaturated aqueous glycine produces unexpected gamma-polymorph. *Crystal Growth & Design* **2001**, 1, (1), 5–8.

39. Alexander, L. F.; Radacsi, N., Application of electric fields for controlling crystallization. *Crystengcomm* **2019**, 21, (34), 5014–5031.

40. Taleb, M.; Didierjean, C.; Jelsch, C.; Mangeot, J. P.; Aubry, A., Equilibrium kinetics of lysozyme crystallization under an external electric field. *Journal of Crystal Growth* **2001**, 232, (1–4), 250–255.

41. Koizumi, H.; Uda, S.; Fujiwara, K.; Nozawa, J., Control of Effect on the Nucleation Rate for Hen Egg White Lysozyme Crystals under Application of an External ac Electric Field. *Langmuir* **2011**, 27, (13), 8333–8338.

42. Parks, C.; Koswara, A.; Tung, H.-H.; Nere, N.; Bordawekar, S.; Nagy, Z. K.; Ramkrishna, D., Molecular Dynamics Electric Field Crystallization Simulations of Paracetamol Produce a New Polymorph. *Crystal Growth & Design* **2017**, 17, (7), 3751–3765.

43. Hou, D.; Chang, H.-C., ac field enhanced protein crystallization. *Applied Physics Letters* **2008**, 92, (22).

44. Pareja-Rivera, C.; Cuellar-Cruz, M.; Esturau-Escofet, N.; Demitri, N.; Polentarutti, M.; Stojanoff, V.; Moreno, A., Recent Advances in the Understanding of the Influence of Electric and Magnetic Fields on Protein Crystal Growth. *Crystal Growth & Design* **2017**, 17, (1), 135–145.

45. Koizumi, H.; Fujiwara, K.; Uda, S., Control of Nucleation Rate for Tetragonal Hen-Egg White Lysozyme Crystals by Application of an Electric Field with Variable Frequencies. *Crystal Growth & Design* **2009**, 9, (5), 2420–2424.

46. Li, F.; Lakerveld, R., Influence of Alternating Electric Fields on Protein Crystallization in Microfluidic Devices with Patterned Electrodes in a Parallel-Plate Configuration. *Crystal Growth & Design* **2017**, 17, (6), 3062–3070.

47. Liu, T.-H.; Uwada, T.; Sugiyama, T.; Usman, A.; Hosokawa, Y.; Masuhara, H.; Chiang, T.-W.; Chen, C.-J., Single femtosecond laser pulse-single crystal formation of glycine at the solution surface. *Journal of Crystal Growth* **2013**, 366, 101–106.

48. Yuyama, K.-i.; Chang, K.-D.; Tu, J.-R.; Masuhara, H.; Sugiyama, T., Rapid localized crystallization of lysozyme by laser trapping. *Physical Chemistry Chemical Physics* **2018**, 20, (9), 6034–6039.

49. Yuyama, K.-i.; Wu, C.-S.; Sugiyama, T.; Masuhara, H., Laser trapping-induced crystallization of L-phenylalanine through its high-concentration domain formation. *Photochemical & Photobiological Sciences* **2014**, 13, (2), 254–260.

50. Nakamura, K.; Hosokawa, Y.; Masuhara, H., Anthracene crystallization induced by single-shot femtosecond laser irradiation: Experimental evidence for the important role of bubbles. *Crystal Growth & Design* **2007**, 7, (5), 885–889.

51. Matic, J.; Sun, X. Y.; Garetz, B. A.; Myerson, A. S., Intensity, wavelength, and polarization dependence of nonphotochemical laser-induced nucleation in supersaturated aqueous urea solutions. *Crystal Growth & Design* **2005**, 5, (4), 1565–1567.

52. Tsuri, Y.; Maruyama, M.; Fujimoto, R.; Okada, S.; Adachi, H.; Yoshikawa, H. Y.; Takano, K.; Murakami, S.; Matsumura, H.; Inoue, T.; Tsukamoto, K.; Imanishi, M.; Yoshimura, M.; Mori, Y., Crystallization of aspirin form II by femtosecond laser irradiation. *Applied Physics Express* **2019**, 12, (1).

53. Nalesso, S.; Bussemaker, M. J.; Sear, R. P.; Hodnett, M.; Lee, J., A review on possible mechanisms of sonocrystallisation in solution. *Ultrasonics Sonochemistry* **2019**, 57, 125–138.

54. Lee, J.; Yasui, K.; Ashokkumar, M.; Kentish, S. E., Quantification of Cavitation Activity by Sonoluminescence To Study the Sonocrystallization Process under Different Ultrasound Parameters. *Crystal Growth & Design* **2018**, 18, (9), 5108–5115.

55. Jia, J.; Wang, W.; Gao, Y.; Zhao, Y., Controlled morphology and size of curcumin using ultrasound in supercritical CO2 antisolvent. *Ultrasonics Sonochemistry* **2015**, 27, 389–394.

56. Iyer, S. R.; Gogate, P. R., Ultrasound assisted crystallization of mefenamic acid: Effect of operating parameters and comparison with conventional approach. *Ultrasonics Sonochemistry* **2017**, 34, 896–903.

57. Nii, S.; Takayanagi, S., Growth and size control in anti-solvent crystallization of glycine with high frequency ultrasound. *Ultrasonics Sonochemistry* **2014**, 21, (3), 1182–1186.

58. Vishwakarma, R. S.; Gogate, P. R., Intensified oxalic acid crystallization using ultrasonic reactors: Understanding effect of operating parameters and type of ultrasonic reactor. *Ultrasonics Sonochemistry* **2017**, 39, 111–119.

59. Bhangu, S. K.; Ashokkumar, M.; Lee, J., Ultrasound Assisted Crystallization of Paracetamol: Crystal Size Distribution and Polymorph Control. *Crystal Growth & Design* **2016**, 16, (4), 1934–1941.

60. Ike, Y.; Hirasawa, I., Polymorph Control of L-Phenylalanine in Cooling Crystallization by Ultrasonication. *Chemical Engineering & Technology* **2018**, 41, (6), 1093–1097.

61. Zeiger, B. W.; Suslick, K. S., Sonofragmentation of Molecular Crystals. *Journal of the American Chemical Society* **2011**, 133, (37), 14530–14533.

62. Gracin, S.; Uusi-Penttila, M.; Rasmuson, A. C., Influence of ultrasound on the nucleation of polymorphs of p-aminobenzoic acid. *Crystal Growth & Design* **2005**, 5, (5), 1787–1794.

63. Sander, J. R. G.; Zeiger, B. W.; Suslick, K. S., Sonocrystallization and sonofragmentation. *Ultrasonics Sonochemistry* **2014**, 21, (6), 1908–1915.
64. Jordens, J.; Gielen, B.; Xiouras, C.; Hussain, M. N.; Stefanidis, G. D.; Thomassen, L. C. J.; Braeken, L.; Van Gerven, T., Sonocrystallisation: Observations, theories and guidelines. *Chemical Engineering and Processing-Process Intensification* **2019**, 139, 130–154.
65. Gogate, P. R.; Patil, P. N., Sonochemical Reactors. *Topics in Current Chemistry* **2016**, 374, (5).
66. Mastan, T. H.; Lenka, M.; Sarkar, D., Nucleation kinetics from metastable zone widths for sonocrystallization of L-phenylalanine. *Ultrasonics Sonochemistry* **2017**, 36, 497–506.
67. Sazaki, G.; Moreno, A.; Nakajima, K., Novel coupling effects of the magnetic and electric fields on protein crystallization. *Journal of Crystal Growth* **2004**, 262, (1–4), 499–502.
68. Yan, E.-K.; Zhang, C.-Y.; He, J.; Yin, D.-C., An Overview of Hardware for Protein Crystallization in a Magnetic Field. *International Journal of Molecular Sciences* **2016**, 17, (11).
69. Yin, D.-C.; Lu, H.-M.; Geng, L.-Q.; Shi, Z.-H.; Luo, H.-M.; Li, H.-S.; Ye, Y.-J.; Guo, W.-H.; Shang, P.; Wakayama, N. I., Growing and dissolving protein crystals in a levitated and containerless droplet. *Journal of Crystal Growth* **2008**, 310, (6), 1206–1212.
70. Huang, L.-J.; Cao, H.-L.; Ye, Y.-J.; Liu, Y.-M.; Zhang, C.-Y.; Lu, Q.-Q.; Hou, H.; Shang, P.; Yin, D.-C., A new method to realize high-throughput protein crystallization in a superconducting magnet. *Crystengcomm* **2015**, 17, (6), 1237–1241.
71. Sundaram, N. M.; Girija, E. K.; Ashok, M.; Anee, T. K.; Vani, R.; Suganthi, R. V.; Yokogawa, Y.; Kalkura, S. N., Crystallisation of hydroxyapatite nanocrystals under magnetic field. *Materials Letters* **2006**, 60, (6), 761–765.
72. Madsen, H. E. L., Crystallization of heavy-metal phosphates in solution - IV: growth of Cd5H2(PO4)(4),4H(2)O in magnetic field. *Journal of Crystal Growth* **2004**, 263, (1–4), 564–569.
73. Gao, Y. Y.; Xie, C.; Wang, J. K., Effects of low magnetic field on batch crystallisation of glycine. *Materials Research Innovations* **2009**, 13, (2), 112–115.
74. Lawton, S.; Steele, G.; Shering, P.; Zhao, L.; Laird, I.; Ni, X.-W., Continuous Crystallization of Pharmaceuticals Using a Continuous Oscillatory Baffled Crystallizer. *Organic Process Research & Development* **2009**, 13, (6), 1357–1363.
75. Jolliffe, H. G.; Gerogiorgis, D. I., Process modelling, design and technoeconomic evaluation for continuous paracetamol crystallisation. In *28th European Symposium on Computer Aided Process Engineering*, Friedl, A.; Klemes, J. J.; Radl, S.; Varbanov, P. S.; Wallek, T., Eds. 2018; Vol. 43, pp 1637–1642.
76. Ricardo, C.; Ni, X., Evaluation and Establishment of a Cleaning Protocol for the Production of Vanisal Sodium and Aspirin Using a Continuous Oscillatory Baffled Reactor. *Organic Process Research & Development* **2009**, 13, (6), 1080–1087.
77. Ni, X.; Liao, A., Effects of cooling rate and solution concentration on solution crystallization of L-glutamic acid in an oscillatory baffled crystallizer. *Crystal Growth & Design* **2008**, 8, (8), (8), 2875–2881.
78. Callahan, C. J.; Ni, X.-W., On the investigation of the effect of apparatus configurations on the nucleation mechanisms in a cooling crystallization of sodium chlorate. *Canadian Journal of Chemical Engineering* **2014**, 92, (11), 1920–1925.
79. Brown, C. J.; Adelakun, J. A.; Ni, X.-w., Characterization and modelling of antisolvent crystallization of salicylic acid in a continuous oscillatory baffled crystallizer. *Chemical Engineering and Processing-Process Intensification* **2015**, 97, 180–186.
80. Zhao, L.; Raval, V.; Briggs, N. E. B.; Bhardwaj, R. M.; McGlone, T.; Oswald, I. D. H.; Florence, A. J., From discovery to scale-up: alpha-lipoic acid : nicotinamide co-crystals in a continuous oscillatory baffled crystalliser. *Crystengcomm* **2014**, 16, (26), 5769–5780.
81. Park, S.-A.; Lee, S.; Kim, W.-S., Polymorphic Crystallization of Sulfamerazine in Taylor Vortex Flow: Polymorphic Nucleation and Phase Transformation. *Crystal Growth & Design* **2015**, 15, (8), 3617–3627.

82. Anh-Tuan, N.; Yu, T.; Kim, W.-S., Couette-Taylor crystallizer: Effective control of crystal size distribution and recovery of L-lysine in cooling crystallization. *Journal of Crystal Growth* **2017**, 469, 65–77.

83. Nguyen, A.-T.; Kim, J.-M.; Chang, S.-M.; Kim, W.-S., Phase Transformation of Guanosine 5-Monophosphate in Continuous Couette-Taylor Crystallizer: Experiments and Numerical Modeling for Kinetics. *Industrial & Engineering Chemistry Research* **2011**, 50, (6), 3483–3493.

84. Nguyen, A.-T.; Joo, Y. L.; Kim, W.-S., Multiple Feeding Strategy for Phase Transformation of GMP in Continuous Couette-Taylor Crystallizer. *Crystal Growth & Design* **2012**, 12, (6), 2780–2788.

85. Wu, Z.; Seok, S.; Kim, D. H.; Kim, W.-S., Control of Crystal Size Distribution using Non-Isothermal Taylor Vortex Flow. *Crystal Growth & Design* **2015**, 15, (12), 5675–5684.

86. Benitez-Chapa, A. G.; Nigam, K. D. P.; Alvarez, A. J., Process Intensification of Continuous Antisolvent Crystallization Using a Coiled Flow Inverter. *Industrial & Engineering Chemistry Research* **2020**, 59, (9), 3934–3942.

87. Hohmann, L.; Gorny, R.; Klaas, O.; Ahlert, J.; Wohlgemuth, K.; Kockmann, N., Design of a Continuous Tubular Cooling Crystallizer for Process Development on Lab-Scale. *Chemical Engineering & Technology* **2016**, 39, (7), 1268–1280.

88. Hohmann, L.; Greinert, T.; Mierka, O.; Turek, S.; Schembecker, G.; Bayraktar, E.; Wohlgemuth, K.; Kockmann, N., Analysis of Crystal Size Dispersion Effects in a Continuous Coiled Tubular Crystallizer: Experiments and Modeling. *Crystal Growth & Design* **2018**, 18, (3), 1459–1473.

89. Koyama, M.; Kudo, S.; Amari, S.; Takiyama, H., Development of novel cascade type crystallizer for continuous production of crystalline particles. *Journal of Industrial and Engineering Chemistry* **2020**, 89, 111–114.

90. Majumder, A.; Nagy, Z. K., Fines Removal in a Continuous Plug Flow Crystallizer by Optimal Spatial Temperature Profiles with Controlled Dissolution. *Aiche Journal* **2013**, 59, (12), 4582–4594.

91. Zhao, Y.; Kamaraju, V. K.; Hou, G.; Power, G.; Donnellan, P.; Glennon, B., Kinetic identification and experimental validation of continuous plug flow crystallisation. *Chemical Engineering Science* **2015**, 133, 106–115.

92. Besenhard, M. O.; Neugebauer, P.; Scheibelhofer, O.; Khinast, J. G., Crystal Engineering in Continuous Plug-Flow Crystallizers. *Crystal Growth & Design* **2017**, 17, (12), 6432–6444.

93. Cogoni, G.; de Souza, B. P.; Frawley, P. J., Particle Size Distribution and yield control in continuous Plug Flow Crystallizers with recycle. *Chemical Engineering Science* **2015**, 138, 592–599.

94. Alvarez, A. J.; Myerson, A. S., Continuous Plug Flow Crystallization of Pharmaceutical Compounds. *Crystal Growth & Design* **2010**, 10, (5), 2219–2228.

95. Ferguson, S.; Morris, G.; Hao, H.; Barrett, M.; Glennon, B., Characterization of the anti-solvent batch, plug flow and MSMPR crystallization of benzoic acid. *Chemical Engineering Science* **2013**, 104, 44–54.

96. Ma, Y.; Wu, S.; Macaringue, E. G. J.; Zhang, T.; Gong, J.; Wang, J., Recent Progress in Continuous Crystallization of Pharmaceutical Products: Precise Preparation and Control. *Organic Process Research & Development* **2020**.

97. Domokos, A.; Nagy, B.; Gyurkes, M.; Farkas, A.; Tacsi, K.; Pataki, H.; Liu, Y. C.; Balogh, A.; Firth, P.; Szilagyi, B.; Marosi, G.; Nagy, Z. K.; Nagy, Z. K., End-to-end continuous manufacturing of conventional compressed tablets: From flow synthesis to tableting through integrated crystallization and filtration. *International journal of pharmaceutics* **2020**, 581, 119297.

98. Diab, S.; Gerogiorgis, D. I., Technoeconomic Optimization of Continuous Crystallization for Three Active Pharmaceutical Ingredients: Cyclosporine, Paracetamol, and Aliskiren. *Industrial & Engineering Chemistry Research* **2018**, 57, (29), 9489–9499.

99. Bart Rimez, R. D., Jennifer Conte, Edith Lecomte-Norrant, Christophe Gourdon,; Patrick Cognet, a. B. S., Continuous-Flow Tubular Crystallization To Discriminate between Two Competing Crystal Polymorphs. 1. Cooling Crystallization. *Cryst. Growth Des.* **2018**, 6431–6439.

100. Besenhard, M. O.; Neugebauer, P.; Scheibelhofer, O.; Khinast, J. G., Crystal Engineering in Continuous Plug-Flow Crystallizers. *Cryst Growth Des* **2017**, 17, (12), 6432–6444.

101. Agnew, L. R.; McGlone, T.; Wheatcroft, H. P.; Robertson, A.; Parsons, A. R.; Wilson, C. C., Continuous Crystallization of Paracetamol (Acetaminophen) Form II: Selective Access to a Metastable Solid Form. *Crystal Growth & Design* **2017**, 17, (5), 2418–2427.

102. Benitez-Chapa, A. G.; Nigam, K. D. P.; Alvarez, A. J., Process Intensification of Continuous Antisolvent Crystallization Using a Coiled Flow Inverter. *Industrial & Engineering Chemistry Research* **2019**, 59, (9), 3934–3942.

103. Tang, Z.; Kim, W.-S.; Yu, T., Studies on morphology changes of copper sulfide nanoparticles in a continuous Couette-Taylor reactor. *Chemical Engineering Journal* **2019**, 359, 1436–1441.

104. Zhang, D.; Xu, S.; Du, S.; Wang, J.; Gong, J., Progress of Pharmaceutical Continuous Crystallization. *Engineering* **2017**, 3, (3), 354–364.

105. Cameron Brown, T. M. a. A. F., Continuous Crystallisation. **2018**.

106. Ferguson; S.; Morris; G.; Hao; H.; Barrett; M.; Glennon; B., In-situ monitoring and characterization of plug flow crystallizers. *CHEMICAL ENGINEERING SCIENCE* **2012**.

107. Gorny; Ramona; Hohmann; Lukas; Ahlert; Jonas; Kockmann; Norbert; Klaas; Oliver, Design of a Continuous Tubular Cooling Crystallizer for Process Development on Lab-Scale. *Chemical Engineering & Technology Industrial Chemistry Plant Equipment Process Engineering Biotechnology* **2016**.

108. Eder, R. J. P.; Radl, S.; Schmitt, E.; Innerhofer, S.; Maier, M.; Gruber-Woelfler, H.; Khinast, J. G., Continuously Seeded, Continuously Operated Tubular Crystallizer for the Production of Active Pharmaceutical Ingredients. *Crystal Growth & Design* **2010**, 10, (5), 2247–2257.

109. Siddique, H.; Brown, C. J.; Houson, I.; Florence, A. J., Establishment of a Continuous Sonocrystallization Process for Lactose in an Oscillatory Baffled Crystallizer. *Organic Process Research & Development* **2015**, 19, (12), 1871–1881.

110. Gutwald, T.; Mersmann, A., Evaluation of kinetic parameters of crystallization from batch and continuous experiments. *Separations Technology* **1994**, 4, (1), 2–14.

111. Neugebauer, P.; Khinast, J. G., Continuous Crystallization of Proteins in a Tubular Plug-Flow Crystallizer. *Cryst Growth Des* **2015**, 15, (3), 1089–1095.

112. Ferguson, S.; Morris, G.; Hao, H.; Barrett, M.; Glennon, B., In-situ monitoring and characterization of plug flow crystallizers. *Chemical Engineering Science* **2012**, 77, 105–111.

113. Marie Stihl, B. L. h., and ike C. Rasmuson, Reaction Crystallization Kinetics of Benzoic Acid. *AIChE Journal* **2001**.

114. Lai, T.-T. C.; Ferguson, S.; Palmer, L.; Trout, B. L.; Myerson, A. S., Continuous Crystallization and Polymorph Dynamics in the l-Glutamic Acid System. *Organic Process Research & Development* **2014**, 18, (11), 1382–1390.

115. Lai, T.-T. C.; Cornevin, J.; Ferguson, S.; Li, N.; Trout, B. L.; Myerson, A. S., Control of Polymorphism in Continuous Crystallization via Mixed Suspension Mixed Product Removal Systems Cascade Design. *Crystal Growth & Design* **2015**, 15, (7), 3374–3382.

116. Quon, J. L.; Zhang, H.; Alvarez, A.; Evans, J.; Myerson, A. S.; Trout, B. L., Continuous Crystallization of Aliskiren Hemifumarate. *Crystal Growth & Design* **2012**, 12, (6), 3036–3044.

117. Powell, K. A.; Bartolini, G.; Wittering, K. E.; Saleemi, A. N.; Wilson, C. C.; Rielly, C. D.; Nagy, Z. K., Toward Continuous Crystallization of Urea-Barbituric Acid: A Polymorphic Co-Crystal System. *Crystal Growth & Design* **2015**, 15, (10), 4821–4836.

118. Powell, K. A.; Saleemi, A. N.; Rielly, C. D.; Nagy, Z. K., Periodic steady-state flow crystallization of a pharmaceutical drug using MSMPR operation. *Chemical Engineering and Processing: Process Intensification* **2015**, 97, 195–212.

119. Chaaban, J. H.; Dam-Johansen, K.; Skovby, T.; Kiil, S., Separation of Enantiomers by Continuous Preferential Crystallization: Experimental Realization Using a Coupled Crystallizer Configuration. *Organic Process Research & Development* **2013,** 17, (8), 1010–1020.
120. Rougeot, C.; Hein, J. E., Application of Continuous Preferential Crystallization to Efficiently Access Enantiopure Chemicals. *Organic Process Research & Development* **2015,** 19, (12), 1809–1819.
121. Sulttan, S.; Rohani, S., Coupling of CFD and population balance modelling for a continuously seeded helical tubular crystallizer. *Journal of Crystal Growth* **2019,** 505, 19–25.
122. Gao, Z.; Wu, Y.; Gong, J.; Wang, J.; Rohani, S., Continuous crystallization of α-form L-glutamic acid in an MSMPR-Tubular crystallizer system. *Journal of Crystal Growth* **2019,** 507, 344–351.
123. Yang, Y.; Song, L.; Gao, T.; Nagy, Z. K., Integrated Upstream and Downstream Application of Wet Milling with Continuous Mixed Suspension Mixed Product Removal Crystallization. *Crystal Growth & Design* **2015,** 15, (12), 5879–5885.
124. Wood, B.; Girard, K. P.; Polster, C. S.; Croker, D. M., Progress to Date in the Design and Operation of Continuous Crystallization Processes for Pharmaceutical Applications. *Organic Process Research & Development* **2019,** 23, (2), 122–144.
125. Polster, C. S.; Cole, K. P.; Burcham, C. L.; Campbell, B. M.; Frederick, A. L.; Hansen, M. M.; Harding, M.; Heller, M. R.; Miller, M. T.; Phillips, J. L.; Pollock, P. M.; Zaborenko, N., Pilot-Scale Continuous Production of LY2886721: Amide Formation and Reactive Crystallization. *Organic Process Research & Development* **2014,** 18, (11), 1295–1309.

Method of Characteristics for the Efficient Simulation of Population Balance Models

Xiaoxiang Zhu, Lifang Zhou, and Richard D. Braatz

1 Introduction

Particulate processes are ubiquitous in chemical engineering and include crystallization [1], aerosols [2], living cell dynamics [3], and polymerization [4, 5]. Population balance models (PBMs) are commonly used to describe the dynamics of such processes. The product quality typically depends on the particle size distribution (PSD), and considerable efforts have been devoted to engineering of the PSD [1, 6]. Among the various particular processes, probably one of the most heavily studied in recent years is the modeling, prediction, and control of the size distribution for crystallization processes, given its importance in the development of pharmaceutical products [7, 8].

In the modeling of particulate processes, population balance models nearly always include a hyperbolic partial differential equation of the form [9]:

$$\frac{\partial f(x,t)}{\partial t} + \frac{\partial \left(G(x,t) f\left(x,t\right)\right)}{\partial x} = h\left(f\left(x,t\right), x, t\right) \tag{1}$$

where $f(x, t)$ is the population distribution (density) function, $G(x, t)$ is the growth rate function, t is time, x is the internal coordinate (e.g., length, volume, mass, age), and h is the rate of generation or disappearance of particles, which typically involve nucleation, aggregation, agglomeration, coalescence, and/or breakage. The algebraic functions G and h usually have an additional dependency, not shown explicitly in Eq. (1) to simplify the notation, on the concentration of one or more

X. Zhu · L. Zhou · R. D. Braatz (✉)
Department of Chemical Engineering, Massachusetts Institute of Technology, Cambridge, MA, USA
e-mail: braatz@mit.edu

© The Author(s), under exclusive license to Springer Nature Switzerland AG 2022
A. Fytopoulos et al. (eds.), *Optimization of Pharmaceutical Processes*, Springer Optimization and Its Applications 189, https://doi.org/10.1007/978-3-030-90924-6_2

species in solution whose dynamics are described by nonlinear ordinary differential equations.

Several types of solution techniques have been developed for solving the population balance models, including the method of moments [10–12], discretization methods [9, 13–15], and Monte Carlo methods [16, 17]. The standard method of moments (SMM) and the quadrature method of moments (QMOM) convert the partial integrodifferential equation into a set of ordinary differential equations (ODEs). Very often these moment equations do not form a closed finite number of ODEs. The QMOM is a popular method for deriving a closed set of ODEs in the method of moments, by applying a quadrature approximation of the distribution function [11]. The moment equations alone only allow average properties of the particles to be computed (such as mean length), and techniques for reconstruction of the size distribution from moments have been developed [18, 19]. Discretization methods such as finite difference and finite volume methods solve the PBMs directly and can simulate the size distribution dynamically, but are usually computationally expensive and can exhibit numerical diffusion or dispersion [9]. More advanced numerical schemes such as the parallel high-resolution finite volume method have been developed to reduce the computational time and increase numerical accuracy [13, 14, 20]. Another well-known discretization method is the method of classes [21, 22], which is a variation of a first-order-accurate finite volume method and the numerical method of lines. While some discretization methods are much faster and/or more accurate than others, such methods still exhibit some distortion in the shape of the distribution.

Advances in particle sensor technology have enabled the online acquisition of data that has inspired an increase in efforts to utilize such information in real-time optimization and control [7]. Real-time simulation and optimization of the PSD would be facilitated by having even faster PBM solvers, which has resulted in a resurge in interest in a classical method known as the *method of characteristics* (MOCH) [18, 23–27]. An early work that employed MOCH discretized the size into bins and integrated the population density function within each bin to generate a set of ODEs [23]. This combined MOCH-discretization approach had improved accuracy compared with some finite discretization methods that had been previously proposed in the literature [24, 28]. Another approach combines the MOCH and finite volume methods for modeling processes with nucleation, growth, and aggregation [29]. Those studies assumed constant supersaturation (and, as a result, growth rates). In growth-only crystallization processes with size-independent growth, the MOCH was used to solve a PBM that included the effect of impurities [25]. To take into account the mass conservation constraint, MOCH has also been combined with SMM to simulate crystallizations with size-independent growth and nucleation [26]. An extension combined the QMOM and the MOCH for simulating crystallizations with size-dependent growth and nucleation [18, 27]. Such combined moments-MOCH approaches require two steps: pre-solve the moment equations to obtain the supersaturation and the lower order moments, and subsequently use the supersaturation information in the MOCH simulation.

This paper revisits the implementation of the method-of-characteristics approach for efficiently modeling the size distribution evolution in typical crystallization processes without combination with other methods such as finite volume methods, SMM, and QMOM. The PBM is converted into a differential-algebraic equation (DAE) system that allows the simultaneous simulation of both the entire size distribution and the solute concentration. The solution technique is demonstrated with examples of representative mechanisms that arise in particulate systems, including multidimensional growth, size-dependent growth and nucleation, and growth with agglomeration.

2   Transforming the PBMs into a DAE System with the Method of Characteristics

The method of characteristics requires finding the *characteristics* in the x–t plane such that the partial differential equation (PDE) can be converted into a set of ordinary differential equations (ODEs). Along the characteristic curves, the ODEs with initial conditions are solved and transformed back to construct the solution of the original PDE [30]. Using the product rule, the population balance Eq. (1) can be rewritten as.

$$\frac{\partial f(x,t)}{\partial t} + G(x,t)\frac{\partial f(x,t)}{\partial x} = -f(x,t)\frac{\partial G(x,t)}{\partial x} + h(f(x,t),x,t) \qquad (2)$$

The identification of the characteristics is straightforward, and the systems of equations are generated as [18, 23, 26].

$$\frac{dx}{dt} = G(x,t) \qquad (3)$$

$$\frac{df(x,t)}{dt} = -f(x,t)\frac{\partial G(x,t)}{\partial x} + h(f(x,t),x,t) \qquad (4)$$

where the initial conditions for x and f are obtained from the initial size distribution, with $x(0) = x_0$ and $f(x,0) = f_0(x)$. For each characteristic x, there is a pairing f.

As mentioned above, the functions G and h are usually dependent on additional variables such as particle size and solution concentration(s). To complete the model equations for the system, mass conservation equations must also be satisfied. This chapter describes the implementation of the mass conservation equations as algebraic constraints that are simultaneously solved with the characteristic Eqs. (3) and (4) as a system of differential-algebraic equations (DAEs). For example, when the length L is chosen as the internal coordinate, the solute concentration can be related to the third-order moment μ_3 by the mass conservation constraint:

$$C(t) = C(0) - \rho k_v \left(\mu_3(t) - \mu_3(0) \right) \tag{5}$$

where ρ is the density of the solid phase and k_v is the shape factor, and consistent units for the solute concentration C and the number density function f are used (e.g., both based on per mass solvent). The third-order moment μ_3 is expressed as an integral of the distribution function:

$$\mu_3(t) = \int_0^\infty f(L, t) L^3 dL \tag{6}$$

where L is the discrete size of the particles. Eq. (5) is coupled to the characteristic Eqs. (3) and (4) by the third-order moment. In most particulate processes, the growth rate G is dependent on the solute concentration. As a result, the model Eqs. (3)–(6) are tightly coupled.

In the combined moment-MOCH approaches, the third moment Eq. (6) and solution concentration Eq. (5) are pre-computed for the entire time range, and the results were subsequently supplied to solve the characteristic equations [18, 26]. For dealing with size-dependent growth, the QMOM method utilizes a quadrature approximation that is evaluated at each time step, using either the product-difference algorithm [11, 31] or a differential-algebraic equation approach [10] (more details referred therein).

In the approach described in this chapter, the third-order moment Eq. (6) is calculated during real-time simulation of the evolution of the size distribution. By choosing N length characteristics (which give N pairs of L and f equations), the size distribution at any time is fully described by the N points, and the distribution information can be directly utilized to obtain the third-order moment (or any other moments) accurately using any quadrature methods, with the simplest being.

$$\mu_3(t) = \sum_{i=1}^{N} f(L_i, t) L_i^3 \Delta L_i \tag{7}$$

The DAE-based MOCH approach solves the population balance models efficiently, without simulating any moment equations and without approximating any derivatives of the distribution function f. The next section describes the implementation details, as well as the utilization of the alternative differential forms of the conservative Eq. (5) with its potential drawbacks.

3   Algorithms of the DAE-Based MOCH Approach

The idea of MOCH is usually illustrated by plotting the length characteristics (L–t relationships) [18, 25, 26]. The length characteristics could be grouped into two types (Fig. 1), which correspond to different mechanisms in the population balance

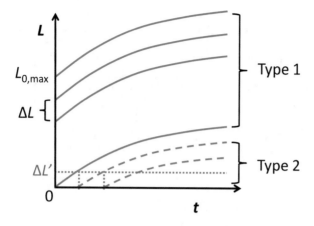

Fig. 1 Evolution of characteristic lines originating from the length L-axis (for initial particles, denoted as Type 1) and time t-axis (for newborn particles, denoted as Type 2) [18]

models. In a system with growth and nucleation, the characteristic curve of the first type starts on the length L-axis and corresponds to the growth of any initial particles present in the system (such as crystal seeds). The characteristic curve of the second type originates from the time t-axis, and represents the generated new particles (via mechanisms such as nucleation) followed by growth. The characteristic curves on the t-axis are not used in simulations when the mechanism of new particle formation (e.g., nucleation) is absent in the system.

The algorithm for constructing the system of equations is illustrated in Fig. 2. For an initial distribution f, the initial length is sampled with N_1 points by using a length interval ΔL. An equal length interval ΔL is not required by the MOCH method, but could be chosen for convenience of implementation. Typically, the value of ΔL can be chosen much larger than those in finite difference or finite volume methods (as demonstrated later in Example 1). Those points correspond to the first-type characteristics on the L-axis in Fig. 1. Each sampled point gives two differential equations associated with the length and distribution function (Eqs. (3) and (4)), and as a result the N_1-sampled points of the initial distribution give $2N_1$ ODEs with corresponding initial conditions.

If nucleation exists in the system, N_2 characteristics are generated for the second-type characteristic curve. The second-type characteristics will add another $2N_2$ ODEs to the DAE system. For the N_2 second-type characteristics, the initial values of the length and density function are initialized as zero (consider that those characteristics are inactive until certain time points during the crystallization). The value of N_2 can be predetermined by dividing an expected lower bound on the final size of the initial crystal seeds with a length interval $\Delta L'$, which specifies that a characteristic curve becomes active (meaning a point is added to describe the size distribution) when the previous characteristic grows to the size of $\Delta L'$ (Fig. 1). The values of $\Delta L'$ are user-defined depending on how frequent the nucleation points are

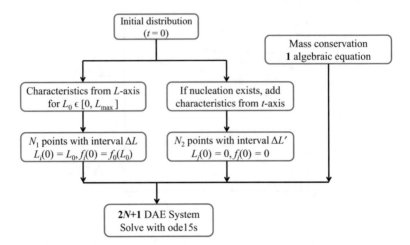

Fig. 2 Procedure for construction of the DAE system for simulation of the population balance model with the method of characteristics illustrated with a growth-nucleation system

created compared with the initial particles. One choice for $\Delta L'$ that is convenient for implementation is the maximum size of nuclei r_0 [18].

The generated $2N$ ODEs ($N = N_1 + N_2$) together with the mass conservation Eq. (5) constitute a differential-algebraic equation system with index 1. Such a system is conveniently handled by available commercial solvers, and ode15s in Matlab was chosen in this study for its general availability.

Calling ode15s involves defining the mass matrix in the DAE system, $M\dot{y} = F(t, y)$, which is.

$$M = \begin{bmatrix} I_{2N} & 0 \\ 0 & 0 \end{bmatrix}$$

where I_{2N} is the $2N$-by-$2N$ identity matrix. The solution of a DAE system using ode15s requires a consistent initial condition; for our particular system with index 1, the consistent initial condition is satisfied by the initial mass balance.

Our method employs conservation equations as algebraic constraints rather than as differential equations, to produce an index-1 DAE system to be solved. Eqs. (3)–(5) and (7) define an index-1 DAE system to be solved where the mass conservation Eq. (5) is the algebraic constraint. Taking a time derivative of Eq. (5) would convert the DAE system into an ODE system, as

$$\frac{dC}{dt} = -\rho k_v \frac{d\mu_3}{dt} \tag{8}$$

When the growth rate function G has either no or linear dependency on size, the moment equations close and the $d\mu_3/dt$ term can be reduced, as commonly seen in the literature for PBMs [1]. For example, in size-independent growth case, Eq. (8) reduces to the heavily used expression:

$$\frac{dC}{dt} = -3\rho k_v G \mu_2 \qquad (9)$$

where μ_2 is the second-order moment. However, with a more complicated size dependency in the growth rate, a reduction such as Eq. (9) no longer holds. The $d\mu_3/dt$ term in Eq. (8) could be explicitly computed from the method of moments, which introduces error in the solute balance due to the approximations used to enforce closure [10–12, 18], or could be computed from a discretized equation such as Eq. (7), which introduces time-discretization error that results in loss of mass conservation in the system unless the time interval Δt is very small. These types of numerical error associated with time discretization used to numerically solve Eq. (8) are not present in the algebraic Eq. (5), and a DAE solver automatically sets its tolerances on the algebraic equations to be very small, so that mass conservation holds nearly exactly even for large values of the time interval Δt.

4   Numerical Examples

The proposed DAE-based MOCH approach for simulating PBMs is demonstrated on several examples of typical crystallization and other particulate processes with representative mechanisms. The method itself is general and can be potentially extended to other mechanisms. The first example illustrates the accuracy and efficiency of the DAE-based MOCH approach. Then growth and nucleation are simulated for cooling crystallization processes, where both size-independent growth and size-dependent growth are demonstrated. A multidimensional crystal growth process with size dependencies is illustrated in Example 3. In the last example, extension of the method to a simultaneous growth and aggregation process for aerosol system is simulated and discussed.

4.1   Example 1: Crystallization with Size-Dependent Growth Rate

The size-dependent crystal growth rate is nearly always assumed in the literature to have the form:

$$G = k_g S^g (1 + \gamma L)^p \qquad (10)$$

where S is the supersaturation (defined as ΔC, the difference between the concentration and solubility) and k_g, g, γ, and p are growth parameters. Size-independent

Table 1 Simulation parameters for the crystallization with size-dependent growth rate in Example 1

Parameter		Value
Density of solid	ρ	10^{-12} g/μm^3
Shape factor	k_v	0.6
Initial concentration	C_0	0.1 g/g solvent
Lumped growth constant	$k_g S^g$	0.02 μm/s
Size dependency of growth	γ	0.005
Size dependency power	p	1
Length interval for N_1	ΔL	1.5 μm

growth is a special case included in the expression by simply setting γ to zero. Using feedback control, the supersaturation over the whole batch could be controlled accurately [32–34]. For such a process, the analytical solutions of the length characteristics and population density function can be obtained [18]. In particular, when $p = 1$,

$$L(t) = \frac{1}{\gamma} \left((1 + \gamma L_0) \exp \left(\gamma k_g S^g t \right) - 1 \right) \tag{11}$$

$$f(t) = f_0 (L_0) \exp \left(-\gamma k_g S^g t \right)$$

which is equivalently written as.

$$f(t, L) = f_0 \left(\frac{(1 + \gamma L) \exp \left(-\gamma k_g S^g t \right) - 1}{\gamma} \right) \exp \left(-\gamma k_g S^g t \right) \tag{12}$$

In this example, a Gaussian distribution was used as the initial number density f, with mean size of 90 μm and standard deviation of 8 μm. The constraint of a constant supersaturation was implemented by using a lumped growth constant $k_g S^g$ of 0.02 μm/s. The crystal size distribution simulated using the DAE-based MOCH approach overlaps with the analytical results for the system (see Fig. 3, with simulation parameters in Table 1). The only difference between the MOCH and exact analytical solution would be associated with numerical roundoff and the numerical solution of a DAE system; numerical roundoff errors are vanishingly small for a double-precision calculation, and the error in the numerical solution can be adjusted by setting the error tolerance on the DAE solver ($<10^{-6}$).

As a result of the size dependency of the growth, the number density distribution flattens as the crystals grow (see Fig. 3). The simulation technique using the method of characteristics completely avoids numerical dispersion or diffusion, which occurs in some extent in the other methods which utilize discretization of the internal coordinates, such as the method of classes, finite difference, and finite volume methods. To illustrate the idea, the standard finite volume method is simulated and plotted in Fig. 3, where significant numerical error is observed even with mesh size

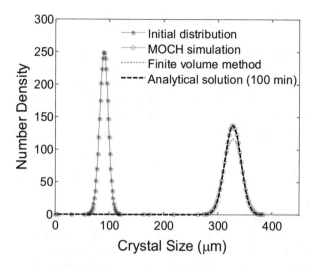

Fig. 3 Simulation of the crystallization in Example 1 overlaps with the analytical solution and is much more accurate than a standard finite volume method

that is 1/8 of the ΔL used in the DAE-based MOCH approach. The finite volume method discretized the length coordinate and resulted in a set of ODEs that are solved [28].

In the MOCH approach, the discretization of the length is only needed for the initial length range where f is nonzero, and the red circle and blue star markers have one-on-one correspondence in Fig. 3. In the finite volume method, the discretization was performed on the entire length coordinate (up to a maximum crystal size of interest by the end of the simulation) with a much smaller length interval. The finite volume method generated significantly more equations (2400) compared with that of the MOCH approach (111), which results in the greatly increased computational cost. As a result, the DAE-based MOCH approach is highly computationally efficient (computation time is 0.024 s for the DAE-based MOCH approach and 51.3 s for the finite volume method in Example 1, with the latter being >2000 times more expensive and having larger numerical error).

4.2 Example 2: Growth and Nucleation for Cooling Crystallization

Growth and new particle generation are common in many particulate systems, especially in crystallization processes. This example considers both size-independent and size-dependent growth, and demonstrates the capability and convenience of the approach for handling size dependency. Secondary nucleation is considered, with a typical expression given by.

$$h = k_b S^b \mu_3 \delta (r_0, L) \tag{13}$$

where the h is the right-hand side of Eq. (4) and k_b and b are nucleation parameters. The δ function is the Dirac delta function at r_0 [14], or a modified delta function (1 if L is less than or equal to r_0 and 0 elsewhere) [18]. While such treatments could simplify the nucleation modeling, they exclude the fact that, in reality, the nuclei may be formed with a more general size distribution. To accommodate this consideration, a smooth size distribution of the nuclei was assumed as.

$$h = \alpha k_b S^b \mu_3 \left(-\frac{4}{r_0^2} \left(L - \frac{r_0}{2} \right)^2 + 1 \right) \text{ for } 0 \le L \le r_0 \tag{14}$$

where α is a constant that ensures the consistency of the total generated seeds in Eq. (13). For a Dirac delta function in Eq. (13), α is 3/2. Compared with the commonly used delta function approximations of the nucleation distribution, this smooth representation also allows a fast convergence in the DAE solver by eliminating possible discontinuities in the ODEs of number density functions of the second-type characteristics.

A cooling crystallization process is considered in this example, in which the liquid solution is cooled with a constant rate from 30 °C to 10 °C, and the solubility of the crystallizing compound decreases linearly with temperature over the range (see solid line in Fig. 4). (The same approach applies to any solubility curve and temperature profile.) The simulation is formulated and implemented as described in Fig. 2, and the parameters are summarized in Table 2. The parameter values for growth and nucleation are based on the published values for potash alum in water [18]. Both simulated systems with size-dependent or size-independent growth started at the same initial conditions. The trends in the concentration evolution in Fig. 4 are quite similar, with an initial large supersaturation that reduced quickly as a result of crystal growth and nucleation. The size-dependent growth case experienced a faster drop in concentration and supersaturation. For size-independent growth, the initial number density distribution peak migrates toward higher length values while maintaining the exact shape (see Fig. 5a). A second peak of crystals is generated by nucleation and growth. The number density of the crystals generated by nucleation greatly exceeds the number density of initial crystals. When converted to the volume fraction distribution, the volume of nucleated crystals is comparable to that of the initial crystals after growth (Fig. 5b). The conversion of the number density distribution to volume distribution is carried out by.

$$f_{v,i} = f_{n,i} L_i^3 / \sum_{j=1}^{N} \left(f_{n,j} L_j^3 \Delta L_j \right) \tag{15}$$

The distribution of the nucleated crystals for the size-dependent growth case has a much lower peak value (see Fig. 6a), which indicates that a lower number of

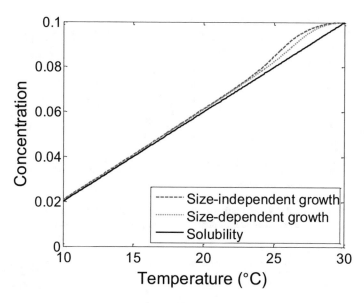

Fig. 4 Concentration evolution curve along with the temperature change for size-independent growth (*blue dash*) and size-dependent growth (*red dot*) in Example 2

Table 2 Simulation parameters for the growth-nucleation systems in Example 2

Parameter		Value
Crystal density	ρ	10^{-12} g/μm^3
Shape factor	k_v	0.6
Initial concentration	C_0	0.1 g/g solvent
Growth rate constant	k_g	10 μm/s
Growth order constant	g	1
Size dependency of growth	γ	0 (size-independent),0.005 (size-dependent)
Size dependency power	p	1
Nucleation rate constant	αk_b	0.038 (μm^{-3} s^{-1})
Nucleation order constant	b	3.4174
Length interval for N_1	ΔL	3 μm
Length interval for $N_2\ (= r_0)$	$\Delta L'$	3 μm

crystals were nucleated compared with the size-independent case. The reduction in the nucleation rate occurred as an immediate result of the lower supersaturation levels in the size-dependent growth case (Fig. 4). The size dependency of growth has a negative feedback on the supersaturation level that leads to a faster supersaturation drop. This effect also leads to a redistribution of the crystallized solute mass among the initial crystals and nucleated crystals. The volume fraction of crystals due to secondary nucleation is much smaller for the size-dependent growth case (cf. Figs. 5b and 6b).

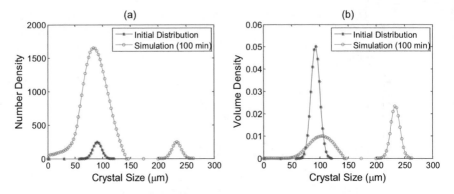

Fig. 5 Simulated crystal size distribution of the growth-nucleation system in Example 2 with size-independent growth: (**a**) number density distribution and (**b**) volume distribution

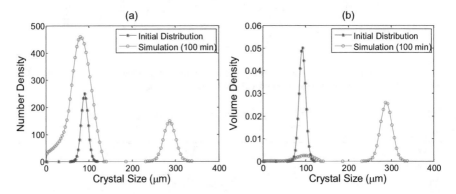

Fig. 6 Simulated crystal size distribution of the growth-nucleation system in Example 2 with size-dependent growth: (**a**) number density distribution and (**b**) volume distribution

The time evolution of the length characteristics for both cases is plotted in the L–t plane in Fig. 7. For size-independent growth, the characteristic curve of the initial crystals evolves at the same rate and keeps the same distance from each other (Fig. 7a). Such a constant distance is not maintained for size-dependent growth, with stretching being more significant at higher lengths (see Fig. 7b). Very sparse sampling (only a few characteristic curves) for the initial crystal size between 0 and 60 μm was used, considering that the number density functions are zero for the region. For the characteristic curves generated on the time axis, the spacing was enlarged along the time axis, due to the slowdown of crystal growth at later times. This behavior of enlarging time intervals among the characteristics on the time axis was also observed in the combined QMOM-MOCH approach [18].

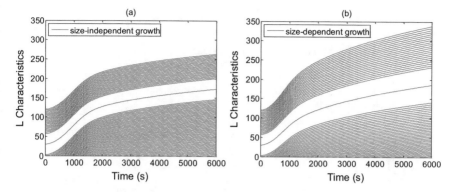

Fig. 7 Length characteristics for secondary nucleation and (**a**) size-independent growth and (**b**) size-dependent growth (Example 2)

4.3 Example 3: Multidimensional Crystallization

In particulate processes with multiple internal coordinates (typically said to be *multidimensional* in the literature), methods based on discretization of the internal coordinates [13, 14] are typically too computationally expensive to enable their use in many real-time control applications, and are even relatively slow for parameter estimation applications. The extension of the MOCH to multidimensional PBMs is demonstrated in this example. For an population balance model with any dimension N,

$$\frac{\partial f(\mathbf{x}, t)}{\partial t} + \sum_{i=1}^{N} \frac{\partial \left(G_i(\mathbf{x}, t) f(\mathbf{x}, t) \right)}{\partial x_i} = h\left(f(\mathbf{x}, t), \mathbf{x}, t \right) \qquad (16)$$

the ordinary differential equations describing the characteristics are

$$\frac{dx_i}{dt} = G_i(\mathbf{x}, t) \ \text{ for } i = 1, \ldots, N \qquad (17)$$

$$\frac{df(\mathbf{x}, t)}{dt} = -f(\mathbf{x}, t) \left(\sum_{i=1}^{N} \frac{\partial G_i(\mathbf{x}, t)}{\partial x_i} \right) + h\left(f(\mathbf{x}, t), \mathbf{x}, t \right) \qquad (18)$$

The algorithmic steps described in this paper (Fig. 2) apply to the multidimensional PBM in the same way, whereas the number of equations will change due to the additional dimension(s). In this demonstration, Example 1 is extended to a 2D case where the seed crystals have mean length of 150 μm and mean width of 90 μm. The simulation uses the same parameters from Example 1 for the two dimensions, and both size-independent growth and size-dependent growth are

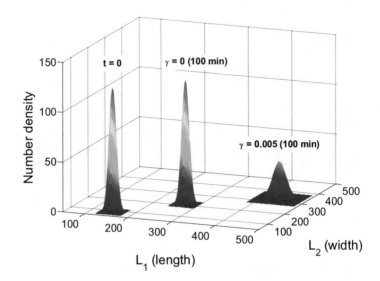

Fig. 8 Extension of Example 1 to illustrate 2D growth with constant supersaturation control for both size-independent ($\gamma = 0$) and size-dependent ($\gamma = 0.005$) growth

demonstrated in Fig. 8. Both simulations took very little computational cost (~2 s). For size-independent growth, the entire peak maintained exactly the same shape and shifted the same distance in both the length and width directions. For size-dependent growth, the size distribution peak broadened and moved further, with more growth in the length direction due to the size dependency.

This methodology also applies to the simulation of multidimensional particulate processes where the system alternates between periods of growth and dissolution, where dissolution is described by the same population balance (23) but with a negative G. An application of the MOCH approach to a 2D crystal growth and dissolution system for parameter estimation has been published by the authors [35].

4.4 Example 4: Growth with Agglomeration

The agglomeration (or aggregation) of particles is a more complicated phenomenon that often occurs during particulate processing. For such processes, the particle volume is usually used as the internal coordinate in the population balance model, although length could be used by converting from the volume [15]. A convenience of using volume is that the total volume is conserved during particle agglomeration rather than the length. The mathematical form of agglomeration is expressed as the generation of larger particles from smaller particles and the disappearance of small particles that participated in the process:

$$B(v, t) = \frac{1}{2} \int_0^v \beta(v - \varepsilon, \varepsilon) f(v - \varepsilon, t) f(\varepsilon, t) d\varepsilon \tag{19}$$

$$D(v, t) = f(v, t) \int_0^\infty \beta(v, \varepsilon) f(\varepsilon, t) d\varepsilon \tag{20}$$

This example considers particles that grow and aggregate at the same time. For the purpose of numerical demonstration, an aerosol example is chosen for which an analytical solution is available for comparison [2]. The same example has been used in previous PBM simulation studies using a high-resolution finite volume method [9]. The initial number density distribution is.

$$f_0(v) = \frac{N_0}{v_0} e^{-v/v_0} \tag{21}$$

where N_0 and v_0 are parameters that specify the initial total number of crystals and mean volume, respectively. At a constant growth rate with size-independent agglomeration kernel, an analytical solution of Eq. (19) is [2].

$$f(v, t) = \frac{M_0^2/M_1}{1 - 2\Lambda v_0} \exp\left[-\frac{\frac{M_0}{M_1}\left(v - 2\Lambda\left(\frac{N_0}{M_0} - 1\right)\right)}{1 - 2\Lambda v_0\left(\frac{N_0 - M_0}{M_1}\right)} \right] \tag{22}$$

$$\Lambda = \frac{G_0}{\beta_0 N_0 v_0}$$

$$M_0 = \frac{2N_0}{2 + \beta_0 N_0 t}$$

$$M_1 = N_0 v_0 \left[1 - \frac{2G_0}{\beta_0 N_0 v_0} \ln\left(\frac{2}{2 + \beta_0 N_0 t}\right) \right]$$

The number density of the growth-agglomeration example was simulated with the parameters in Table 3. In this example, a volume interval Δv instead of a length interval is used to generate the sampled points on a size range that includes the expected maximum particle size. Because of the equal interval between the sampled points, the convolution integral in Eq. (19) is conveniently handled by using a built-in command in Matlab (conv) that operates on the vector with f_i as its elements. The simulated size distribution overlaps with the analytical results (see Fig. 9). This example demonstrates again the advantage of being free from

Table 3 Simulation parameters for the growth-agglomeration systems in Example 3

Parameter		Value
Initial distribution parameter	N_0	1000
Initial distribution parameter	v_0	100 μm^3
Constant growth rate	G_0	1 μm^3/s
Constant agglomeration kernel	β_0	1 s^{-1}
Volume interval for N_1	Δv	2 μm^3

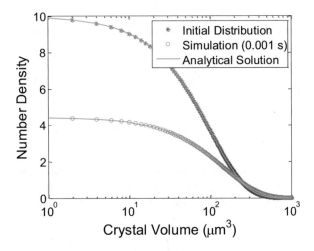

Fig. 9 The simulated number density distribution of the growth-agglomeration system in Example 3 overlaps with the analytical solution

numerical diffusion or dispersion with the DAE-based MOCH approach, which is especially important in handling distributions that have discontinuities, which typically requires special techniques in discretization methods [9]. Due to the constant agglomeration kernel, the volume distribution flattens out very fast (see Fig. 10). The example demonstrates the potential of the MOCH approach to be suitable for agglomeration processes.

5 Conclusions

The method-of-characteristics (MOCH) approach is described for the efficient simulation of the particle size distribution in particulate processes, and demonstrated in several case studies. The approach transforms the population balance models and the mass conservation equation into a differential-algebraic equation (DAE) system, which is able to handle particulate processes that have complicated size dependency of growth rate, multidimensional growth (and/or dissolution), and nucleation. The approach was also demonstrated for an application to a particular process with agglomeration was also demonstrated, in which the population balance

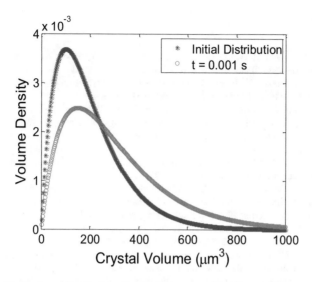

Fig. 10 Simulated volume distribution of the growth-agglomeration system (Example 3)

model includes integrals among its terms. Such population balance models are computationally expensive to solve using finite difference, volume, and element methods.

The DAE-based MOCH implementation is accurate (comparable to analytical solutions) and computationally efficient, and the method only requires the solution of a DAE system of relatively low dimension. The DAE-based MOCH approach has a computational efficiency that is fast enough for real-time applications such as nonlinear model predictive control. The particular DAE solver used in the examples was an adaptive time stepper with a very low error tolerance; in applications where six decimal places of accuracy are not required, such as in real-time feedback control, the computational times could be further reduced by relaxing the error tolerance. These simulation times indicate that employing the MOCH approach makes online parameter estimation, state estimation, and feedback control feasible for particulate processes with complicated characteristics (such as arbitrary side-dependent growth) that could hamper alternative simulation methods such as the method of moments.

Considering the high accuracy and easier implementation compared with other methods, the DAE-based MOCH approach is a promising approach for use in the parameter estimation, design, and control of the size distribution for particulate processes having a very wide range of phenomena.

Acknowledgments Financial support provided by Novartis is acknowledged. Joseph K. Scott and Ali Mesbah at the Massachusetts Institute of Technology and Michael L. Rasche at the University of Illinois at Urbana-Champaign are acknowledged for related discussions.

References

1. A. D. Randolph and M. A. Larson, Theory of Particulate Processes: Analysis and Techniques of Continuous Crystallization. New York: Academic Press, 1971.
2. T. E. Ramabhadran, T. W. Peterson, and J. H. Seinfeld, "Dynamics of aerosol coagulation and condensation," AIChE Journal, vol. 22, p. 840-851, 1976.
3. N. V. Mantzaris, J.-J. Liou, P. Daoutidis, and F. Srienc, "Numerical solution of a mass structured cell population balance model in an environment of changing substrate concentration," Journal of Biotechnology, vol. 71, p. 157-174, 1999.
4. T. J. Crowley, E. S. Meadows, E. Kostoulas, and F. J. Doyle Iii, "Control of particle size distribution described by a population balance model of semibatch emulsion polymerization," Journal of Process Control, vol. 10, p. 419-432, 2000.
5. X. X. Zhu, B. G. Li, L. B. Wu, Y. G. Zheng, S. P. Zhu, K. D. Hungenberg, S. Mussig, and B. Reinhard, "Kinetics and modeling of vinyl acetate graft polymerization from poly(ethylene glycol)," Macromolecular Reaction Engineering, vol. 2, p. 321-333, 2008.
6. U. Teipel, "Particle technology: design of particulate products and dispersed systems," Chemical Engineering & Technology, vol. 27, p. 751-756, 2004.
7. Z. K. Nagy and R. D. Braatz, "Advances and new directions in crystallization control," Annual Review of Chemical and Biomolecular Engineering, vol. 3, p. 55-75, 2012.
8. R. D. Braatz, "Advanced control of crystallization processes," Annual Reviews in Control, vol. 26, p. 87-99, 2002.
9. R. Gunawan, I. Fusman, and R. D. Braatz, "Parallel high-resolution finite volume simulation of particulate processes," AIChE Journal, vol. 54, p. 1449-1458, 2008.
10. J. Gimbun, Z. K. Nagy, and C. D. Rielly, "Simultaneous quadrature method of moments for the solution of population balance equations, using a differential algebraic equation framework," Industrial & Engineering Chemistry Research, vol. 48, p. 7798-7812, 2009.
11. R. McGraw, "Description of aerosol dynamics by the quadrature method of moments," Aerosol Science and Technology, vol. 27, p. 255-265, 1997.
12. D. L. Marchisio, J. T. Pikturna, R. O. Fox, R. D. Vigil, and A. A. Barresi, "Quadrature method of moments for population-balance equations," AIChE Journal, vol. 49, p. 1266-1276, 2003.
13. D. L. Ma, D. K. Tafti, and R. D. Braatz, "High-resolution simulation of multidimensional crystal growth," Industrial & Engineering Chemistry Research, vol. 41, p. 6217-6223, 2002.
14. R. Gunawan, I. Fusman, and R. D. Braatz, "High resolution algorithms for multidimensional population balance equations," AIChE Journal, vol. 50, p. 2738-2749, 2004.
15. M. J. Hounslow, R. L. Ryall, and V. R. Marshall, "A discretized population balance for nucleation, growth, and aggregation," AIChE Journal, vol. 34, p. 1821-1832, 1988.
16. M. Smith and T. Matsoukas, "Constant-number Monte Carlo simulation of population balances," Chemical Engineering Science, vol. 53, p. 1777-1786, 1998.
17. Y. Lin, K. Lee, and T. Matsoukas, "Solution of the population balance equation using constant-number Monte Carlo," Chemical Engineering Science, vol. 57, p. 2241-2252, 2002.
18. E. Aamir, Z. K. Nagy, C. D. Rielly, T. Kleinert, and B. Judat, "Combined quadrature method of moments and method of characteristics approach for efficient solution of population balance models for dynamic modeling and crystal size distribution control of crystallization processes," Industrial & Engineering Chemistry Research, vol. 48, p. 8575-8584, 2009.
19. A. E. Flood, "Thoughts on recovering particle size distributions from the moment form of the population balance," Developments in Chemical Engineering and Mineral Processing, vol. 10, p. 501-519, 2002.
20. S. Qamar, M. P. Elsner, I. A. Angelov, G. Warnecke, and A. Seidel-Morgenstern, "A comparative study of high resolution schemes for solving population balances in crystallization," Computers & Chemical Engineering, vol. 30, p. 1119-1131, 2006.
21. P. Marchal, R. David, J. P. Klein, and J. Villermaux, "Crystallization and precipitation engineering .1. An efficient method for solving population balance in crystallization with agglomeration," Chemical Engineering Science, vol. 43, p. 59-67, 1988.

22. F. Puel, G. Fevotte, and J. P. Klein, "Simulation and analysis of industrial crystallization processes through multidimensional population balance equations. Part 2: a study of semi-batch crystallization," Chemical Engineering Science, vol. 58, p. 3729-3740, 2003.
23. S. Kumar and D. Ramkrishna, "On the solution of population balance equations by discretization—III. Nucleation, growth and aggregation of particles," Chemical Engineering Science, vol. 52, p. 4659-4679, 1997.
24. S. Qamar, A. Ashfaq, I. Angelov, M. P. Elsner, G. Warnecke, and A. Seidel-Morgenstern, "Numerical solutions of population balance models in preferential crystallization," Chemical Engineering Science, vol. 63, p. 1342-1352, 2008.
25. F. Fevotte and G. Fevotte, "A method of characteristics for solving population balance equations (PBE) describing the adsorption of impurities during crystallization processes," Chemical Engineering Science, vol. 65, p. 3191-3198, 2010.
26. M. J. Hounslow and G. K. Reynolds, "Product engineering for crystal size distribution," AIChE Journal, vol. 52, p. 2507-2517, 2006.
27. S. Qamar, S. Mukhtar, A. Seidel-Morgenstern, and M. P. Elsner, "An efficient numerical technique for solving one-dimensional batch crystallization models with size-dependent growth rates," Chemical Engineering Science, vol. 64, p. 3659-3667, 2009.
28. A. Mesbah, H. J. M. Kramer, A. E. M. Huesman, and P. M. J. Van den Hof, "A control oriented study on the numerical solution of the population balance equation for crystallization processes," Chemical Engineering Science, vol. 64, p. 4262-4277, 2009.
29. S. Qamar and G. Warnecke, "Numerical solution of population balance equations for nucleation, growth and aggregation processes," Computers & Chemical Engineering, vol. 31, p. 1576-1589, 2007.
30. S. J. Farlow, Partial Differential Equations for Scientists and Engineers. New York: Dover, 1993.
31. R. G. Gordon, "Error bounds in equilibrium statistical mechanics," Journal of Mathematical Physics, vol. 9, p. 655-663, 1968.
32. V. Liotta and V. Sabesan, "Monitoring and feedback control of supersaturation using ATR-FTIR to produce an active pharmaceutical ingredient of a desired crystal size," Organic Process Research & Development, vol. 8, p. 488-494, 2004.
33. H. Grön, P. Mougin, A. Thomas, G. White, D. Wilkinson, R. B. Hammond, X. Lai, and K. J. Roberts, "Dynamic in-process examination of particle size and crystallographic form under defined conditions of reactant supersaturation as associated with the batch crystallization of monosodium glutamate from aqueous solution," Industrial & Engineering Chemistry Research, vol. 42, p. 4888-4898, 2003.
34. G. X. Zhou, M. Fujiwara, X. Y. Woo, E. Rusli, H. H. Tung, C. Starbuck, O. Davidson, Z. H. Ge, and R. D. Braatz, "Direct design of pharmaceutical antisolvent crystallization through concentration control," Crystal Growth & Design, vol. 6, p. 892-898, 2006.
35. M. Jiang, X. Zhu, M. C. Molaro, M. L. Rasche, H. Zhang, K. Chadwick, D. M. Raimondo, K.-K. K. Kim, L. Zhou, Z. Zhu, M. H. Wong, D. O'Grady, D. Hebrault, J. Tedesco, and R. D. Braatz, "Modification of crystal shape through deep temperature cycling," Industrial & Engineering Chemistry Research, vol. 53, p. 5325-5336, 2014.

Linearized Parameter Estimation Methods for Modeled Crystallization Phenomena Using In-Line Measurements and Their Application to Optimization of Partially Seeded Crystallization in Pharmaceutical Processes

Izumi Hirasawa, Joi Unno, and Ikuma Masaki

1 Modeling and Parameter Estimation

In pharmaceutical processes, crystallization affects the final product quality such as bioavailability, crystal stability, and filtration efficiency, among other important attributes. The product quality depends on the crystal size distribution (CSD), and hence it is important to control the CSD. The CSD may be determined according to a balance between nucleation and growth and is influenced by breakage and agglomeration. This balance or influence can be modeled by mathematical expressions with some model parameters. By using these models, the critical quality attributes on the crystal size, such as size distribution, mean size, standard deviation, and coefficient of variation (CV), can be predicted by simulation.

In Sect. 1, we make comments on the mathematical models for each crystallization phenomenon and linearized or simplified parameter estimation methods. In Sect. 1.1, we show the fundamental equations on the balances and the kinetics of crystallization. These include so complicated a partial differential equation (PDE) that the computation cannot be performed without much more time-consuming numerical integration than ordinary differential equations (ODEs) usually take. In Sect. 1.2, we mention a few examples and the advantages of in-line measurements. In addition, general remarks on parameter estimation is given in Sect. 1.3. Finally, the parameter estimation methods and concrete examples of each kinetics, such as growth, secondary nucleation, primary nucleation, breakage, and agglomeration, are explained in Sects. 1.4 to 1.8, respectively.

I. Hirasawa (✉) · J. Unno · I. Masaki
Department of Applied Chemistry, Waseda University, Tokyo, Japan
e-mail: izumih@waseda.jp; j.unno@fuji.waseda.jp; i-190-m@akane.waseda.jp

© The Author(s), under exclusive license to Springer Nature Switzerland AG 2022
A. Fytopoulos et al. (eds.), *Optimization of Pharmaceutical Processes*, Springer
Optimization and Its Applications 189, https://doi.org/10.1007/978-3-030-90924-6_3

1.1 Mathematical Model

In mathematical modeling, it is necessary to quantify the crystallization phenomena, such as nucleation, growth, agglomeration, and breakage kinetics, and to apply the three conservation laws of mass, energy, and crystal population. Randolph and Larson [1] reported pioneering works on the population balance. In this whole chapter, the batch crystallization process is modeled with the following population and mass balance equations:

$$\frac{\partial (W_s n)}{\partial t} + G \frac{\partial (W_s n)}{\partial L} = W_s (B_1 + B_2) \delta (L - L_0) + W_s (B_a - D_a + B_b - D_b)$$

(1)

$$R_h \frac{dW_a}{dt} = -3 W_s \rho_c k_v G \mu_2 - W_s \rho_c k_v (B_1 + B_2) L_0^3$$

(2)

Here t is time, L is characteristic crystal size, n is population density, W_s and W_a are mass of solvent and solute, L_0 is size of nucleus, ρ_c is solid density, k_v is volume shape factor, R_h is ratio of molecular weight of hydrate to one of anhydrate, δ is Dirac delta function, and the energy balance is neglected. Primary nucleation rate B_1, secondary nucleation rate B_2, and growth rate G are represented as follows:

$$B_1 = k_{b1} S^{b1}$$

(3)

$$B_2 = k_{b2} S^{b2} \mu_3$$

(4)

$$G = k_g S^g$$

(5)

Here k_{b1} and $b1$ are primary nucleation rate parameters, k_{b2} and $b2$ are second nucleation rate parameters, and k_g and g are growth rate parameters. S is a numerical expression related to the driving force for each phenomenon or the difference in chemical potential. Supercooling ΔT, supersaturation $\Delta C = C - C_{sat}$, and relative supersaturation $\sigma = \Delta C / C_{sat}$ are often employed as S, where C is the concentration of solute and C_{sat} is the solubility. Among them, supercooling is easy to handle in engineering, but supersaturation and relative supersaturation are sometimes used instead of supercooling. In Eq. (1), agglomeration has a birth term B_a and a death one D_a. Likewise, breakage has a birth one B_b and a death one D_b. The population balance equation (PBE) represented by Eq. (1) consists of nucleation, growth, breakage, and agglomeration rates, while the mass balance equation (MBE) by Eq. (2) only of nucleation and growth ones, without considering breakage and agglomeration. This is because the total mass will be conserved during the breakage or agglomeration process. The models of breakage and agglomeration kinetics are mentioned in Sects. 1.7 and 1.8, respectively. μ_i is the ith moment of CSD and defined by the following equation:

$$\mu_i = \int_0^\infty n L^i dL \qquad (6)$$

From the moments of several orders, the crystallization process can be characterized at any time. For instance, μ_0 is the crystal particle number, μ_1 is the sum of crystal sizes, μ_2 multiplied by surface shape factor represents the total surface area of crystals, and μ_3 multiplied by volume shape factor represents the total volume of crystals, all of which are the quantities per unit solvent mass. In addition, by using the method of moments (MOM), in which several lower-order moments are considered, the PDE depending on time and crystal size can be converted into the simultaneous ODEs depending only on time. The MOM was originally developed for the crystallization problems by Hulburt and Katz [2].

1.2 In-Line Measurements

In-line measurements with process analytical technologies (PATs) in pharmaceutical processes may help one analyze the phenomena and the kinetics and stabilize the process control with some feedback loops. As for crystallization, the PAT tools for CSD, concentration, polymorphism, and so on may offer much useful information to researchers and manufacturers. In Sect. 1.2, we make a few comments especially on the in-line measurements of CSD and concentration.

In classical measurements of CSD, the suspension in the crystallizer is sampled to measure the sizes of crystals with microscopy or sieving. This method is called off-line measurement, in which there are an influence of extraction and a limit on the number of times of sampling. On the contrary, in-line measurements are automatically performed in situ and output the data regularly.

For example, focused beam reflectance measurement (FBRM) is often utilized for the in-line measurements of CSD. In the processes, the FBRM apparatus measures chord length distribution (CLD), which is different from CSD because chord length is the length for which the beam irradiated to a crystal goes across the projection area of the crystal. However, CLD can be converted into CSD with the statistical methods as follows. At first, the chord length depends on the particle shape and the detective position. For example, when the crystal is a cube, in some cases the chord length is shorter than the edge length with the proximity of the vertex detected, and in others longer with the diagonal line detected. Therefore, the probability that a crystal is measured at a given chord length is considered. Then, this probability is calculated over the whole range of chord length and crystal size and discretized according to both of the histograms. The calculation can be carried out by Monte Carlo method, in which angles of rotation, a detective position, and so on are randomly distributed in a domain, to make shape transformation matrix **S**, which may convert a given CSD vector into a CLD vector. In addition, the inverse problem of this conversion can derive CSD from CLD. However, this inverse problem is often ill-posed and may easily cause noises and negative values in calculated CSD.

Therefore, for example, this problem will be solved as a nonnegative least-squares one as follows:

$$
\begin{cases}
\vec{y}_{CSD} = \underset{\vec{y}}{\arg\min} \left\| \mathbf{S}\,\vec{y} - \vec{x}_{CLD} \right\| \\
\vec{y}_{CSD,i} \geq 0 \quad \text{for all } i
\end{cases}
\tag{7}
$$

Here, x is the CLD vector and y is the CSD one. Worlitschek et al. [3] pioneered this type of CSD restoration, and the application for L-arginine (Arg) crystallization, where the crystal shape may change with the crystal growth, was reported by Unno et al. [4].

For in-line measurements of concentration, attenuated total reflectance Fourier-transform infrared (ATR-FT-IR) spectroscopy is useful. In ATR-FT-IR spectroscopy, the peak intensity or area specific to each material depends not only on solution composition but also on solution temperature. For example, Zhang et al. [5] built a calibration model, in which the concentration is represented by the linear combination of the absorbances at every wavelength and of the solution temperature, based on ATR-FT-IR spectroscopy for the crystallization of L-glutamic acid.

1.3   Parameter Estimation

Each kinetic parameter can be estimated from the observed quantities, such as crystal number, concentration, mean crystal size, and CSD itself. However, every rate equation usually has more than one parameter, and hence overfitting may occur when all the kinetic parameters are estimated at the same time. As a result, the physical implications of the estimated parameters fade away, and the suitability for the unseen data different from the data used for the parameter fitting will not be good. Thus, it is preferable to perform parameter fitting in the restricted measurement range or in the limited experimental system where only target phenomenon will occur or stand out. Moreover, by limiting the other phenomena, the PBE is simplified and the linear fitting is facilitated. As a method of the parameter fitting, some researchers often utilize the non-linear least-squares method, in which the parameters are determined so that the error of some observed quantities will be minimized. However, in the non-linear fitting, the numerical solution might be changed by the settings of solver and the initial values, which are rarely published in papers. Thus, in consideration of reproducibility, a linear or simplified fitting is preferable for the parameter estimation. The estimation methods for each kinetic parameter are described below.

1.4 Growth Kinetics

The growth rate of crystals can be derived from in-line measurements of the CSD and the concentration. In the parameter estimation of the growth kinetics, it is preferable that neither breakage nor agglomeration happens significantly. If we select the range where the nucleation terms are negligibly small, the MBE of Eq. (2) can be simplified as follows:

$$\frac{dW_h}{dt} = 3W_s \rho_c k_v G \mu_2 \tag{8}$$

In Eq. (8), the mass of crystals W_h is calculated from ATR-FT-IR, and the second moment of CSD μ_2 from ATR-FT-IR and FBRM. Thus, growth rate is calculated by the following equation:

$$G \approx \frac{\Delta W_h}{\Delta t} / (3W_s \rho_c k_v \mu_2) \tag{9}$$

Finally, the regression analysis is carried out based on the following equation derived from Eq. (5):

$$\log G = g \log S + \log k_g \tag{10}$$

As a concrete example, the plot of $\log G$ vs. $\log \sigma$ is shown in Fig. 1, which was originally reported by Unno and Hirasawa [6]. Here, target substance was Arg. A saturated amount of Arg anhydrate was dissolved in 300 mL of water at an initial temperature higher than the saturated temperature. Then, the solution was linearly cooled down to the final temperature and stirred with a four-blade agitator (φ40) at the rotation speed of 400 rpm. In cooling, an adequate quantity of seed crystals was added when the solution temperature reached the saturated temperature. The value of growth order was estimated to be 2.32 and that of growth coefficient 4.15 μm/s by this linear fitting. In fact, depending on the diffusion process of solute in the solution and on the surface accumulation process, the value of growth order is assumed to be 1–2.

1.5 Secondary Nucleation Kinetics

When an adequate quantity of seed crystals is added to the batch crystallizer, rapid secondary nucleation may become the dominant phenomenon, and nucleation might not be a stochastic process. Consequently, secondary nucleation kinetics can be estimated with comparative ease. In Eq. (4), B_2 is proportional to μ_3, and hence it is necessary to determine a reasonable mean value of μ_3 from seeding to cloud detection point, at which the PAT tools detect that the magma density or the crystal

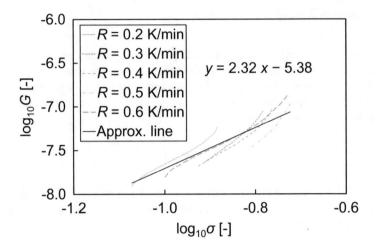

Fig. 1 Regression analysis for estimation of kinetic parameters of growth. (Reproduced from Ref. [6])

number has reached a predetermined threshold value. First, the following equations are presumed to be established:

$$\mu_3 = k'\mu_0 \tag{11}$$

$$\mu_{0m} \approx r\mu_{0s} \gg \mu_{0s} \tag{12}$$

Here r is the number ratio of cloud detection point to seeding. Subscripts s and m mean seed crystal and threshold value of crystal number. When ΔT is employed as S, the relation between r and waiting time t_m at the cooling rate of R is expressed as follows:

$$B_2 = \frac{d\mu_0}{dt} = k_{b2}(\Delta T)^{b2}\mu_3 = k_{b2}(Rt)^{b2}\mu_3 = k\mu_0 t^{b2}$$

$$\Longleftrightarrow \ln\frac{\mu_{0m}}{\mu_{0s}} = \ln r = \frac{k}{b2+1}t_m^{b2+1} \tag{13}$$

Here, average value of μ_0 in the time interval of the integral calculus is denoted by $\mu_{0,\text{avg}}$; then, it is expressed as the following equation:

$$B_2 = \frac{d\mu_0}{dt} = k\mu_{0,\text{avg}}t^{b2} \Longleftrightarrow \mu_{0m} - \mu_{0s} \approx \mu_{0m} \approx r\mu_{0s} = \mu_{0,\text{avg}}\frac{k}{b2+1}t_m^{b2+1}$$

$$= \mu_{0,\text{avg}}\ln r$$

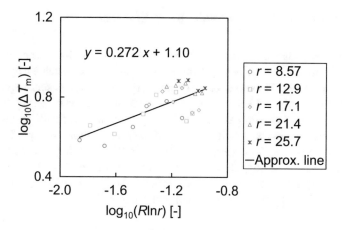

Fig. 2 Regression analysis for estimation of kinetic parameters of secondary nucleation. (Reproduced from Ref. [6])

$$\Longleftrightarrow \ \mu_{0,\text{avg}} = \frac{r}{\ln r}\mu_{0s} \ \Longleftrightarrow \ \mu_{3,\text{avg}} = \frac{r}{\ln r}\mu_{3s} \qquad (14)$$

Equations (13) and (14) are substituted into Eq. (4) and organized, and the following equation can be obtained:

$$B_2 = k_{b2}(\Delta T)^{b2}\mu_{3,\text{avg}} = k_{b2}(\Delta T)^{b2}\frac{r}{\ln r}\mu_{3s} = \frac{d\mu_0}{dt} = R\frac{d\mu_0}{d(\Delta T)}$$

$$\Longleftrightarrow \ \log(\Delta T_m) = \frac{1}{b2+1}\log(R\ln r) + \frac{1}{b2+1}\log\frac{\mu_{0s}(b2+1)}{k_{b2}\mu_{3s}} \qquad (15)$$

Therefore, secondary nucleation parameters can be estimated by the slope and the intercept of $\log(\Delta T_m)$ vs. $\log(R\ln r)$. This type of parameter estimation was originally reported by Unno et al. [7], and a concrete example is shown in Fig. 2, which was originally reported by Unno and Hirasawa [6]. Here, target substance was Arg. A saturated amount of Arg anhydrate was dissolved in 300 mL of water at an initial temperature higher than the saturated temperature. Then, the solution was linearly cooled down to the final temperature and stirred with a four-blade agitator (φ40) at the rotation speed of 400 rpm. In cooling, an adequate quantity of seed crystals was added when the solution temperature reached the saturated temperature. The value of secondary nucleation order was estimated to be 2.67 and that of secondary nucleation coefficient $1.65 \times 10^{10} \ \text{s}^{-1}\text{m}^{-3}\text{K}^{-2.67}$ by this linear fitting.

1.6 Stochastic Primary Nucleation Kinetics

In general, secondary nucleation may occur so frequently that it can be regarded as deterministic, which means that the same result can be obtained by repeating the same operation. However, primary nucleation may not occur frequently but rather stochastically, which means that the results will vary with some trend even if the same operation is repeated. Therefore, it is difficult to control the crystallization processes which involve primary nucleation. For predicting this type of crystallization processes, the PBE and MBE including stochastic primary nucleation need to be solved. The probability that the number of crystals newly nucleated from t to $t + \tau$ will equal k follows the Poisson distribution with the parameter of the expected nuclei number and is denoted as follows:

$$P(t, \tau; k) = \Pr\left\{\int_t^{t+\tau} W_s B^* d\tau' = k\right\} = \frac{\left(\int_t^{t+\tau} W_s B^* d\tau'\right)^k}{k!} \exp\left[-\int_t^{t+\tau} W_s B^* d\tau'\right]$$

(16)

$$\int_t^{t+\tau} W_s B^* d\tau' \sim \mathrm{Po}\left[\int_t^{t+\tau} W_s B d\tau'\right]$$

(17)

Here, the superscript "*" emphasizes that the value is a stochastic variable, and Eq. (17) means that the left side of the equation follows the Poisson distribution. Then, τ is replaced by a reasonably short time Δt to derive an approximate equation as follows:

$$B^*(t) \sim \frac{\mathrm{Po}\left[W_s(t) B(t) \Delta t\right]}{W_s(t) \Delta t}$$

(18)

In Eq. (18), Δt should be so short a time that the change in the expectation of the nucleation rate and the increase in the crystal size can be ignored during Δt. The stochastic nucleation rate expressed by Eq. (18) is substituted into Eqs. (1) and (2) to derive stochastic differential equations (SDEs), which is solved once to obtain one of sample paths. The SDEs should be solved so many times that one can estimate the statistical properties of them. Maggioni and Mazzotti [8] have recently investigated the modeling of stochastic primary nucleation and reviewed the relevant literature.

Unno and Hirasawa [6] reported the concrete method for the parameter estimation which involves stochastic nucleation. At first, for the data acquisition, the means and standard derivations of the waiting times were measured in the same system as the concrete examples in Sects. 1.4 and 1.5 until the total crystal number reached 6×10^5 and 1.5×10^6 in unseeded crystallization. Next, parameter space was made by simulation using stochastic primary nucleation rates represented as follows:

$$B_1 = E\left[B_1^*\right] = k_{b1} \exp\left[-b1(\ln S)^{-2}\right]$$

(19)

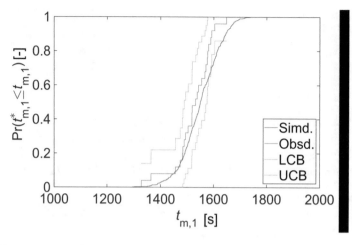

Fig. 3 Simulated and observed cumulative distribution functions of waiting times until the total crystal number of 6×10^5. (Reproduced from Ref. [6])

Finally, the primary nucleation parameters were estimated so that the means and standard derivations corresponded with experimental values. The value of primary nucleation order was estimated to be 2.28 and that of primary nucleation coefficient 69.7 kg-solvent^{-1} s^{-1} by this parameter estimation. Using estimated parameters, the simulated waiting times until the total crystal number of 6×10^5 are compared to the observed ones. The relation between the waiting time and the cumulative distribution function is illustrated in Fig. 3. The number of observations was 25 while that of simulations 500.

1.7 Breakage Kinetics

As mentioned in Sect. 1.1, breakage has a birth term B_b and a death term D_b, which are represented as follows:

$$B_b(L, t) = \int_L^\infty f_{\text{bre}}(L|\lambda) k_{\text{bre}}(\lambda) n(\lambda, t) d\lambda \qquad (20)$$

$$D_b(L, t) = k_{\text{bre}}(L) n(L, t) \qquad (21)$$

Here, k_{bre} is the breakage kernel and f_{bre} is the fragment distribution function. In Eq. (20), a single crystal with a size of λ breaks to yield two crystals, one of which has a size of L. The mathematical expressions for k_{bre} and f_{bre} of various models presented by Marchisio et al. [9], Hasseine et al. [10], Bari and Pandit [11], and Li and Yang [12] are listed in Tables 1 and 2, respectively. The kinetic parameters of breakage

Table 1 Functions of breakage kernel

Mechanism	Function
Constant	q_1
Power law	$q_1 L^{q_2}$
Exponential	$q_1 \exp(q_2 L^3)$

Table 2 Fragment distribution functions

Mechanism	Fragment distribution function
Erosion L_1 is minimum size	$\delta (L - L_1) + \delta \left(L - \left(\lambda^3 - L_1^3 \right)^{\frac{1}{3}} \right)$
Constant ratio fragmentation Mass ratio $1{:}r_m$ Symmetric fragmentation at $r_m = 1$	$\delta \left(L - \lambda \left(\frac{1}{1+r_m} \right)^{1/3} \right) + \delta \left(L - \lambda \left(\frac{r_m}{1+r_m} \right)^{1/3} \right)$
Parabolic distribution Uniform at $C = 2$	$\frac{3CL^2}{\lambda^3} + \left(1 - \frac{C}{2} \right) \left[\frac{72L^8}{\lambda^9} - \frac{72L^5}{\lambda^6} + \frac{18L^2}{\lambda^3} \right]$

in these models are estimated using the PBE. For example, "power law" model and "mass ratio" model are applied to the breakage kinetics, and PBE is expressed as follows if only breakage happens in the crystallizer:

$$\frac{\partial (W_s n)}{\partial t} = W_s (B_a - D_a) \tag{22}$$

Applying the MOM to Eq. (22) derives the following equation:

$$\frac{d (W_s \mu_k)}{dt} = W_s R_k q_1 \mu_{k+q_2} \tag{23}$$

Here, R_k is represented as follows for "mass ratio" model:

$$R_k = \frac{1 + r_m^{k/3}}{(1 + r_m)^{k/3}} - 1 \tag{24}$$

In Eqs. (23) and (24), breakage parameters are q_1, q_2, and r_m. Eq. (23) is the ODE only about breakage. The mass conservation during breakage can be utilized to derive the following relation and to estimate q_2 based on the moment order α, which satisfies the relation:

$$\frac{d (W_s \mu_\alpha)}{dt} = W_s R_\alpha q_1 \mu_{\alpha+q_2} = \text{const.}$$

$$W_s \mu_3 = \text{const.}$$

$$\Longleftrightarrow q_2 = 3 - \alpha \tag{25}$$

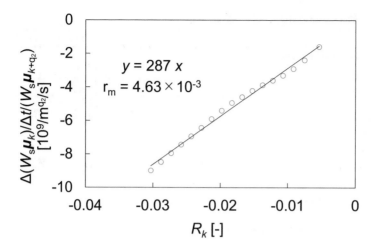

Fig. 4 Parameter estimation of breakage kinetics

In addition, finite differences in Eq. (23) are computed for some moment orders k to derive the following equation and to estimate q_1 and r_m:

$$\frac{\Delta\left(W_s\mu_k\right)}{\Delta t} / \left(W_s\mu_{k+q_2}\right) = R_k q_1 \tag{26}$$

Here, both numerator and denominator of the left side are vectors for a time horizon, and the right side is a scalar. If R_k is represented by a linear function of parameter(s), the other parameters excluding q_2 can be estimated by linear least-squares method. Otherwise, as in Eq. (24), they can be estimated only by non-linear least-squares method. As a concrete example, the parameter estimation of breakage kinetics was performed in the same system as in Sects. 1.4 and 1.5. The resulting relation between $\Delta(W_s\mu_k)/\Delta t/(W_s\mu_{k+q2})$ and R_k is depicted in Fig. 4. In this parameter estimation, at first q_2 was determined at 4.0, and then q_1 and r_m were estimated at 2.87×10^{11} m$^{-4.0}$ s^{-1} and 4.63×10^{-3}, respectively.

1.8 Agglomeration Kinetics

As mentioned in Sect. 1.1, agglomeration has a birth term B_a and a death term D_a, which are represented as follows:

$$B_a(L, t) = \frac{L^2}{2} \int_0^L \frac{k_{agg}\left(\lambda, (L^3 - \lambda^3)^{\frac{1}{3}}\right)}{(L^3 - \lambda^3)^{\frac{2}{3}}} n\left((L^3 - \lambda^3)^{\frac{1}{3}}, t\right) n(\lambda, t)\, d\lambda \tag{27}$$

Table 3 Basis functions of aggregation kernel

Mechanism	Basis function
ConstantSize independent	1
Size independent	
Brownian motion	$\frac{(L+\lambda)^2}{L\lambda}$
Sum	$L^3 + \lambda^3$
Hydrodynamic	$(L+\lambda)^3$
Laminar shear	
Isotropic turbulence	
Differential forceTurbulent inertiaDifferential sedimentation	$(L+\lambda)^2\|L^2 - \lambda^2\|$
Turbulent inertia	
Differential sedimentation	

Table 4 Coefficients of aggregation kernel

Mechanism	Coefficient	Symbols used
Constant and so on	a_1	a_1 = constant [equation-dependent]
Size independent and so on	$a_1 G^{a_{1G}} \varepsilon^{a_{1\varepsilon}}$	G = growth rate [m/s] ε = turbulent dissipation rate [m^2/s^3] a_{1G} = exponent of G [−] $a_{1\varepsilon}$ = exponent of ε [−]
Brownian motion	$\frac{2k_B T}{3\mu}$	k_B = Boltzmann constant [J/K] T = thermodynamic temperature [K] μ = viscosity [pa s]
Laminar shear	$\frac{4\gamma}{3}$	γ = velocity gradient [s^{-1}]
Isotropic turbulence	$\sqrt{\frac{8\pi\varepsilon}{15\nu}}$	ν = kinematic viscosity [m^2/s]
Turbulent inertia	$\frac{1.27(\rho_p - \rho_f)}{\mu}\sqrt[4]{\frac{\varepsilon^3}{\nu}}$	ρ_p = particle density [kg/m^3] ρ_f = fluid density [kg/m^3]
Differential sedimentation	$\frac{0.7g(\rho_p - \rho_f)}{\mu}$	g = gravitational acceleration [m/s^2]

$$D_a(L, t) = n(L, t) \int_0^\infty k_{agg}(\lambda, L) n(\lambda, t) \, d\lambda \qquad (28)$$

Here k_{agg} is the agglomeration kernel. In Eq. (27), two crystals, one of which has a size of λ, agglomerate to yield a single crystal with a size of L, and in Eq. (28), the reverse relation is established. The mathematical expressions of the basis functions and the coefficients for k_{agg} of various models presented by Vanni [13], Marchisio et al. [9], Laloue et al. [14], Ó'Ciardhá et al. [15], and Gencaslan et al. [16] are listed in Tables 3 and 4, respectively. In Tables 3 and 4, a basis function multiplied by a corresponding coefficient is an agglomeration kernel. When agglomeration is dependent on supersaturation, nucleation and growth must occur at the same time in the crystallizer. Thus, it is difficult to prepare the experimental system where only agglomeration may stand out. In this case, we have no choice but to substitute the other parameters into Eq. (1).

2 Application of Modeling to Optimization

Mathematical models for crystallization are usually described with the differential equations, which may include the parameters depending on materials and have the initial, boundary, and other conditions determined by procedures. The quantities resulting from crystallization or related to its process can be simulated by solving the differential equations. In mathematical modeling, the parameters are estimated to minimize the error between the simulated quantities and the observed ones. On the other hand, in optimization after mathematical modeling, some procedures are determined to minimize the difference between the simulated quantities and the desired ones. Therefore, both modeling and optimization can be regarded as the minimization problems via the differential equations, and in optimization similar algorithms can be applied as in modeling.

In seeded batch cooling crystallization, the seeding method and the cooling method may be optimized for improving the quantities related to the crystal product quality. In Sect. 2, several seeding policies classified based on seed loading quantity are discussed at first, and among them partial seeding is focused on as a good choice for pharmaceutical processes. Secondly, in partially seeded crystallization of a model substance, the seeding and cooling methods are simultaneously optimized for the best product quality. Thirdly, the crystallization process designed optimally for the model substance is postulated to be implemented. Fourthly, we show the case study of partially seeded crystallization of Arg and the optimization of the seeding method. Finally, we make a few comments on the effect of stochastic nucleation mentioned above on quality stability or fluctuation of the crystallization products.

2.1 Seeding Policies

In the batch crystallization, the surface area of the suspended crystals and the supersaturation of the solution need to be controlled for obtaining the product crystals with the desired quality. The initial surface area of the suspended crystals can be controlled with the seeding method, while the supersaturation may be controlled with the cooling method in the cooling crystallization. The seeding and cooling policies have been studied by many researchers since the pioneering work of Griffiths [17] on industrial crystallization.

In manufacturing pharmaceuticals, large and uniform crystals are desired for high efficiency of downstream processes, such as filtering and drying. The seeding methods have been developed for the optimization of the crystal size. The seeding policies can be roughly classified into internal seeding and external seeding.

In internal seeding, seed crystals are not added to the solution in cooling, and primary nuclei and secondary ones following them grow up to yield the product crystals. In this process, the resulting products are not contaminated by the external seed crystals, and hence the internal seeding attracts attention as a good method for manufacturing the added-value crystal products such as pharmaceuticals. The applications of internal seeding have been reported by Doki et al. [18], Kim et al. [19], Lenka and Sarkar [20], and so on. However, in internal seeding the extra nuclei need to be dissolved by temperature cycling in order to obtain large and uniform crystals. Finally, a reasonable number of nuclei survive and are treated as seed crystals in typical seeding. The heater and the cooler may expend much time and energy on this temperature cycling in large industrial plants. In addition, the process containing internal seeding may be strongly affected by the stochastic nature of primary nucleation, and hence the batch time or the product quality can fluctuate under a certain controlling condition.

In external seeding, seed crystals are added to the solution for some purpose. The external seeding may be classified into full seeding and partial seeding, based on the purpose of seeding.

In full seeding, a large quantity of seed crystals is added to consume and lower the supersaturation by the crystal growth and to suppress nucleation. The full seeding was first investigated with the statistical method by Doki et al. [21], and then has been widely studied from laboratory scale to industrial plant. The full seeding is so robust a method that it may yield the crystal products of very high quality and be hardly affected by the cooling method. Meanwhile, in full seeding, it may be preferable to add a sufficient quantity of small and uniform seed crystals because the product crystal quality strongly depends on the seed one. However, a large quantity of seed crystals is avoided in the production of added-value crystals due to the impurities from filtrated, dried, milled, and sieved seed crystals, and to the risk of exposure to their dust. Moreover, unlike the crystals nucleated in the solution, the dry seed ones may not necessarily grow successfully.

On the other hand, in partial seeding, a small quantity of seed crystals is added to induce secondary nucleation. And then, the nuclei grow to yield the products of moderate quality. Roughly speaking, partial seeding has been applied unintentionally to the actual plants so far, which means that some seeded crystallizers may not be fully seeded for inhibiting nucleation practically. Lee et al. [22] referred to the partial seeding as a reasonable method which might contribute to a high reproducibility. In partial seeding, the seed crystals may not act as children which are going to grow up to be the product crystals but as catalysts for secondary nucleation, and hence the quality of the seed crystals does not necessarily affect the product quality. The simulated results supporting this claim, which were originally reported by Unno and Hirasawa [23], are shown in Sect. 2.2. Therefore, the seed crystals may not need milling and sieving, and they can be replaced with the seed slurry, which may contribute to a significant reduction in impurities and dust.

The concept of classification of seeding policies is outlined in Fig. 5. From the above, partial seeding can be considered to be a relatively good choice for the seeding policy for pharmaceutical processes. However, the process containing partial seeding can be strongly affected by the cooling method, which is attributed to the dependency of secondary nucleation kinetics on supersaturation. For the optimal control of partially seeded crystallization, a moderate number of secondary nuclei should be induced at an early stage, and then they should grow to be the product

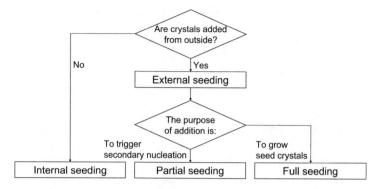

Fig. 5 Concept of classification of seeding policies

crystals with extra nucleation inhibited. Very few studies on this type of optimization problem have been reported, and the optimization of the cooling method is still debatable. Simulation examples of the optimal process design are shown in Sect. 2.3.

2.2 Optimization of Partial Seeding

In Sect. 2.2, the simulated results of seeded batch cooling crystallization in the model system, which were originally reported by Unno and Hirasawa [23], are discussed to characterize partial seeding.

At first, an aqueous solution of potassium sulfate is selected as a target substance, and the following preconditions are assumed to be established: a suspension in the crystallizer is well-mixed, there is no crystal breakage nor agglomeration, crystal growth follows the McCabe ΔL law, which means that neither growth rate dispersion nor size-dependent crystal growth occurs, primary nucleation and secondary nucleation are considered to be deterministic processes, the rate of each phenomenon is expressed as the power function of the supercooling degree, and the secondary nucleation rate is proportional to the magma density, or the third moment of CSD. The physical properties and the kinetic parameters are listed in Table 5.

Next, the experimental procedure is considered as follows. Seed crystals are added to saturated potassium sulfate aqueous solution at 50 °C, and the solution is cooled down to 30 °C. Then, the solution is kept at 30 °C for an hour.

Finally, the PBE and MBE, which contain differential equations, are solved to deduce several lower-order moments of the product CSD. Using the resulting moments, the mean size and the CV are calculated to evaluate the product quality. Here the mean size should be defined or weighted according to the purpose of optimization. The mean size $L_{i,j}$, which will be the size of the crystal with the mean

Table 5 Physical properties and kinetic parameters of potassium sulfate

Name	Symbol	Unit	Value
Density of crystal	ρ_c	[kg/m^3]	2662
Volumetric shape factor	k_v	[−]	1.5
Constant of solubility curve	α_{sat}	[−]	6.29×10^{-2}
Constant of solubility curve	β_{sat}	[−]	2.46×10^{-3}
Constant of solubility curve	γ_{sat}	[−]	-7.14×10^{-6}
Primary nucleation coefficient	k_{b1}	[#/(s kg-solvent K^{b1})]	1.0×10^{-6}
Primary nucleation order	b1	[−]	5.96
Secondary nucleation coefficient	k_{b2}	[#/(s K^{b2} m^3)]	1.0×10^6
Secondary nucleation order	b2	[−]	3.00
Linear growth coefficient	k_g	[m/(s K^g)]	1.0×10^{-7}
Linear growth order	g	[−]	0.9
Nucleated crystal size	L_0	[μm]	1.00

Solubility curve is represented by $C/(\text{g/g-solvent}) = \alpha_{sat} + \beta_{sat} (\theta / °C) + \gamma_{sat} (\theta/°C)^2$, where C is the concentration of saturated solution and θ is the solution temperature.
Reproduced from Ref. [24]

value of the quantity proportional to L^i if $j = 0$ or be the L^j-weighted mean size if $i − j = 1$, is represented using the moments as follows:

$$L_{i,j} = \left(\frac{\mu_i}{\mu_j} \right)^{\frac{1}{i-j}} \tag{29}$$

For example, mean volume size, which is the size of the crystal with the mean volume, is denoted by $L_{3,0}$ and volume mean size, which is the volume-weighted mean size, by $L_{4,3}$. The mean volume size is often used when the full seeding is investigated because only the total volume of crystals is increased without changing the total number in successful full seeding. The CV may also be weighted by L^j and is given as follows:

$$CV_j = \sqrt{\frac{\mu_j \mu_{j+2}}{\mu_{j+1}^2} - 1} \tag{30}$$

For example, the volume-weighted CV is denoted by CV_3. The CV originally means the ratio of the standard deviation in CSD to the mean size, and hence the CV of the size distribution of large and uniform crystals is small. Therefore, the minimization of the CV can correspond to the optimization of partial seeding. These statistics defined or weighted are deduced from the histogram in which the horizontal axis indicates the quantity proportional to L^{i-j} and the vertical axis does that proportional to L^j. In the typical histogram, i is set to 1 and j to 0. Moreover, in simulations, one can distinguish the origins of product crystals. In Sect. 2, based on the origin, the product crystals are classified as seed-grown, seed-originated, or primary nuclei-originated. Grown seed crystals, of which the product crystals are composed in the successful full seeding, are defined as seed-grown crystals. Grown secondary nuclei originated from seed-grown crystals and their grown descendants, of which the product crystals may be mainly composed in the partial seeding, are defined as seed-originated crystals. Grown primary nuclei, grown secondary nuclei originated from grown primary nuclei, and their grown descendants, of which the product crystals are completely composed in the internal seeding, are defined as primary nuclei-originated crystals. Mass fractions from each origin are computed in Sect. 2.

Consequently, the statistics mentioned above versus seed loading ratio, or ratio of seed loading mass to theoretical crystal yield, are computed and illustrated several other materials.

This trend indicates that partial seeding is most effectively performed at the first local minimum point of the CV. Therefore, the seed loading ratio at which the CV takes the first local minimum can be regarded as the optimal one under a certain condition of the seed quality and the cooling method. Then, the optimum seed loading ratio is estimated for some cooling rates and some seed crystal sizes, and the resulting relation among optimum seed loading ratio, cooling rate, and seed crystal size is illustrated in Fig. 7. In addition, the resulting relation among local minimum CV, cooling rate, and seed crystal size is shown in Fig. 8. Here, the local minimum CVs correspond to the first local minima, and the optimum seed loading ratios to the arguments of the first local minima, in the charts of CV versus seed loading ratio. In Fig. 7, the optimum seed loading ratio is affected both by the seed quality and by the cooling method. On the other hand, in Fig. 8, the local minimum CV is not affected by the seed crystal size but by the cooling rate, which might be attributed to the role of the seed crystals in the partial seeding as the catalysts for secondary nucleation. In short, the seed quality will not affect the optimal product quality but the optimal control.

2.3   Process Design

In Sect. 2.3, a simple method for the crystallization process design is developed for the optimization of partially seeded crystallization of the model substance. As mentioned in Sect. 2.2, the seed quality will not affect the optimal product quality, which enables the seed slurry to replace the seed crystals filtrated, dried, milled, and sieved. The seed slurry can be prepared by recycling the product slurry or in the other unseeded crystallizer. The crystal quality of the seed slurry cannot be controlled but monitored with the PAT tools. The acquired data will be utilized for determining the optimal control procedure.

The seed quality may be determined by the size and the standard deviation in the size. However, in the simulation, the standard deviation affects neither the minima nor the arguments and may not matter to the partial seeding. As for the cooling method, one can change the cooling period and the temperature profile for

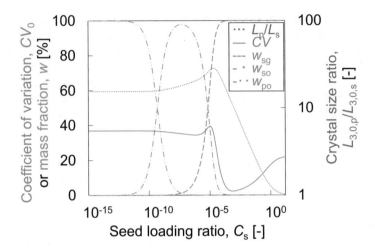

Fig. 6 Mean volume size ratio of product crystal to seed one, CV, and mass fractions of crystals from each origin versus ratio of seed loading mass to theoretical crystal yield at the cooling rate of 3.3 K/h and at the seed size of 31.6 μm. Seed, product, seed-grown, seed-originated, and primary nuclei-originated are denoted by the subscripts s, p, sg, so, and po, respectively. (Reproduced from Ref. [23])

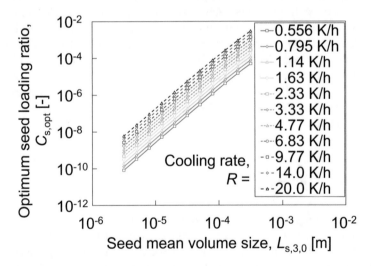

Fig. 7 Optimum seed loading ratio for partial seeding versus seed mean volume size and versus cooling rate. (Reproduced from Ref. [23])

controlling the product quality. For example, in Fig. 6, the cooling period is fixed to 6 h, and the solution is cooled linearly, which means that the decrease in temperature is proportional to the first power of time. Therefore, the product CVs in Fig. 8 may be improved by changing the temperature profiles, such as the exponent of time. In other words, the cooling may be programmed for optimization of the partial

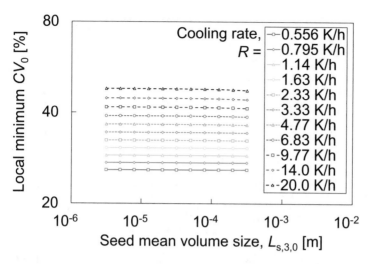

Fig. 8 Local minimum value of CV versus seed mean volume size and versus cooling rate. (Reproduced from Ref. [23])

seeding. Then, the exponent of time for temperature profile is optimized for partial seeding under several conditions of the cooling period, and the optimum exponent and the resulting minimum CV versus the cooling period are depicted in Fig. 9. At the same time, the re-optimized seed loading ratio for the programmed cooling is shown in Fig. 10. Here, typical mean size, or $L_{1,0}$, is used, both the exponent and the seed loading ratio need to be optimized simultaneously, and the regression equations are also shown. As is mentioned in Sect. 2.3, these regression equations will be utilized for the process design. Nevertheless, it should be noted that there is room for improvement in the temperature profile in this case, where the decrease in temperature is set to be proportional to the power function of time.

Before a concrete example is provided, the several conditions of the experimental procedure are added to those considered in Sect. 2.2 as follows. At first, mass of solvent is set to 3 kg, which fixes the theoretical crystal yield to 113 g. Next, the seed slurry, in which the seed mean size is measured at 100 μm, is prepared in the other unseeded crystallizer and then added to the main crystallizer. Finally, in order to improve productivity, the product crystals are required to have the CV not more than 40%. Under these conditions, cooling and seeding methods are optimized to meet the demand for the product quality and to minimize the cooling period.

This type of optimization involves complex non-linear problems, but they can be solved as a simplified linear programming problem of the regression equations mentioned in Sect. 2.2. The regression equations used for the process design are shown below:

$$CV_{0,\text{opt}}/\% = -18.5 \log_{10}(\tau_1/s) + 113 \tag{31}$$

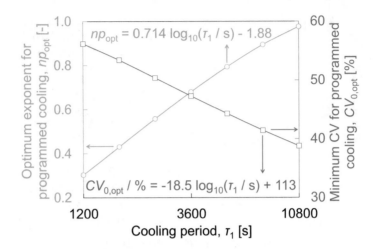

Fig. 9 Optimum exponent for programmed cooling and resulting minimum product CV versus cooling period for the partial seeding

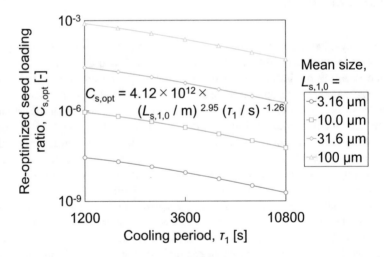

Fig. 10 Re-optimized seed loading ratio for programmed cooling versus cooling period for the partial seeding

$$np_{opt} = 0.714 \log_{10}(\tau_1/s) - 1.18 \tag{32}$$

$$C_{s,opt} = 4.12 \times 10^{12} (L_{s,1,0}/m)^{2.95} (\tau_1/s)^{-1.26} \tag{33}$$

Here, $CV_{0,opt}$ is local minimum CV, np_{opt} is optimum exponent for programmed cooling, $C_{s,opt}$ is optimum seed loading ratio, and τ_1 is cooling period. Eq. (31) is concerned with the satisfaction of the demand for the quality and with the minimization of the production time, Eq. (32) with the optimization of the cooling method, and Eq. (33) with the optimization of the seeding method.

These equations are utilized for the process design as follows. At first, the demand for the quality is substituted into Eq. (31), and the resulting inequity is solved to derive the minimum cooling period required to meet the demand. This method supposes the tendency that higher product quality requires longer cooling period. Next, the minimum cooling period obtained is substituted into Eq. (32) to derive the optimum temperature profile. Finally, the minimum cooling period and the seed mean size measured are substituted into Eq. (33) to derive the optimum seed loading quantity.

In the case of the model substance, at first, $CV_{0,opt} \leq 40\%$ is substituted into Eq. (31) to derive $\tau_1 \geq 2.51$ h. Then, $\tau_1 = 2.51$ h into Eq. (32) to derive $np_{opt} = 0.948$, where, like in natural cooling, the cooling is a little faster at an early stage than at a late stage. In partial seeding, this type of cooling might be work well, because the faster cooling at an early stage might induce the secondary nuclei, and because the slower one at the last stage might enlarge the nuclei. Finally, $\tau_1 = 2.51$ h and $L_{s,1,0} = 100\,\mu$m into Eq. (33) to derive $C_{s,opt} = 6.96 \times 10^{-5}$, and the optimum seed loading ratio multiplied by the theoretical crystal yield is the optimum seed loading quantity of 7.86 mg. These control variables completely define the optimized method of cooling and seeding for partially seeded crystallization.

2.4   Case Study: L-Arginine Crystallization

In Sect. 2.2, seeded crystallization in the model system is investigated to characterize partial seeding. In Sect. 2.4, we show the case study of partially seeded crystallization of Arg, which were originally reported by Unno and Hirasawa [25].

An aqueous solution of Arg is selected as a target substance. The experimental procedure was as follows. At first, the seed suspension to which the seed crystals had been sieved and added was prepared and kept at 30 °C. Then, a saturating quantity of Arg was dissolved in 300 mL of water at 35 °C, which was higher than saturation temperature of 30 °C. Finally, the solution was linearly cooled down to 20 °C, stirred at 300 rpm, and monitored with the PAT tools. In cooling, the seed suspension was added when the solution temperature reached 30 °C. After the cooling, the solution temperature was kept for half an hour. The seed loading ratios were set to around the optimum ratio predicted by simulation. As for the simulation, the physical properties and the kinetic parameters reported by Unno et al. [7] were utilized, and similar preconditions as in Sect. 2.2 were assumed to be established with such exceptions as follows: primary nucleation was neglected, the coefficients of each rate varied with temperature according to the Arrhenius equations, and the growth rate was expressed as the function of the relative supersaturation.

As a result, simulated and measured charts of CV of the product crystals versus seed loading ratio are illustrated in Fig. 11. In Fig. 11, the simulated optimum seed loading ratio is reasonably close to the measured one. However,

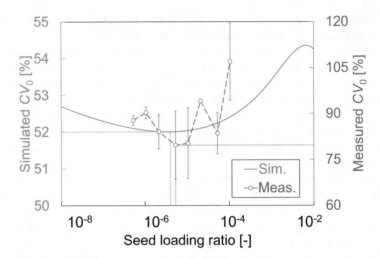

Fig. 11 Simulated and measured relations between seed loading ratio and product CV at the cooling period of 1.67 h and with the seed crystals sieved to 44–74 μm. The error bar is standard error of three measurements. (Reproduced from Ref. [7])

the minimum CV is not predicted successfully due to the ignorance of primary nucleation, agglomeration, and breakage. In addition, the error bars are so long that one can hardly recognize significant differences among the plots, which might be attributed to the stochastic nature of nucleation in a laboratory scale and to the measurement errors of the very small suspension volume added. These results suggest the difficulties in validation of the optimal partial seeding in laboratories.

2.5 Quality Stability

In Sect. 1.6, we show how to solve the SDEs including stochastic nucleation, and the experimental results in Sect. 2.4 imply that the stochastic nature of nucleation may affect the fluctuation of the product quality under a certain controlling condition. In Sect. 2.5, we discuss the simulation for the effect of stochastic nucleation on the product quality in seeded crystallization.

As in Sect. 2.2, an aqueous solution of potassium sulfate is selected as a target substance, and similar preconditions are assumed to be established with the exception that primary nucleation and secondary nucleation are considered to be stochastic processes. Then, the same experimental procedure as in Sect. 2.2 is considered, and the product CV is calculated 50 times per 1 condition.

Consequently, the simulated relation between seed loading ratio and product CV is illustrated by the box plot in Fig. 12 under an example condition. The deterministic CVs are also shown in Fig. 12. These results may imply that in some cases, the fluctuation of the product quality caused by the stochastic nature of nucleation is not negligible. For example, at the seed loading ratio of 10^{-2} in Fig.

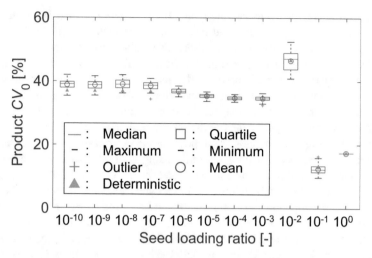

Fig. 12 Stochastic and deterministic relations simulated between seed loading ratio and product CV at the cooling period of 6 h, the seed mean size of 316 μm, and the solvent mass of 10 g. In the box plot, the maximum whisker length is 1.5 times of each box length

12, the box length of the quartile is 5 percentage points despite the median of a little less than 50%.

In addition, another simulation suggests that primary nucleation may occur in the range of the seed loading ratio not more than 10^{-4} and that secondary nucleation not more than 10^{-1}. Compared to these ranges, Fig. 12 might indicate that stochastic nucleation, both primary and secondary, causes the fluctuation of measured values and that stochastic primary nucleation specially causes the error between the deterministic value and the mean of stochastic ones.

The stochastic behavior of nucleation, which will make it difficult to control the crystallization process, may be inevitable if nucleation happens. However, the fluctuation and the error can be reduced by means of nucleation at high speed or scale-up of the crystallizer. Moreover, one can predict them in the simulation mentioned above. This prediction will have to be taken into account for the process design. For instance, the optimal control which can produce the crystals with high quality but may cause the significant fluctuation will have to be avoided or improved.

3 Conclusions

At first, the mathematical models for the crystallization phenomena, such as growth, nucleation, breakage, and agglomeration, are introduced to describe pharmaceutical crystallization processes, and parameter estimation methods are developed for the parameters of these models. For the simple parameter estimation, in-line measurements with PATs, such as FBRM and ATR-FT-IR, may be helpful. By using these PAT tools, the kinetic parameters of growth and secondary nucleation for Arg crystallization can be estimated simply and linearly. As for primary nucleation, the stochastic nature is significant, and hence the SDEs including stochastic primary nucleation should be solved so many times, as well as repeated measurements, that the kinetic parameters can be estimated. With the PAT tools, some parameters of breakage may be estimated simply and linearly, but others may non-linearly. It is difficult to analyze solely the agglomeration kinetics due to the dependence of agglomeration on supersaturation, but the kinetic parameters of agglomeration may be estimated when the parameters of the other phenomena are known.

Then, the developed models are applied to the optimization of pharmaceutical crystallization processes. Among several seeding policies classified based on seed loading quantity, partial seeding may be a good choice for pharmaceutical processes. In partially seeded crystallization of a model substance, the seeding and cooling methods are simultaneously optimized for the best product quality, which results in the design formulae of the seeding and cooling conditions. By using the design formulae, the detailed operating conditions of the crystallization process designed optimally can be calculated for the model substance. This optimization method was applied to partially seeded crystallization of Arg. Consequently, the simulated optimum seed loading ratio was reasonably close to the measured one. However, the minimum CV was not predicted successfully due to the ignorance of primary nucleation, agglomeration, and breakage, and the results may have been affected by the stochastic nature of nucleation. As for the stochastic nature of nucleation, the simulated result in seeded crystallization of a model substance suggests that the stochastic behavior of both primary and secondary nucleation may cause the fluctuation of the product crystal quality. Therefore, the stochastic behavior of nucleation will have to be considered for the process design.

References

1. Randolph AD, Larson MA (1962) Transient and steady state size distributions in continuous mixed suspension crystallizers. AIChE J 8(5): 639–645. doi:https://doi.org/10.1002/aic.690080515
2. Hulburt HM, Katz S (1964) Some problems in particle technology: A statistical mechanical formulation. Chem Eng Sci 19(8): 555–574. doi:https://doi.org/10.1016/0009-2509(64)85047-8
3. Worlitschek J, Hocker T, Mazzotti M (2005) Restoration of PSD from chord length distribution data using the method of projections onto convex sets. Part Part Syst Charact 22(2): 81–98. doi:https://doi.org/10.1002/ppsc.200400872
4. Unno J, Umeda R, Hirasawa I (2018) Computing crystal size distribution by focused-beam reflectance measurement when aspect ratio varies. Chem Eng Technol 41(6): 1147–1151. doi:https://doi.org/10.1002/ceat.201700615
5. Zhang F, Liu T, Wang XZ et al (2017) Comparative study on ATR-FTIR calibration models for monitoring solution concentration in cooling crystallization. J Cryst Growth 459: 50–55. doi:https://doi.org/10.1016/j.jcrysgro.2016.11.064
6. Unno J, Hirasawa I (2020a) Parameter estimation of the stochastic primary nucleation kinetics by stochastic integrals using focused-beam reflectance measurements. Crystals 10(5): 380. doi:https://doi.org/10.3390/cryst10050380

7. Unno J, Kawase H, Kaneshige R et al (2019) Estimation of kinetics for batch cooling crystallization by focused-beam reflectance measurements. Chem Eng Technol 42(7): 1428–1434. doi:https://doi.org/10.1002/ceat.201800646
8. Maggioni GM, Mazzotti M (2015) Modelling the stochastic behaviour of primary nucleation. Faraday Discuss 179: 359–382. doi:https://doi.org/10.1039/c4fd00255e
9. Marchisio DL, Vigil RD, Fox RO (2003) Quadrature method of moments for aggregation-breakage processes. J Colloid Interface Sci 258(2): 322–334. doi:https://doi.org/10.1016/S0021-9797(02)00054-1
10. Hasseine A, Senouci S, Attarakih M et al (2015) Two analytical approaches for solution of population balance equations: Particle breakage process. Chem Eng Technol 38(9): 1574–1584. doi:https://doi.org/10.1002/ceat.201400769
11. Bari AH, Pandit AB (2018) Sequential crystallization parameter estimation method for determination of nucleation, growth, breakage, and agglomeration kinetics. Ind Eng Chem Res 57(5): 1370–1379. doi:https://doi.org/10.1021/acs.iecr.7b03995
12. Li H, Yang B-S (2019) Model evaluation of particle breakage facilitated process intensification for Mixed-Suspension-Mixed-Product-Removal (MSMPR) crystallization. Chem Eng Sci 207: 1175–1186. doi:https://doi.org/10.1016/j.ces.2019.07.030
13. Vanni M. (2000) Approximate population balance equations for aggregation-breakage processes. J Colloid Interface Sci 221(2): 143–160. doi:https://doi.org/10.1006/jcis.1999.6571
14. Laloue N, Couenne F, Le Gorrec Y et al (2007) Dynamic modeling of a batch crystallization process: A stochastic approach for agglomeration and attrition process. Chem Eng Sci 62(23): 6604–6614. doi:https://doi.org/10.1016/j.ces.2007.07.039
15. Ó'Ciardhá CT, Hutton KW, Mitchell NA et al (2012) Simultaneous parameter estimation and optimization of a seeded antisolvent crystallization. Cryst Growth Des 12(11): 5247–5261. doi:https://doi.org/10.1021/cg3006822
16. Gencaslan A, Sayan P, Titiz-Sargut S (2018) Effects of L-serine and L-proline on crystallization kinetics of calcium pyrophosphate dihydrate. Chem Eng Technol 41(6): 1211–1217. doi:https://doi.org/10.1002/ceat.201700671
17. Griffiths H (1925) Mechanical crystallization. J Soc Chem Ind 44: 7T–18T
18. Doki N, Kubota N, Yokota M et al (2002a) Production of sodium chloride crystals of uni-modal size distribution by batch dilution crystallization. J Chem Eng Jpn 35(11): 1099–1104. doi:https://doi.org/10.1252/jcej.35.1099
19. Kim J-W, Kim J-K, Kim H-S et al (2011) Application of internal seeding and temperature cycling for reduction of liquid inclusion in the crystallization of RDX. Org Process Res Dev 15(3): 602–609. doi:https://doi.org/10.1021/op100334y
20. Lenka M, Sarkar D (2018) Improving crystal size distribution by internal seeding combined cooling/antisolvent crystallization with a cooling/heating cycle. J Cryst Growth 486: 130–136. doi:https://doi.org/10.1016/j.jcrysgro.2018.01.029
21. Doki N, Kubota N, Yokota M et al (2002b) Determination of critical seed loading ratio for the production of crystals of uni-modal size distribution in batch cooling crystallization of potassium alum. J Chem Eng Jpn 35(7): 670–676. doi:https://doi.org/10.1252/jcej.35.670
22. Lee M, Geertman R, Rauls M et al (2014) Challenges in industrial crystallization. In: Proceedings of the 19th international symposium on industrial crystallization, Congress center Pierre Baudis, Toulouse, France, 16–19 Sept 2014
23. Unno J, Hirasawa I (2019) Partial seeding policy for controlling size distribution of product crystal by batch cooling crystallization. J Chem Eng Jpn 52(6): 501–507. doi:https://doi.org/10.1252/jcej.18we272
24. Kobari M, Kubota N, Hirasawa I (2011) Computer simulation of metastable zone width for unseeded potassium sulfate aqueous solution. J Cryst Growth 317(1): 64–69. doi:https://doi.org/10.1016/j.jcrysgro.2010.12.069
25. Unno J, Hirasawa I (2020b) Partial seeding policy for controlling the crystal quality in batch cooling crystallization. Chem Eng Technol 43(6): 1065–1071. doi:https://doi.org/10.1002/ceat.201900618

Mathematical Modeling of Different Breakage PBE Kernels Using Monte Carlo Simulation Results

Ashok Das and Jitendra Kumar

1 Introduction

The production of particles with some specific internal and external properties is crucial in pharmaceutical, chemical, mineral, food processing, and other material processing industries. Some of the important particulate processes used in these industries are crystallization, agglomeration, milling, grinding, polymerization, etc. In these processes, particles change their internal and external properties (e.g., size, shape, porosity, enthalpy, etc.), and one can observe aggregation, fragmentation, nucleation, rupture, and growth of particles. The most popular method to track the macroscopic behavior of the system is to use the population balance equations (PBEs) [1]. The PBE is an integro-differential equation, which tracks the evolution of the number density function with respect to time. The PBE uses certain mathematical kernels to describe the particulate processes, such as aggregation, breakage, growth, and nucleation. However, the sole focus of this chapter will be to discuss the PBE kernels corresponding to different types of breakage processes.

Due to the integro-differential nature, PBEs are analytically solvable for some extremely trivial classes of kernels only. That is why PBEs are often solved numerically. In the literature, several numerical techniques are available to solve the PBE, such as sectional method [2–5], method of moments [6, 7], finite element method [8–10], finite volume technique [11–14], etc. Most of these numerical techniques discretize the domain of concern to solve the equations. Additionally, the researchers have also used the stochastic and discrete nature of the Monte Carlo technique to solve the PBE [15–17]. However, the ubiquitous use of population balance modeling is hindered in practical situations due to the unavailability of

A. Das · J. Kumar (✉)
Department of Mathematics, Indian Institute of Technology Kharagpur, Kharagpur, West Bengal, India
e-mail: jkumar@maths.iitkgp.ac.in

© The Author(s), under exclusive license to Springer Nature Switzerland AG 2022
A. Fytopoulos et al. (eds.), *Optimization of Pharmaceutical Processes*, Springer Optimization and Its Applications 189, https://doi.org/10.1007/978-3-030-90924-6_4

macroscopic physically motivated PBE kernels. Over the years, the researchers have used empirical or semi-empirical kernels, which generally use fitted constants to predict the experimental outcomes for some particular set of operating conditions. Furthermore, although the PBE kernels are dependent of material properties and time simultaneously, most of the studies available in the literature omitted either the time dependency or the dependency on material properties. It is still a challenging task to incorporate the physics of the particulate process (e.g., process parameters, material properties, etc.) and propose the PBE kernels that can track the variations in the material properties under concern and time simultaneously. In recent years, Das et al. [18–20] have developed PBE kernels for some processes, which are dependent on particle dimensions and process time simultaneously. The focus of this chapter will be to discuss the development and verification of those PBE kernels.

On the other hand, the Monte Carlo (MC) technique became popular as a replication tool to experimental particulate systems. In a series of studies, Terrazas-Velarde et al. [21–23] developed a constant volume MC algorithm to simulate the aggregation mechanism in a spray fluidized bed granulator. The simulation results predicted the lab-scale experimental results qualitatively for porous and non-porous particles. In later years, Dernedde et al. [24, 25] developed an efficient concept of positions and sectors on the agglomerate surfaces to model the spray fluidized bed aggregation process and to determine the moisture content on agglomerate surfaces. In 2019, Bhoi et al. [26] developed a constant number MC algorithm which predicted the sonofragmentation experimental observations accurately. Recently, Singh and Tsotsas [27, 28] developed a tunable constant volume MC model of fluidized bed granulation process using different morphological descriptors. Instead of working with experimental results, working with the MC technique may be advantageous for the development of PBE kernels. For instance, access to many properties, which are challenging or impossible to measure in an experimental setup, is easily available. Additionally, the user achieves the control to switch on and off any specific event in the MC simulation in order to evaluate its impact on the whole simulation [26, 29]. Due to these reasons, in this chapter, we have used the MC technique as a replacement of experimental setup.

In this chapter, at first, we will discuss the MC algorithm in detail and then will discuss the development of some breakage PBE kernels which depend on particle dimensions and process time simultaneously. Finally, the validation of the discussed models will be done with the help of MC simulation results.

2   Monte Carlo Algorithm

The Monte Carlo (MC) method is a probabilistic approach which uses the generation of random numbers to estimate the values of entities under consideration. Metropolis and Ulam [30] introduced the MC method in 1949. The uncomplicated concepts and the discrete nature of Monte Carlo help to naturally adapt itself in dynamic processes [30, 31]. The MC algorithm works with a representative sample of the whole system, which is considered to have identical properties as the original system, and after simulation, a scale-up factor is used to predict the original results [26, 32].

The MC algorithms are divided into two categories given the time step length, which are "time-driven MC" and "event-driven MC." In the time-driven approach, at first, we assign a time step and then implement all possible events within the time step. However, in the event-driven approach, first, an event is selected to occur, and then the time is advanced accordingly. The event-driven MC has an upper hand over the time-driven MC, as an event is guaranteed in each time step of the event-driven MC, which is not the case for the time-driven MC [31].

Another critical aspect of the MC method is about the size of the simulation box, i.e., the considered total number of particles in the MC simulation box. The number of particles in the simulation box changes according to the nature of the process. In the case of aggregation process, the number of particles decreases with time and eventually reduces to only one after prolonged simulation. This compromises the accuracy of the process. On the contrary, the number of particles increases with time in case of breakage processes. This situation increases the computational cost of the MC simulation process. To counter this scenario and to regulate the number of particles in the simulation, MC methods can also be divided into two types in view of the size of the simulation box, which are "constant number MC" (CNMC) and "constant volume MC" (CVMC). In CVMC, the total volume of the MC simulation box is kept fixed until some drastic change occurs in the total number of particles. By convention, the CVMC method doubles or halves the simulation box size, respectively, when its size has reduced (in case of aggregation process) or expanded (in case of breakage process) by a factor of two. This method balances the accuracy and computational efficiency of the simulation. On the other hand, in the CNMC method, we fix the total number of particles in the simulation box at each time step by either duplicating one particle of the simulation box (in case of aggregation) or deleting one particle randomly from the simulation box (in case of breakage process) [15–17, 33].

Zhao et al. [31] suggested that the CVMC method works better in case of aggregation processes, whilst CNMC performs better in case of breakage processes. That is why we have used the event-driven CNMC algorithm to replicate different breakage mechanisms. The general flowchart of a CNMC algorithm is depicted in Fig. 1. At the start, we initialize the process conditions and simulation parameters. We also fix the size of the simulation box, i.e., the number of particles in the simulation box (N_{MC}), which has identical properties to the original system. We further represent the concerned particle properties in terms of arrays in the MC system. If the process has I number of events, which are occurring simultaneously, we calculate the frequency of each individual events (λ_i). Then, the total number of events per unit time is given as

$$\lambda = \sum_{i=1}^{I} \lambda_i \qquad (1)$$

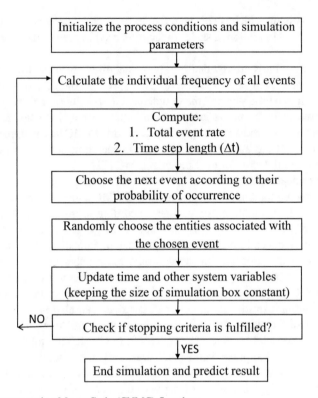

Fig. 1 Constant number Monte Carlo (CNMC) flowchart

Then, we calculate the time step length of the next event as

$$\Delta t = \frac{-1}{\lambda} \ln(1 - \zeta) \tag{2}$$

where ζ is a uniformly distributed random number between 0 and 1. To select the next event depending on their event rates, we first calculate the cumulative frequencies using Eq. (3).

$$R_i = \sum_{k=1}^{i} \lambda_k, \quad \text{for } i = 1, 2, \ldots, 5 \tag{3}$$

Then, we select the ith state for the next event if the below equation is satisfied.

$$R_{i-1} < r\lambda \leq R_i \tag{4}$$

where r is another uniformly distributed random number in $(0, 1)$. Furthermore, using a similar technique, the corresponding entities associated with the selected event were chosen. Then, we execute the event and update the system accordingly. Since no particulate processes have been discussed here, we have not discussed about the events and their frequencies. We will discuss this in the respective sections.

3 Mathematical Modeling of PBE Kernels

This section will focus on developing and verifying the PBE kernels which depend on particle dimensions and process time simultaneously. The considered particulate processes are linear breakage, nonlinear collisional breakage, and sonofragmentation of rectangular crystals. Particle breakage can occur in various ways. However, in view of the process conditions, the breakage process can be broadly classified into two major classes: linear and nonlinear breakage. Linear breakage process occurs only due to some internal stresses of particles or some process-specific conditions, for example, thermal or mechanical conditions of the particulate process. In addition to that, if the breaking behavior of particles is also influenced due to collisions (or, interactions) between particles, then we classify it as the nonlinear breakage. A particular class of nonlinear breakage process is binary collisional breakage, where the fragmentation occurs solely through instantaneous binary collisions among particles. Sonofragmentation is one special type of linear breakage process, which is very popular in crystallization process. It uses the ultrasound to break crystal structures. In this chapter, we will discuss about the PBE kernels corresponding to the abovementioned fragmentation mechanisms.

3.1 Linear Breakage

The continuous one-dimensional linear breakage PBE is the following [18]:

$$\frac{\partial n(x, t)}{\partial t} = \underbrace{\int_x^\infty b(x, y)S(y, t)n(y, t)\,\mathrm{d}y}_{\text{birth of particle } x} - \underbrace{S(x, t)n(x, t)}_{\text{death of particle } x} \tag{5}$$

with the given initial data

$$n(x, 0) = n_0(x), \quad x \in \mathbb{R}^+ \tag{6}$$

where $n(x, t)$ is the number density function, $S(x, t)$ is the breakage selection function, and $b(x, y)$ is the breakage distribution function. This breakage distribution function $b(x, y)$ illustrates the breakage rate for formation of particles of volume x from a particle of volume y and satisfies the following two properties:

1. $\int_0^y b(x, y)\, dx = \nu(y)$, where $\nu(y)$ is the number of daughter particles produced due to breakage of the particle of volume y.

2. $\int_0^y x\, b(x, y)\, dx = y$,$\forall y > 0$. This property is called the mass conservation property.

Modeling of Linear Breakage Selection Function

The rate of successful linear breakage events is expressed by the selection function $S(x, t)$. In the literature [34, 35], $S(x, t)$ is usually partitioned into a product of volume-dependent and volume independent (i.e., time-dependent) components. However, the occurrence of a successful breakage event depends on the particle's internal bonding strength. If the applied stress upon the surface of the particle is higher than the internal bonding strength of the particle, then the particle breaks into fragments. This indicates that the rate of successful breakage events is also dependent on the probability of successful events ($\psi(x, t)$). For this, Das et al. [18] proposed the following factorization of the breakage selection function:

$$S(x, t) = S^*(x)\, S_0(t)\, \psi(x, t) \tag{7}$$

where the pre-factor $S^*(x)$ describes the particle volume dependency on breakage process, i.e., how the particle selection depends on the particle volume. The second factor $S_0(t)$ is the time dependency in particle breakage process. The last factor $\psi(x, t)$ is the probability of successful breakage events and can be defined as the ratio of the frequency of successful breakage events (f_s) to the stressing frequency per particle (f_{str}), i.e.,

$$\psi(x, t) = \frac{f_s}{f_{str}} \tag{8}$$

In the process, particle selection for the stressing events mainly depends on the volume-dependent part of the selection function $S^*(x)$ and their availability in the system. Therefore, the selection probability of any particle at time t is

$$P(x, t) = \frac{S^*(x)\, n(x, t)}{\int_0^\infty S^*(x)\, n(x, t)\, dx} \tag{9}$$

If $N_p(t)$ denotes the total number of particles present in the system, then the frequency of total number of stressing events is $f_{str}(t) N_p(t)$. Furthermore, in the event of a particle of volume x breaking into $v(x)$ number of smaller fragments, the increase in the total number of particles is $(v(x) - 1)$. Then, the rate of change in the total number of particles (N_p) can be written as

$$
\frac{dN_p(t)}{dt} = \int_0^\infty (v(x) - 1) \, [f_{str}(t) \, N_p(t)] \, P(x, t) \, \psi(x, t) \, dx
$$

$$
= \frac{f_{str}(t) \, N_p(t)}{\int_0^\infty S^*(x) \, n(x, t) \, dx} \int_0^\infty [v(x) - 1] \, S^*(x) \, \psi(x, t) \, n(x, t) \, dx \quad (10)
$$

On the other hand, integrating equation (5) with respect to x, we get the rate of change of total number of particles as

$$
\frac{dN_p(t)}{dt} = S_0(t) \int_0^\infty [v(x) - 1] \, S^*(x) \, \psi(x, t) \, n(x, t) \, dx \quad (11)
$$

Now, comparing Eqs. (10) and (11), we get

$$
S_0(t) = f_{str}(t) \frac{N_p(t)}{\int_0^\infty S^*(x) \, n(x, t) \, dx} \quad (12)
$$

Finally, using Eqs. (7), (8), and (12), we get the mathematical formulation of the volume and time-dependent linear breakage selection function as

$$
S(x, t) = S^*(x) \, S_0(t) \, \psi(x, t) = f_s(x, t) \, N_p(t) \frac{S^*(x)}{\int_0^\infty S^*(x) \, f(x, t) \, dx} \quad (13)
$$

Monte Carlo Simulation Details

To verify the accuracy of the discussed model, a CNMC algorithm is used to replicate a simple linear breakage process. Since the whole algorithm is discussed before, here we will only discuss the requisites of the simulation. The selection of particles for stressing events is the only event that takes place in this MC simulation. In each of the stressing event, we choose one particle using the probability function in Eq. (9). After selection of the particle, we use the predefined $\psi(x, t)$ to check whether the particle will break or not.

Verification of the Model

For the verification of the developed model of linear breakage selection function, the breakage PBE (Eq. (5)) was numerically solved using the developed model (13), and the numerical results were compared with the results obtained from the CNMC simulations. A detailed discussion on the model verification can be found in Das et al. [18]. For this chapter, the verification has been conducted for the following two simple test cases:

- **Case 1:** $\psi_1(x, t) = 1$, i.e., every stressing event on particles results in breakage event.
- **Case 2:** $\psi_2(x, t) \propto x$, i.e., the probability of successful stressing event varies with the volume of the chosen particle, but it is independent of time t. For this case, we consider $\psi_2(x, t) = \dfrac{x}{x_{max}}$.

The simulation parameters and material properties that were kept constant for the simulations are given in Table 1. For simplicity, we have considered a fixed value of the stressing frequency per particle (f_{str}). Furthermore, we have considered that particles get selected for the stressing events depending on their volume (i.e., $S^*(x) = x$), and in case of breakage events, particles randomly break into two smaller fragments (i.e., $b(x, y) = \frac{2}{y}$).

To start any MC simulation or to solve any PBE, we need to have the initial size distribution of particles beforehand. For this linear breakage process, a normally distributed particle size distribution (PSD) was considered with a mean $400v_{pp}$ and variance $20\,v_{pp}$ (see Fig. 2). Here, v_{pp} denotes the volume of a primary particle (monomer). For the verification of the model, the comparisons of the total number of particles and the final PSD are considered. The comparisons for both the considered cases are illustrated in Fig. 3. The evolution of normalized total number of particles for both the cases is presented in Fig. 3a. Furthermore, the comparison of PSDs is illustrated in Fig. 3b. From the figures, it is clear that the results obtained from solving the PBE predicted the MC simulation results with good agreement. For the case $\psi_1 = 1$, every stressing event results in breakage. That is why we can observe

Table 1 Process parameters and material properties for the linear breakage system

Parameter/Property	Symbol	Value	Unit
Bed mass	M_{bed}	1	kg
Primary particle (monomer) diameter	d_{pp}	4×10^{-4}	m
Particle density	ρ_p	2400	kg/m^3
Stressing frequency per particle	f_{str}	0.0125	s^{-1}
Number of particles in MC simulation box	N_{MC}	50,000	–
Total process time	$t_{process}$	100	s
Volume-dependent part of the selection function	$S^*(x)$	x	–
Breakage distribution function	$b(x, y)$	$\frac{2}{y}$	–

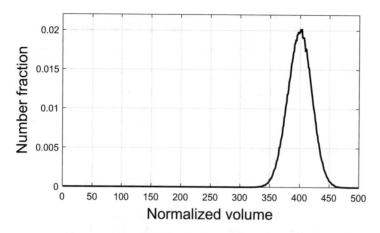

Fig. 2 Normally distributed initial size distribution of particles with normalized mean volume 400 and variance 20

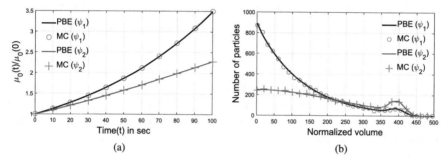

(a)

(b)

Fig. 3 Comparison of (**a**) normalized total number of particles and (**b**) particle size distributions obtained from PBE and MC results after 100 s

rapid increase in the number of particles compared to the other case in Fig. 3a. Due to this, we can observe that more particles have accumulated in the smaller volume region in this case (Fig. 3b).

3.2 Nonlinear Collisional Breakage

If particle fragmentation occurs only due to the impacts from particle collision, we term it as nonlinear collisional breakage. Cheng and Redner [36] mathematically formulated the one-dimensional binary collisional breakage in terms of an integro-differential equation as

$$\frac{\partial n(x,t)}{\partial t} = \underbrace{\int_0^\infty \int_x^\infty K(y,z,t)b(x,y;z)n(y,t)n(z,t)\mathrm{d}y\mathrm{d}z}_{\text{birth of particle of volume } x}$$

$$\underbrace{- n(x,t)\int_0^\infty K(x,y,t)n(y,t)\mathrm{d}y}_{\text{death of particle of volume } x} \tag{14}$$

along the initial distribution,

$$n(x,0) = n_0(x), \quad x \in \mathbb{R}^+ \tag{15}$$

where $K(x,y,t)$ is the collisional breakage kernel and denotes the rate of successful collisions between particles of volume x and y at time t. Here, a successful collision means those collisions where at least one of the colliding particles breaks into smaller fragments. In practice, the collision between a particle pair of volumes x and y is equivalent to the collision between the pair of volumes y and x. Therefore, the collision kernel is assumed to be symmetric in its last two arguments, i.e.,

$$K(x,y,t) = K(y,x,t), \quad \text{for all } x,y \in \mathbb{R}^+ \text{ and } t > 0 \tag{16}$$

Also, $b(x,y;z)$ is the breakage distribution function, which illustrates the rate of formation of particles of volume x by breakage of particle of volume y, due to collision between y and z. The breakage distribution function $b(x,y;z)$ satisfies the following two properties:

1. $\int_0^y b(x,y;z)\,\mathrm{d}x = v(y;z)$, where $v(y;z)$ is the number of daughter particles produced due to breakage of the particle of volume y after its collision with a particle of volume z.

2. $\int_0^y x\,b(x,y;z)\,\mathrm{d}x = y, \quad \forall y > 0, z > 0,$ and $x \le y$. This property is called the mass conservation property. This condition confirms that the total volume of daughter particles generated due to the breakup process is equal to the volume of the mother particle.

Modeling of Nonlinear Collisional Breakage Kernel

Following a similar line to the previous model, Das et al. [20] proposed the following factorization of the collisional breakage kernel:

$$K(x,y,t) = K^*(x,y)\,K_0(t)\,\psi(x,y,t) \tag{17}$$

where $K^*(x, y)$ is the volume dependency in particle collisions, $K_0(t)$ is the time dependency in collisional breakage process, and the last factor $\psi(x, y, t)$ is the probability of successful collisions and can be defined as the ratio of the frequency of successful breakage events (f_s) to the collision frequency per particle (f_c), i.e.,

$$\psi(x, y, t) = \frac{f_s}{f_c} \tag{18}$$

Generally, in a collision event, two particles of the system get selected according to their volume dependency and collide with each other. At the time of collision, particles exert force on each other, and if the collision energy is more than the particle's internal bonding strength (for example, dynamic-yield strength, shear strength, etc.), then one or both of the colliding particles break into two or more fragments of smaller volume depending upon the breakage distribution function.

The total number of collision events per second is $\frac{1}{2} f_c(t) N_p(t)$, where $N_p(t)$ is the total number of particles of the system at time t. The factor $\frac{1}{2}$ is considered to avoid the double counting of collisions. Also, particles in the system are selected for collision events depending on the volume-dependent part of collision kernel $K^*(x, y)$ and the availability of particles of those particular volumes in the system. Then, the collision probability of particles of volume x and y at any instance t can be written as

$$P(x, y, t) = \frac{K^*(x, y)\, n(x, t)\, n(y, t)}{\frac{1}{2} \int_0^\infty \int_0^\infty K^*(x, y)\, n(x, t)\, n(y, t)\, dxdy} \tag{19}$$

The fraction $\frac{1}{2}$ in the denominator is considered to avoid the double counting of particles. If the breakage criterion satisfies, then the colliding particles break into smaller fragments. If the breakup events of volume x and y result in $v(x; y)$ and $v(y; x)$ number of daughter particles, respectively, then the increase in the total number of particles due to this collisional breakage event is $(v(x; y) + v(y; x) - 2)$. Consequently, the rate of change of total number of particles can be represented by the following equation:

$$\frac{dN_p(t)}{dt} = \frac{1}{2} \int_0^\infty \int_0^\infty (v(x; y) + v(y; x) - 2) \left[\frac{1}{2} f_c(t) N_p(t) \right]$$
$$\times P(x, y, t)\, \psi(x, y, t)\, dx\, dy$$

$$= f_c(t)\, N_p(t)$$
$$\times \frac{\int_0^\infty \int_0^\infty [v(x; y) - 1]\, K^*(x, y)\, \psi(x, y, t)\, n(x, t)\, n(y, t)\, dxdy}{\int_0^\infty \int_0^\infty K^*(x, y)\, n(x, t)\, n(y, t)\, dx\, dy} \tag{20}$$

The collision probability of volume pair (x, y) is the same as the collision probability of volume pair (y, x). For this, we considered the fraction $\frac{1}{2}$ in the right-hand side of Eq. (20).

On the contrary, the rate of change of total number of particles in the nonlinear breakage PBE can be computed by integrating Eq. (14) with respect to x and y from 0 to ∞.

$$\frac{dN_p(t)}{dt} = K_0(t) \int_0^\infty \int_0^\infty [\nu(x; y) - 1] K^*(x, y) \psi(x, y, t) n(x, t) n(y, t) \, dx \, dy \tag{21}$$

Comparing Eqs. (20) and (21), we get

$$K_0(t) = \frac{f_c(t) N_p(t)}{\displaystyle\int_0^\infty \int_0^\infty K^*(x, y) n(x, t) n(y, t) \, dx \, dy} \tag{22}$$

Then, using Eqs. (17), (18), and (22), we have the volume and time-dependent collision kernel for nonlinear breakage process as

$$K(x, y, t) = f_s(x, y, t) N_p(t) \frac{K^*(x, y)}{\displaystyle\int_0^\infty \int_0^\infty K^*(x, y) n(x, t) n(y, t) \, dx \, dy} \tag{23}$$

Monte Carlo Simulation Details

In this case also, particle collision is the only possible event which takes place in the MC simulation. For each collision event, we use the probability function of Eq. (19) to choose two different particles. Then, we break the colliding particles according to the breakage behavior and update the system accordingly.

Verification of the Model

Similar to the case of linear breakage process, we will use the MC simulation results to verify the developed model of collisional breakage kernel. The collisional breakage PBE (Eq. (14)) was solved numerically using the developed model (23), and the results were compared against the results obtained from the MC simulations. The weighted finite volume scheme to solve the PBE can be found in Das et al. [20]. To test the authenticity of the model, we have considered a collisional breakage process where, in cases of successful collision events, both the colliding particles break into two smaller fragments with volumes 60% and 40% of the parent particles, respectively. Then, in this case, the breakage distribution function can be written as [20]

$$b(x, y; z) = \delta(x - 0.4\,y) + \delta(x - 0.6\,y) \tag{24}$$

Furthermore, we considered that the collisions are independent of their volumes, i.e., $K^*(x, y) = 1$. Other simulation parameters that were kept constant during the simulations are the same as the case of linear breakage process (see Table 1). The initial size distribution of particles is also provided in Fig. 2. The verification process was conducted for the following cases of ψ:

- $\psi_1(x, y, t) = 1$, i.e., every collision event between particles results in a breakage event.

- $\psi_2(x, y, t) = \begin{cases} 0 \text{ if } v \le 200 \\ 1 \text{ if } v > 200 \end{cases}$, where $v = \dfrac{2xy}{x + y}$ is the characteristic volume of the colliding particles, and breakage event occurs only if the characteristic volume of the colliding particles is greater than 200.

To verify the developed model accuracy, the evolution of normalized total number of particles and PSDs obtained from solving the collisional breakage PBE and from CNMC simulations were plotted against each other in Figs. 4 and 5. From the figures, it is clear that the model predicted the CNMC results meticulously for both the considered cases. Since the particles were breaking in 60% and 40% of the volume and initially particles were distributed normally around the normalized volume 400, we can observe some discrete normally distributed peaks around some particular sizes, for example, 240, 160, etc. Also, for the case $\psi_1 = 1$, i.e., when every collision results in a breakage event, Fig. 5a illustrated that a greater number of particles are concentrated in the smaller particle zone compared to the other case. In the case of ψ_2, breakage events were occurring only when the characteristic volume of the colliding particles is higher than or equal to 200. For this, a more prominent peak can be observed around the normalized volume 160 in Fig. 5b, since once a particle breaks into this zone, then it is unlikely to break again.

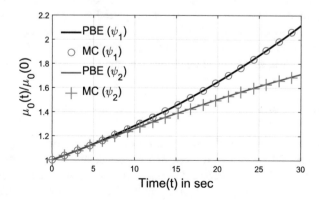

Fig. 4 Evolution of normalized total number of particles

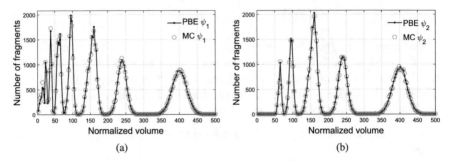

Fig. 5 Comparison of particle size distributions obtained from PBE and MC results after 30 s

The developed model was further verified for several other test cases. For the detailed discussion of the verification process, the readers are referred to see the work of Das et al. [20].

3.3 Sonofragmentation of Rectangular Plate-Like Crystals

The ultrasound assisted sonofragmentation process is well known in chemical and pharmaceutical industries. The use of ultrasound creates cavitation bubbles, and the implosion of the bubbles creates shock waves, which lead to crystal breakage. The use of ultrasound creates lesser impurities compared to other fragmentation techniques. There exist several studies in the literature related to sonofragmentation experiments of one-dimensional crystal particles. However, this is not the case for sonofragmentation of multi-dimensional crystals, as it is mostly unexplored regarding experiments and their mathematical modeling. In 2019, Bhoi et al. [26] performed sonofragmentation experiments on rectangular shaped pyrazinamide crystals and studied the effects of sonication period and sonication power. The authors also developed an MC algorithm to understand the breakage behavior of crystals. Later, Das et al. [19] developed the corresponding bivariate PBM. In this section, we will discuss the abovementioned studies.

Experimental Section

Sonofragmentation experiments were carried out on the δ-form of pyrazinamide crystals in a toluene medium. Experiments were conducted for different sonication periods (30, 60, and 90 s), keeping the ultrasonic amplitude value fixed at 30%. After each experiment, images of filtered and dried crystal fragments were captured using an optical microscope (see Fig. 6). The initial size distribution of crystals along length and width axes is shown in Fig. 7. The key observations from the experimental setup are following:

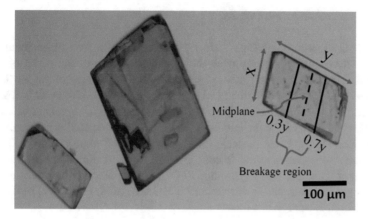

Fig. 6 Optical microscope image of δ-form pyrazinamide crystals (taken from Das et al. [19])

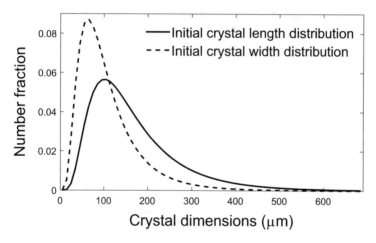

Fig. 7 Initial crystal size distributions along length and width

1. δ-form of pyrazinamide crystals is considered as thin rectangular plate-type particles with constant thickness and the particles break into only two fragments.
2. Due to the rectangular shape of crystals, they mostly break across their width. Further binary breakage of crystals was observed.
3. Crystal particles with length lesser than 20 μm do not break further into smaller fragments.
4. The total frequency of stressing events for the whole system stays constant throughout the experiment ($f_{ev,tot}(t) = $ constant), for a constant ultrasonic amplitude.

Monte Carlo Simulation Details

In the MC algorithm, crystals were represented with a two-dimensional array, and the elements of that array were the characteristic length and width of crystal particles. The trial and error method was used to fix the value of $f_{ev,tot}$ (i.e., the total frequency of events) for the fixed ultrasonic amplitude value at 30%. The fixed value of $f_{ev,tot}$ was 3.15×10^5 [19]. Furthermore, to find the breaking behavior of crystals, several breakage techniques were tested and compared with experimental results. However, the best possible match was observed when crystals break only across the width axis, and the fracture occurs at any random point between 30% and 70% of its length (see Figs. 6 and 8) [26]. These observations are used in the modeling of PBE kernels. Furthermore, the MC simulation results will be discussed in the validation part.

Modeling of Bivariate Breakage PBE Kernels

Since the length of the sides of crystal particles is the only property of concern and the fragmentation mechanism is of linear type, we use the bivariate linear breakage PBE. The continuous bivariate linear breakage PBE is

$$\frac{\partial n(x_1, x_2, t)}{\partial t} = \underbrace{\int_{x_1}^{\infty} \int_{x_2}^{\infty} S(y_1, y_2, t)\, b(x_1, x_2 | y_1, y_2)\, n(y_1, y_2, t)\, \mathrm{d}y_1\, \mathrm{d}y_2}_{\text{birth of crystal particles with dimensions } (x_1, x_2)}$$

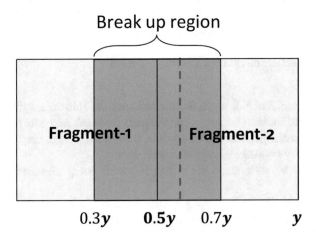

Fig. 8 Schematic diagram of the crystal breakage mechanism, in which rectangular crystals break into two fragments across the minor dimension and the breakup mechanism starts at any random point along the major dimension between 30% and 70% of its length. The dashed line in the figure represents the breakup position on the crystal

$$- \underbrace{S(x_1, x_2, t)\, n(x_1, x_2, t)}_{\text{death of crystal particles with dimensions } (x_1, x_2)} \tag{25}$$

where $n(x_1, x_2, t)$ is the number density function, $S(x_1, x_2, t)$ is the bivariate breakage selection function, and $b(x_1, x_2 | y_1, y_2)$ is the breakage distribution function, respectively. To develop the population balance model accurately, we have to formulate the two kernel functions $S(x_1, x_2, t)$ and $b(x_1, x_2 | y_1, y_2)$.

The bivariate linear breakage selection function $S(x_1, x_2, t)$ defines the rate of successful stressing events, i.e., those events where crystals break due to the implosion of cavitation bubbles. To model the bivariate linear breakage selection function $S(x_1, x_2, t)$, Das et al. [19] proposed the following partition as

$$S(x_1, x_2, t) = S^*(x_1, x_2)\, S_0(t)\, \psi(x_1, x_2, t) \tag{26}$$

Then, performing similar calculations as the monovariate linear breakage process, one can get the following expressions [19]:

$$S_0(t) = \frac{f_{ev,tot}}{\displaystyle\int_0^\infty \int_0^\infty S^*(x_1, x_2)\, n(x_1, x_2, t)\, dx_1\, dx_2} \tag{27}$$

and

$$S(x_1, x_2, t) = f_{ev,tot} \frac{S^*(x_1, x_2)\, \psi(x_1, x_2, t)}{\displaystyle\int_0^\infty \int_0^\infty S^*(x_1, x_2)\, n(x_1, x_2, t)\, dx_1\, dx_2} \tag{28}$$

The breakage distribution function $b(x_1, x_2 | y_1, y_2)$ defines the rate of formation of crystals with dimensions (x_1, x_2) by breakage of crystals with dimension (y_1, y_2). The breakage distribution function satisfies the following properties:

1.

$$\int_0^{y_1} \int_0^{y_2} b(x_1, x_2 | y_1, y_2)\, dx_1\, dx_2 = v(y_1, y_2) \tag{29}$$

where $v(y_1, y_2)$ is the number of smaller fragments created due to the breakage of a crystal with dimensions (y_1, y_2).

2. Since the breakage of the rectangular crystals conserves total area, we have

$$\int_0^{y_1} \int_0^{y_2} x_1\, x_2\, b(x_1, x_2 | y_1, y_2)\, dx_1\, dx_2 = y_1\, y_2 \tag{30}$$

In addition to this, from the experimental observations and MC simulation results, we know that the crystals break across the width into two smaller fragments and the fracture mechanism starts at any random point in the confined region (30%, 70%)

along the length of the crystals (see Fig. 8). Das et al. [19] proposed the following model for the breakage distribution function which follows the abovementioned constraints as

$$
\begin{aligned}
b(x_1, x_2 | y_1, y_2) &= \left[\frac{2}{0.4 y_1} \{ H(x_1 - 0.3 y_1) - H(x_1 - 0.7 y_1) \} \right] \\
&\quad \times \delta(x_2 - y_2) H(y_1 - y_2) \\
&\quad + \left[\frac{2}{0.4 y_2} \{ H(x_2 - 0.3 y_2) - H(x_2 - 0.7 y_2) \} \right] \\
&\quad \times \delta(x_1 - y_1) H(y_2 - y_1) \\
&= \frac{2}{0.4 y_1 y_2} \left[y_1 \delta(x_1 - y_1) H(y_2 - y_1) \right. \\
&\quad \times \{ H(x_2 - 0.3 y_2) - H(x_2 - 0.7 y_2) \} \\
&\quad \left. + y_2 \delta(x_2 - y_2) H(y_1 - y_2) \{ H(x_1 - 0.3 y_1) - H(x_1 - 0.7 y_1) \} \right]
\end{aligned}
$$

$$(31)$$

where δ and H are the Kronecker delta function and Heaviside step function, respectively. In formulation (31), the terms $H(y_1 - y_2)$ and $H(y_2 - y_1)$ help to determine the major dimension (length) of the breaking crystal, and the terms $\delta(x_1 - y_1)$ and $\delta(x_2 - y_2)$ help to keep the length of the minor dimensions (width) intact in the progeny crystal particles. Further, the terms $\{ H(x - 0.3 y) - H(x - 0.7 y) \}$ make sure that the breakup region is the restricted interval $(0.3 y, 0.7 y)$. One can easily verify the correctness of the formulation (31) by satisfying the fundamental properties of any breakage distribution function, i.e., Eqs. (29) and (30). The detailed development of this model is available in Das et al. [19].

Validation of the Model

In this section, we will validate the accuracy and efficiency of the developed models of bivariate breakage selection function (Eq. (28)) and bivariate breakage distribution function (Eq. (31)). The bivariate breakage PBE was solved numerically using the weighted finite volume scheme of Saha et al. [14]. Then, the numerical results were compared against the experimental observations and MC simulation results. The experiments were conducted for a fixed ultrasonic amplitude value (30%), and the sonication period was varied for 30, 60, and 90 s. The initial crystal length and width distributions are depicted in Fig. 7. The following expressions were used while solving the PBE:

$$
S^*(x_1, x_2) = x_1 x_2, \tag{32}
$$

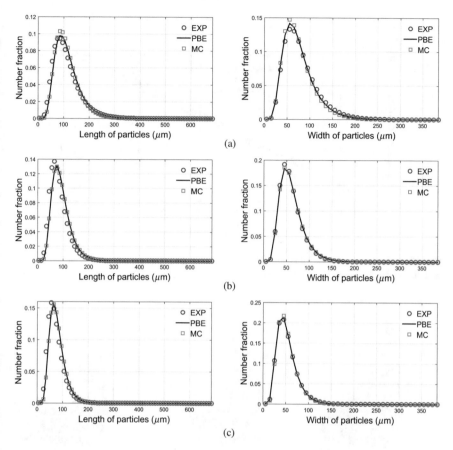

Fig. 9 Comparison of PBE, MC, and experimental results along length and width axes at time (**a**) 30 s, (**b**) 60 s, and (**c**) 90 s. Ultrasonic amplitude of this experiment is set at 30%

$$\text{and} \quad \psi(x_1, x_2, t) = \begin{cases} 1 & \text{if } max(x_1, x_2) \geq 20 \, \mu m, \\ 0 & \text{elsewhere} \end{cases} \tag{33}$$

The comparisons of crystal length and width distributions obtained from solving the PBE, MC simulations, and experimental observations at instances 30, 60, and 90 s are illustrated in Fig. 9. From the figures, it is clear that the PBM results predicted both the experimental results and MC simulation results satisfactorily at all instances. From the figures, it is clear that the average length and width of crystal particles are reducing gradually, and the span of the distributions are getting narrower with higher peak values with increase in sonication time.

The time evolution of the total number of crystal particles in the system was not observed in the experimental setup. However, the time evolution of total number of particles was tracked from solving the PBE and from MC simulations, and the

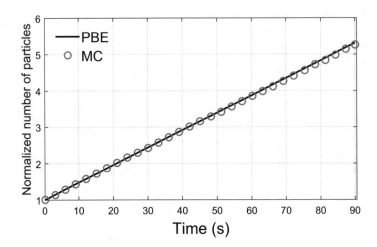

Fig. 10 Comparison of the PBM and MC generated time evolution of normalized number of particles in the system when the ultrasonic amplitude is set at 30 AMP

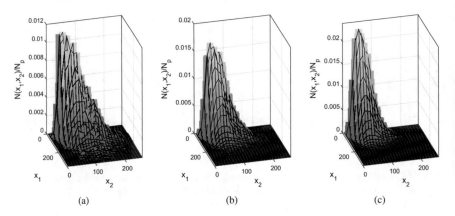

Fig. 11 Population balance model generated crystal size distribution (CSD) of the 30 AMP experimental system at instances (**a**) 30 s, (**b**) 60 s, and (**c**) 90 s

obtained results are illustrated in Fig. 10, which showed meticulous agreement between MC and PBE predictions.

Furthermore, to predict the outcome of the sonofragmentation process in a more accurate manner, crystal size distribution (CSD) of the system was computed by solving the breakage PBE using the developed model of bivariate selection function and breakage distribution function. The computed CSD of the system at instances 30, 60, and 90 s is illustrated in Fig. 11. The time evolution of the crystal size distribution clearly shows how the particles are broken to finer dimensions with increasing sonication time and distribution evolves toward a narrower size distribution.

Table 2 Comparison of the computational efficiency

Sonication time (s)	MC simulation time (s)	PBM simulation time (s)
30	53.98	2.98
60	80.55	3.66
90	138.40	7.65

Furthermore, to check the efficiency of the developed PBM, computation times was calculated for both PBM and MC simulations. The comparison of the computational times is provided in Table 2. From the table, it is clear that the PBM technique is computationally very efficient than the MC simulation technique. In fact, for all the three cases, the PBM simulation time was only 5% (at most) of the MC simulation time.

4 Conclusion

This chapter discusses the development and verification of some breakage PBE kernels, which are dependent on particle dimensions and process time simultaneously. Mathematical models of the volume and time-dependent linear breakage selection function and binary collisional breakage kernel were presented. Furthermore, a comprehensive population balance model of the ultrasound assisted sonofragmentation experiments was developed, which includes the modeling of bivariate breakage selection function, and breakage distribution functions were discussed.

On the other hand, constant number MC simulation algorithms were developed to verify the accuracy of the developed PBMs. The MC simulations verified the accuracy of the developed models (linear breakage selection function and nonlinear collisional breakage kernel). In case of sonofragmentation experiments, MC simulations were first used to understand the breakage mechanism correctly, i.e., by fixing the frequency of stressing events and by fixing the breakup region. Consequently, the developed bivariate PBM and MC simulation results predicted the experimental observations meticulously. Also, it was shown that the population balance modeling techniques are computationally very efficient compared to MC simulations. In conclusion, this chapter promotes the use of population balance equations and the Monte Carlo method to model different breakage processes accurately.

References

1. D. Ramkrishna, Population balances: Theory and applications to particulate systems in engineering, Academic Press, 2000.
2. J. Kumar, G. Warnecke, Convergence analysis of sectional methods for solving breakage population balance equations-II: The cell average technique, Numerische Mathematik 110 (2008) 539–559.

3. M. Kostoglou, A. Karabelas, On sectional techniques for the solution of the breakage equation, Computers & Chemical Engineering 33 (2009) 112–121.
4. J. Kumar, M. Peglow, G. Warnecke, S. Heinrich, L. Mörl, Improved accuracy and convergence of discretized population balance for aggregation: The cell average technique, Chemical Engineering Science 61 (2006) 3327–3342.
5. J. Kumar, M. Peglow, G. Warnecke, S. Heinrich, The cell average technique for solving multi-dimensional aggregation population balance equations, Computers & Chemical Engineering 32 (2008) 1810–1830.
6. C. A. Dorao, H. A. Jakobsen, Numerical calculation of the moments of the population balance equation, Journal of Computational and Applied Mathematics 196 (2006) 619–633.
7. R. Fan, D. L. Marchisio, R. O. Fox, Application of the direct quadrature method of moments to polydisperse gas–solid fluidized beds, Powder Technology 139 (2004) 7–20.
8. S. Rigopoulos, A. G. Jones, Finite-element scheme for solution of the dynamic population balance equation, AIChE Journal 49 (2003) 1127–1139.
9. M. Nicmanis, M. Hounslow, A finite element analysis of the steady state population balance equation for particulate systems: Aggregation and growth, Computers & chemical engineering 20 (1996) S261–S266.
10. V. John, T. Mitkova, M. Roland, K. Sundmacher, L. Tobiska, A. Voigt, Simulations of population balance systems with one internal coordinate using finite element methods, Chemical Engineering Science 64 (2009) 733–741.
11. J. Saha, J. Kumar, A. Bück, E. Tsotsas, Finite volume approximations of breakage population balance equation, Chemical Engineering Research and Design 110 (2016) 114–122.
12. R. Kumar, J. Kumar, Numerical simulation and convergence analysis of a finite volume scheme for solving general breakage population balance equations, Applied Mathematics and Computation 219 (2013) 5140–5151.
13. J. Kumar, J. Saha, E. Tsotsas, Development and convergence analysis of a finite volume scheme for solving breakage equation, SIAM Journal on Numerical Analysis 53 (2015) 1672–1689.
14. J. Saha, N. Das, J. Kumar, A. Bück, Numerical solutions for multidimensional fragmentation problems using finite volume methods, Kinetic Related Models 12 (2018) 79.
15. M. Smith, T. Matsoukas, Constant-number Monte Carlo simulation of population balances, Chemical Engineering Science 53 (1998) 1777–1786.
16. K. Lee, T. Matsoukas, Simultaneous coagulation and break-up using constant-N Monte Carlo, Powder Technology 110 (2000) 82–89.
17. Y. Lin, K. Lee, T. Matsoukas, Solution of the population balance equation using constant-number Monte Carlo, Chemical Engineering Science 57 (2002) 2241–2252.
18. A. Das, A. Bück, J. Kumar, Selection function in breakage processes: PBM and Monte Carlo modeling, Advanced Powder Technology 31 (2020) 1457–1469.
19. A. Das, S. Bhoi, D. Sarkar, J. Kumar, Sonofragmentation of rectangular plate-like crystals: Bivariate population balance modeling and experimental validation, Crystal Growth & Design 20 (2020) 5424–5434.
20. A. Das, J. Kumar, M. Dosta, S. Heinrich, On the approximate solution and modeling of the kernel of nonlinear breakage population balance equation, SIAM Journal on Scientific Computing 42 (2020) B1570–B1598.
21. K. Terrazas-Velarde, M. Peglow, E. Tsotsas, Stochastic simulation of agglomerate formation in fluidized bed spray drying: A micro-scale approach, Chemical Engineering Science 64 (2009) 2631–2643.
22. K. Terrazas-Velarde, M. Peglow, E. Tsotsas, Investigation of the kinetics of fluidized bed spray agglomeration based on stochastic methods, AIChE Journal 57 (2011) 3012–3026.
23. K. Terrazas-Velarde, M. Peglow, E. Tsotsas, Kinetics of fluidized bed spray agglomeration for compact and porous particles, Chemical Engineering Science 66 (2011) 1866–1878.
24. M. Dernedde, M. Peglow, E. Tsotsas, A novel, structure-tracking Monte Carlo algorithm for spray fluidized bed agglomeration, AIChE Journal 58 (2012) 3016–3029.
25. M. Dernedde, M. Peglow, E. Tsotsas, Stochastic modeling of fluidized bed agglomeration: Determination of particle moisture content, Drying Technology 31 (2013) 1764–1771.

26. S. Bhoi, A. Das, J. Kumar, D. Sarkar, Sonofragmentation of two-dimensional plate-like crystals: Experiments and Monte Carlo simulations, Chemical Engineering Science 203 (2019) 12–27.
27. A. K. Singh, E. Tsotsas, Stochastic model to simulate spray fluidized bed agglomeration: a morphological approach, Powder Technology 355 (2019) 449–460.
28. A. K. Singh, E. Tsotsas, A tunable aggregation model incorporated in Monte Carlo simulations of spray fluidized bed agglomeration, Powder Technology 364 (2020) 417–428.
29. A. Das, S. Dutta, M. Sen, A. Saxena, J. Kumar, L. Giri, D. W. Murhammer, J. Chakraborty, A detailed model and Monte Carlo simulation for predicting DIP genome length distribution in baculovirus infection of insect cells, Biotechnology and Bioengineering 118 (2021) 238–252.
30. N. Metropolis, S. Ulam, The Monte Carlo method, Journal of the American Statistical Association 44 (1949) 335–341.
31. H. Zhao, A. Maisels, T. Matsoukas, C. Zheng, Analysis of four Monte Carlo methods for the solution of population balances in dispersed systems, Powder Technology 173 (2007) 38–50.
32. A. Das, J. Kumar, Population balance modeling of volume and time dependent spray fluidized bed aggregation kernel using Monte Carlo simulation results, Applied Mathematical Modelling 92 (2021) 748–769.
33. Y. Tang, T. Matsoukas, A new Monte Carlo methods for simulations of agglomeration and grinding, Fine Powder Processing Technology, Penn State Materials Research Lab, Plenum (1997) 243.
34. H. Liu, M. Li, Population balance modelling and multi-stage optimal control of a pulsed spray fluidized bed granulation, International Journal of Pharmaceutics 468 (2014) 223–233.
35. A. Ding, M. Hounslow, C. Biggs, Population balance modelling of activated sludge flocculation: Investigating the size dependence of aggregation, breakage and collision efficiency, Chemical Engineering Science 61 (2006) 63–74.
36. Z. Cheng, S. Redner, Scaling theory of fragmentation, Physical Review Letters 60 (1988) 2450–2453.

Optimization of Tablet Coating

Preksha Vinchhi and Mayur M. Patel

Abbreviations

API	Active pharmaceutical ingredient
CFD	Computational fluid dynamics
CMAs	Critical material attributes
CMH	Cubic metres per hour
CPPs	Critical processing parameters
CQAs	Critical quality attributes
DEM	Discrete element modelling
DOE	Design of experiment
GPU	Graphical processor unit
HPMC	Hydroxy propyl methylcellulose
NIR	Near-infrared spectroscopy
PAT	Process analytical technology
PQRI	Product quality research institute
QBD	Quality by design
QTPP	Quality target product profile

1 Introduction

1.1 History

Since many centuries, the coating of pharmaceutical formulations has been practised. Late back in the ninth to eleventh century A.D., the first reports related to this topic were affirmed. In the famous book *Al Qanun*, the author 'Avicenna' reported

P. Vinchhi · M. M. Patel (✉)
Department of Pharmaceutics, Institute of Pharmacy, Nirma University, Ahmedabad, India

© The Author(s), under exclusive license to Springer Nature Switzerland AG 2022
A. Fytopoulos et al. (eds.), *Optimization of Pharmaceutical Processes*, Springer
Optimization and Its Applications 189, https://doi.org/10.1007/978-3-030-90924-6_5

coating of pills using silver. Earlier, amongst various solid dosage forms, pills were the primary solid dosage form widely used. Diverse materials were employed to coat the pills, for instance, sugar, honey, talc, gelatin, silver, gold, etc. The primary purpose of pill coating in those days was to mask the unpleasant odour and taste of active pharmaceutical ingredients (APIs). Initially, the coating process was conducted in copper pans hanging by two chains above the fire. In 1840, the first hand-operated coating pan was represented, and in 1844 a patent for the spherical pan was approved [1]. In the nineteenth century, the modern pharmaceutical coating began with sugar coating with the main purpose of increasing the palatability of bitter medicines. However, the sugar coating requires longer processing time, requires a high level of operator expertise, has a possibility of microbial growth in a sugar solution, and has a lack of automation in the process. Thus, alternative coating methods were developed to overcome issues pertaining to sugar-coated tablets. In 1930, noteworthy efforts in tablet coating were done in which polymer films were proposed as an option for substrate coating. Thereafter, in 1954, the first film-coated tablets were introduced into the market by Abbott Laboratories. The film-coated tablets were preferred more than sugar-coated owing to the benefit of a less complex manufacturing process requiring lesser time, cost and labour.

1.2 Definition and Scope

Coating is a widely employed unit operation involved in the manufacturing of solid dosage forms. The procedure by which a solid dry film of coating composition gets smeared over the exterior of desired dosage forms (tablets, pellets or granules) is referred to as coating. The coating composition may involve plasticizer, flavouring and colouring material, polyhydric alcohol, wax, fillers, sugar, resins and gums. In modern pharmaceutical coating, polymers and polysaccharides are principal coaters along with plasticizers and pigments. During the coating process, several precautions should be considered, as coating should be unwavering and sturdy. Avoiding the use of organic solvents is also preferred by ICH guidelines to improve the product safety profile. Film coating (aqueous and non-aqueous) and sugar coating are the two main categories of tablet coating. The tablets that are prone to moisture degradation or oxidation are film-coated in order to increase their shelf life and make them more swallowable by imparting them a smooth finish. Although the step of coating adds up cost and time to the manufacturing of solid dosage forms, it is still highly favoured as it bestows numerous advantages.

1.3 Significance of Coating

Tablet coating is usually intended to mask unpleasant odour or taste, produce an elegant product, increase stability against moisture and light or modify drug release profiles. The drug's shelf life increases by coating as protection from environmental effects such as humidity, light, oxygen, etc. is achieved. Also, the coating acts as an important aspect for high-speed packaging as it reduces the friction between tablets and packaging material. The dust generation from the tablets also reduces due to coating that helps to protect the workers against exposure to harmful drugs while tablet processing. The identification of the tablets also gets easier for the patients as well as healthcare providers due to coating. Tablet coating allows the marketed product a brand identity as well as enhances its aesthetic appeal. A suitable surface for printing is created by coating. Tablet coating is an extensively employed strategy that is regularly selected to control the dissolution rate of the drug in the gastrointestinal tract. The site-specific drug release in the body can also be achieved by coating, for example, enteric coating facilitates drug release in the intestine. Also, the drug release rate can be controlled by coating, for instance, sustained or delayed drug release. Sequential drug release can also be achieved by coating [2].

1.4   Optimization of Tablet Coating

The recent regulatory initiatives outlined in various guidelines, such as ICHQ8, ICHQ9 and ICHQ10, require the science and risk-based manufacturing of product and processes built on 'quality by design' (QBD) principles and process analytical technologies (PAT). The application of QBD approaches is done to enhance the knowledge of product performance influenced by the manufacturing process technique, processing parameters and material attributes. The foremost step for optimizing the coated product is by employing QBD principles in establishing quality target product profile (QTPP) for both the core tablet and coated tablet. Thereafter, the determination of critical quality attributes (CQAs) of both core tablet and coated tablet is done. Furthermore, the critical processing parameters (CPPs) and critical material attributes (CMAs) are identified by risk assessment. Implementation of design of experiments (DOEs) is done to establish the design space of CPPs for the tablet coating procedure. The risk assessment is done on the basis of basic principles, historic knowledge and the data generated from initial experiments. After establishing sufficient understanding of the coating process, identification of design space for CPPs can be conducted by establishing small DOEs for optimizing the process. After optimizing the coating process by applying appropriate modelling strategies and data analysis, the generated information helps to enable real-time processing decisions and processing controls by employing PAT tools for ensuring the manufacturing of consistent product quality. The chapter provides information regarding various tablet coating techniques commonly employed in pharmaceutical industries, types of equipment used in tablet coating, the impact of various material and processing attributes on those techniques, novel tablet coating techniques and PAT tools employed for tablet coating optimization.

2 Tablet Coating Techniques

2.1 Sugar Coating

Originally, tablet coating was developed to mask the bitter taste using sugar and to offer an alluring appearance at the core. Despite increased interest in film coating since 1950, the pharmaceutical technique of sugar coating has been widely performed. Various advantages of sugar coating technique are as follows, (a) It is a simplified technique, (b) It is an extensively accepted technique, (c) It involves use of inexpensive and readily available material, (d) Reworking processes are feasible. The steps involved in sugar-coating technique are explained in Table 1. Though sugar coating provides an elegant and aesthetically delighting coat of even colouration and high gloss, the process also has some drawbacks. The technique is lengthy and also requires proper operator skills. The increase in tablet weight is at least 30–50% which leads to a significant increase in tablet size. Also, on sugar-coated tablets, intangliations cannot be made; thus, there is a need to

Table 1 Steps involved in sugar coating

Steps involved	Description
1. Seal coating	As sugar coating permits water to directly penetrate into the substrate which can affect the product stability and also lead to early tablet disintegration. The aim of seal coating is to provide preliminary protection to the substrate and avert the movement of ingredients of the substrate to the coating layer. Water-resistant material such as zein, cellulose acetate phthalate, polyvinyl acetate phthalate and pharmaceutical shellac is sprayed in alcoholic form to obtain waterproof coat
2. Subcoating	It offers curving of tablet edges and also increases the tablet weight. The subcoating formulation comprises of high quantity of fillers like talc, calcium carbonate, titanium dioxide and kaolin. For improving the structural integrity, the auxiliary film formers like gelatin, acacia and cellulose derivatives can also be incorporated. A rise in weight up to 50–100% occurs after this step. Typically, two key approaches for performing subcoating are suspension subcoating method and lamination method
3. Syrup coating	This step is also known as smoothing or grossing. For formulating a good-quality sugar-coated product, it is essential to make the surface of the substrate smooth before colour coating. To conceal the irregularities on the tablet surface, this step is performed by applying 70% sucrose syrup comprising of titanium dioxide as a whitening agent or opacifier
4. Colour coating	Colour coating is an imperative step as it has a significant visual impact. The desired colour is obtained by adding various colourants either by dissolving them in coating syrup (water-soluble dye) or by dispersing them in coating syrup (water-insoluble pigments)
5. Polishing	To achieve glossy, smoothly finished tablets, this step is done. Various types of polishing systems involve alcoholic slurries wax, waxes in organic solution and dry waxes in a powdered state. It is essential to polish the sugar-coated tablets as they are dull when formulated

print identification marks or logos. Moreover, longer coating time, difficulty in automation and troubles in process standardization have led to the development of improved coating technique [3].

2.2 Film Coating

As sugar-coating technique is very lengthy and dependent on coating operator skills, it is being replaced by film coating technique. Currently, it is the most extensively employed coating method. It allows engraving of logos or any other type of identification on the core of the tablet with intangliations staying readable after coating. Also, the weight gain after the film coating is much lesser compared to sugar coating. For the preparation of controlled release products, the film coating technique is substantially faster and easily adaptable. The film coating process includes spraying of a solution comprising of polymer, plasticizer and pigments on a rotating tablet bed which leads to the formation of a uniform, thin film on the surface of the tablet. The atomized liquid impinges on the substrate's surface, and the film formation takes place as the solvent evaporates. The mechanism of film formation on a substrate is represented in Fig. 1. However, with aqueous dispersions, the film formation is difficult as the polymer spheres dispersed on the substrate must also coalesce. In such cases, to promote the film formation and polymer coalescence, the substrate is stored at elevated temperatures post coating. The duration required for the formation of a proper coalesced film is dependent on numerous variables involving the processing conditions as well as formulation variables [4]. The ideal material for film coating should have the characteristics such as the following: (a) It should produce an elegant coat; (b) it should remain stable in the presence of light, moisture or heat; (c) it must have good solubility in the desired solvent; (d) it must be pharmacologically inert and non-toxic; (e) it should not produce disagreeable taste, odour or colour; and (f) it should be compatible with other coating additives. The polymer selection depends on the desired drug release rate or desired drug release site, i.e. stomach or intestine. Hydroxypropyl methylcellulose (HPMC), povidone, ethylcellulose, methyl hydroxyethylcellulose, etc. are examples of widely used coating polymers. HPMC phthalate, cellulose acetate phthalate and acrylate polymers (Eudragit S and Eudragit L) are the widely employed enteric coating polymers [5].

Types of Film Coating

The film coating can be categorized into two types, viz. organic film coating and aqueous film coating. When the polymer utilized for coating is water-insoluble, usually organic solvent is used to prepare the coating solution. A mixture of water-insoluble polymers, pigments and excipients is solubilized in an organic solvent and then sprayed on the substrate and subsequently dried by providing heat to form a

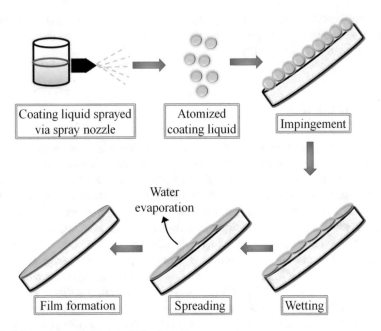

Fig. 1 Schematic representation of film formation mechanism

film on the substrate. Majority of the polymers are soluble in organic solvents so they provide a wide range of polymer alternatives for organic film coating. Employing organic solvents for the coating process reduces the hydrolytic degradation of drug moiety. Also, the use of hydrophobic polymers is advantageous as they provide moisture-protective coating and in turn reduce the water vapour permeability of film. Thus, for moisture-sensitive drug moieties, organic film coating is highly beneficial. However, despite the pharmaceutical requirements, organic film coating has several limitations owing to the issues of flammability, the toxicity of residual solvents and environmental safety concerns. Despite proper ventilation facility in the room, the complete removal of organic solvent vapours is difficult which increases the risk of explosion and toxicity. The production costs increase due to regulatory and environmental issues. Thus, the pharmaceutical industries are focusing more on aqueous film coating. Aqueous film coating provides several advantages over organic film coating in the context of environmental pollution, operation safety and risk of explosion. The aqueous film coating initially requires upgradation in the coating facility owing to the requirement of higher drying capacity as the latent heat of water (2200 kJ) is much higher compared to organic solvents (e.g. methylene chloride latent heat is 550 kJ). Thus, almost four times more energy is required for drying in aqueous film coating compared to organic film coating [5]. Also, in case of preparing aqueous coating solution for water-insoluble polymers, plasticizer or a suitable suspending agent needs to be added for obtaining a homogeneous coating solution. Nevertheless, aqueous film coating is still widely preferred in pharmaceutical industries as it can circumvent the safety issues that are associated with organic film coating [6].

3 Methods for Coating Tablets

Pan coating and fluidized bed coating are the basic techniques extensively employed for applying coating material on substrates. The chapter entails details regarding pan coating and fluidized bed coating process along with factors affecting the process and its optimization.

3.1 Pan Coating

The pan coating is the oldest pharmaceutical coating technique widely used since many years for manufacturing coated tablets, pellets or granules. The key advantage of pan coaters is that they offer relatively less mechanical stress to the core substrate and also ascertain the desired motion of the substrate bed during the coating process. In a conventional pan coater, the tablets are placed in a rotating pan. The coating solution is introduced via an air atomizing spray nozzle. With the rotation of the pan, the tablets' top layers cascade down due to gravitational force which provides another layer of tablets to get coated and dried before entering the tablet bed bulk. Within defined time known as circulation time, the tablets arrive in the spray zone which leads to repetition of coating and drying process. The process of coating in a pan coater is represented in Fig. 2. In pan coating process the tablets movement should occur uniformly via the spraying zone. However, sometimes the tablets enter slow-moving or stagnant regions of the bed which leads to its reduced circulation through the spray zone. Based on pan designs, they can be categorized as standard coating pans (having solid walls) and perforated pans (fully or partially perforated). While based on the kind of process, the pans can be categorized as continuous coating pan or batch process coating pan.

(i) Standard Coating Pan

The standard coating pans also known as conventional coating pans are widely used in pharmaceutical industries. The pan coaters can be categorized based on their rotating axis, i.e. on an inclined axis or horizontal axis. In coater spinning on an inclined axis, the substrate is tumbled in a conventional coating pan which is spinning on an inclined axis. Owing to the inclination, two fundamental motions are superimposed: (a) centrifugal movement on the vertical axis and (b) tumbling movement on the horizontal axis. The coating solution is sprayed on the substrate through a spraying nozzle. Moreover, hot air is blown through the coater that helps in the drying of the coat. At certain time intervals, the substrate enters the spray zone and then cascades down and merges to the

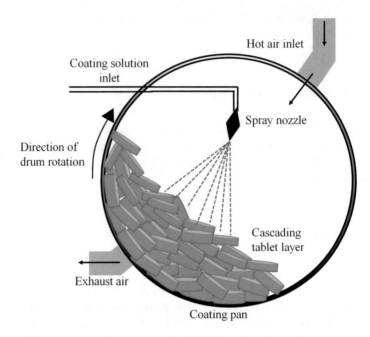

Fig. 2 Schematic representation of pan coating process

core bulk by which the coating and drying process keeps on repeating. However, the inclined axis rotation leads to two disadvantages: (a) inadequate transport of air that leads to improper drying and (b) inefficient movement of particle that results in dead zones which in turn impairs the homogeneous mixing efficiency. For increasing the average contact area between the drying air and the core bed, horizontal rotating pans were developed. In the case of coater rotating on the horizontal axis, the core bed undergoes tumbling motion that results in a reduction of required drying time and provides increased pan volume. However, further refinement was still required for improving the drying efficiency as well as the particle flow. For improving the particle movement in the pan, baffles and blades were introduced in the pan. In 1965, Keil invented single baffle coating pan. Thereafter, Pellegrini invented horizontal axis coating pan with an integral baffle and tapered sidewalls. The sidewalls add an additional lateral movement that increases the particle movement efficiency. The drying air derives the energy essential for moisture evaporation from the coating layers. Therefore, heat and mass transfer efficiency has a significant impact on product quality. The drying efficiency can be improved by increasing mass and heat transfer either by rising rotation speed and temperature or by enhancing the drying air supply. In the conventional drying method, the drying air blows only across the core surface which leads to improper drying of the core materials. This led to the development of different drying gadgets such as immersion sword and immersion tube [1].

(ii) Perforated Coating Pan

Perforated pans are mainly divided into two types: partially perforated pans and fully perforated pans. The coating system contains process airflow controllers and spray nozzles along with a perforated drum placed horizontally. The perforated pan coating unit provides an efficient drying capacity compared to the conventional pans. Utilizing blades and baffles increases friction between pans and the core material that results in a high amount of dust production during coating. Thus, inventors concentrated on the application of perforated pans to enhance air transport to the core material and subsequently upsurge the drying and mixing efficiency. Hostetler developed a side-vented pan in which the peripheral wall was modified with perforations, and at the lower peripheral region, an air supplying inlet was positioned. The modification was intended to enlarge the contact area of the substrate with the coating solution and increase air transfer and core movement [1]. Glatt coater, Hi-coater system, Dria coater pan and Accela Cota system are the main types of perforated coating systems.

The underlying principle of the pan coating process is complex which makes the prediction of the performance of a coated product quite difficult. For achieving desirable coating, several aspects need to be considered such as tablet properties, formulation components of tablets, coating formulation and processing conditions during coating. A proper balance needs to be established between the spray rate of the coating material and the thermodynamic drying settings (temperature, humidity and airflow). Combined determination of liquid flow rate and drying conditions leads to adequate solvent evaporation and helps to obtain aesthetically acceptable and uniform coat. The coating factors affecting the pan coating can be broadly classified as pan coater factors, spraying system factors, thermodynamic factors, coating formulation factors and substrate/core factors [7]. The classification of factors affecting the coating process in a pan coater is represented in Fig. 3.

Coating Formulation Factors

The coating formulation factors affecting the pan coating process are the type of excipient, solvent volatility, solid content, surface tension and viscosity of solution/suspension. The solid content in the coating solution should be higher to lessen the coating time. However, very high solid content also results in a highly viscous coating solution which can cause issues in the coating process. Moreover, with higher solid content, the surface of the film coat might also get affected if the drying conditions or the spray droplet are not adjusted adequately. Conversely, low solid content in coating solution leads to the increased relative humidity in the coating pan that results in poor drying efficiency. The droplet characteristics from the spray gun get affected by the viscosity of the formulation and the changes in solid content; thus, to optimize the spray gun parameters, the solid content needs to be studied. There is a strong interdependency between formulation factors

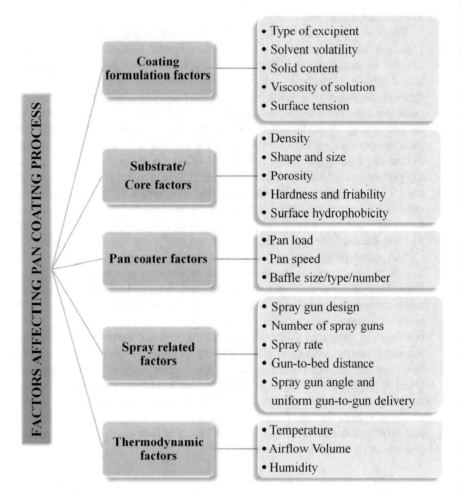

Fig. 3 Factors affecting coating process in a pan coater

and coating process parameters; the DOE approach can be implemented to study the effect of the coating process variable and formulation variables together [8]. Through experiments, the CMAs are recognized, and after the ideal formulation characteristics are established, they can be kept constant.

Core/Substrate Factors

The substrate aspects such as density, size, shape, friability, hardness, porosity, surface hydrophobicity and surface roughness can influence the film coating procedure. The mixing dynamics and ease of coating inside the pan can be affected by the size and shape of the substrate. The coating of a small round-shaped tablet is simpler compared to oval- or oblong-shaped tablets [9]. In the case of odd-shaped substrates, high coating levels are required to ensure the covering of edges properly and achieve uniform coating and desired release. There is a requirement of longer coating runs for tablet surface coverage of odd-shaped substrates [10]. Moreover, to prevent erosion or chipping of tablets during the coating process, the tablet strength parameters such as hardness and friability need to be established. To tolerate the stress throughout the pan coating process, the tablets having adequate strength must be selected. For establishing the tablet strength, measurement of only tablet hardness can be deceptive as it is a measurement based on geometry of the tablet alone. Measurements of parameters such as Young's modulus, tensile strength of tablet and tablet fracture energy are more accurate measurement parameters than the present USP hardness measurement. Tablets having tensile strength ≥ 1 MPa and 15% porosity have desired hardness that can endure several types of pressures underwent by a substrate during the pan coating process. The tablet density, porosity, surface roughness and hydrophobicity influence the film adherence on the tablet surface and the ease of applicability. Selection of the coating solution composition should be done on the basis of tablet surface characteristics. While conducting the coating operation, some of the substrate factors which are the CQAs for the film coating quality should be identified and kept constant.

Pan Coater Factors

Pan Load

Estimation of the batch size is essential when a particular product is to be coated for the first time. The coating pans usually have a definite brim volume capacity. The brim volume is the volume capacity of the pan if loaded to the very bottom of the pan opening. The acceptable operating range for film coating is using a fill volume of 50–95% of the brim volume. A batch size towards higher brim volume range helps to maximize the batch throughput and also enhances the drying capacity as the issue of bypass of inlet air directly to the exhaust plenum is circumvented. The higher batch size aids proper drying as the inlet air passes through the tablet bed in a proper manner. In the case of an underloaded pan, the pan walls and baffles get directly exposed to the spray which leads to a build-up of coating material on these exposed surfaces and sticking of the substrate on them. However, occasionally after for some of the products which undergo high weight gain or change in product movement after coating may demonstrate issues with the acceptable pan load decided initially. Thus, to optimize the pan load is necessary [11].

Pan Speed

For optimizing the coating quality, the mixing of the tablets should be such that each tablet goes under the spray zone for the equal time duration. If there is an issue in tablet mixing, then the first parameter to be evaluated is pan speed. Ideally, the lowest pan speed providing a continuous product flow via the spray zone should be selected. Selecting such speed will keep minimum attrition between the tablets and also allow the uniform application of the film coat. The product mixing can be evaluated by recording the number of tablet pass via spray zone per unit time by using radioactively marked tablets and a counter attached on the spray bar. Also, tablets of different colours can be used to perform the mixing studies. After placing different colour tablets in different zones, the impact of tablet speed can be evaluated by taking tablet samples at set time intervals. After determining the pan speed, the scale-up can be done by duplicating the peripheral edge speed. By multiplying the small pan speed with the ratio of the small pan to large pan diameter, the scale-up can be done.

Baffle Size/Number/Type

The key function of baffles is to move the substrate between the front and back of the pan during the coating process and enable uniform mixing. Usually, the coating pans are designed with a standard design baffle which works properly for major products. There is a requirement of different baffle designs for substrates of unusual sizes or shapes. When working with smaller batches, the use of reduced baffle size is necessary. If the standard baffles are used for small batch, then the product movement will be non-uniform, and the spray gun-to-bed distance will also vary. Whenever the fill volume is lesser than 75% of the brim volume, a small batch baffle usage is recommended.

Spray-Related Factors

Spray Gun Design

The most extensively employed spray gun design is a pneumatic spray gun. In pneumatic spray gun, the atomization takes place by impingement of compressed air stream on liquid stream after emerging from nozzle. The utilization of pneumatic spray guns permits the usage of variable spray rates. Previously, hydraulic spray guns were widely utilized, though they do not provide flexibility in spray rates. For changing the spray rate, an alteration in the fluid nozzle is often required. In some of the spray guns, the spray nozzle configuration and the air cap produce a programmed ratio of atomization to pattern air. In other guns, distinct controls are provided for controlling the pattern air and volume of atomization. This permits adjustment of air pattern or atomization without changing the solution nozzle or air cap. The droplet size of the spray gets controlled by the volume of atomization controls, and the spray width is controlled by the pattern air volume controls. The solution stream breaks into droplet size by atomization air, whereas the pattern air flattens the spray into a fan-shaped pattern.

Quantity of Spray Guns

An adequate quantity of spray guns is required to provide uniform exposure to the entire product bed. To achieve uniform coating, the spray zone must ideally involve the front to the back edge of the product bed. Adding a greater number of spray guns does not assure that an increased spray rate can be attained. The need for adding spray guns is justified only if the prevailing guns are inadequate to cover the entire tablet bed from front to back edge. The set-up of the spray guns must be such that wide spray patterns can be obtained without overlapping. If the spray pattern overlaps, then it can cause overwetting of the product bed [12].

Spray Rate

The spray rate is an imperative processing parameter that has a significant impact on the coating process thermodynamics. If the API or the formulation is sensitive or not very stable in high moisture conditions, then the spray rate is a very important aspect. The tablet bed environment and the rate of solvent evaporation are influenced by the spraying rate of the coating solution. While determining the spray rate, some of the factors such as spray pattern width, solution viscosity and product movement should be considered. The spray pattern width will be similar to the spray gun spacing if the spray pattern width is set up correctly. The spray rate per gun can be increased by choosing the broader spray pattern width (spray width that does not overlap the adjacent spray pattern). The solution viscosity affects droplet size distribution. Higher viscosity leads to decreased ability of spray gun to produce suitable droplet size distribution. Higher viscosity limits the highest spray rate that may be utilized. In the case of product movement, with the faster and more consistent the product movement, higher spray rate is achievable [13].

Gun-to-Bed Distance

The gun-to-bed distance is the total distance amongst the spray nozzle tip and the surface of the cascading bed of substrate. It can be defined as the distance covered by the spray droplets before striking the tablet surface. If the distance between gun and bed is very low, then it may lead to overwetting of the substrate which may result in tablet defects such as twinning and surface dissolution. Contrarily, if the gun-to-bed distance is very high, smaller droplets reach the substrate which may result in lesser processing proficiency and defects such as logo infilling and rough surface.

In a research work done by Pandey et al., various processing parameters were evaluated to investigate their impact on tablet logo bridging. It was concluded in the study that gun-to-bed distance and solid content in the suspension were the highly sensitive process parameters [14]. The typical gun-to-bed distance for production-sized coating pan is 20–25 cm. If the distance is higher than 25 cm, then, ideally, the inlet process temperature must be decreased so that excessive spray drying can be circumvented. On the contrary, if the distance is less than 20 cm, then the issue of shortened evaporation time can be resolved by increasing the inlet or product temperature reducing the spray rate.

Spray Gun Angle and Uniform Gun-to-Gun Solution Delivery

Preferably, the spray gun angle to the moving bed should be 90°, and the spray gun must be placed amidst the leading and trailing edges, i.e. middle of the substrate bed. The substrate may not get proper time to dry if the spray guns are placed too low on the substrate bed. Contrarily, if they are pointed more towards the leading edge of the substrate bed, there is a possibility that the spray gets smeared on the mixing baffles or the pan walls. Moreover, if the spray guns are not positioned at a 90° angle to the substrate bed, the spray solution might build up on the wings of the air cap while exiting from the solution nozzle. All the spray guns should supply an equal amount of coating solution so that uniformity in the coating can be achieved. The latest inclination in coating systems is towards employing a single pump assorted for several spray guns. It is mandatory for such systems that calibration should be executed on fixed intervals for ensuring that all the spray guns will deliver an equal amount of coating solution. It is highly preferred that the calibration should be performed with the coating solution itself rather than water as the viscosity of the coating solution will be significantly higher than that of water.

Thermodynamic Factors

The first law of thermodynamics is the fundamental law that influences the environment of the coating pan. The evaporation rate of coating solution from the surface of the substrate is governed by the thermodynamic factors such as moisture content/humidity, airflow volume and the temperature [15]. A change in any of above-mentioned parameter will affect the operating conditions downstream; thus, to sustain equilibrium throughout the coating process, modification in other processing parameters will be essential. For instance, if the spray rate is increased, the amount of moisture in the pan increases which leads to a decrease in drying capacity. Thus, on increasing the spray rate, to increase the drying capacity, factors such as temperature and airflow volume need to be adjusted. To evaluate the thermodynamic environment, parameters such as tablet bed temperature and relative humidity can be monitored, and the influence of drying or spraying factors can be understood. As changes in thermodynamic parameters often have a noteworthy effect on the coating quality, it is necessary to understand the relationship between coating process parameters and thermodynamic factors.

Temperature

The temperature control in the coating process can be achieved by controlling the exhaust, inlet or substrate/product temperature. Controlling the inlet air temperature is the extensively used process control parameter. The process control established on the product or exhaust temperature often occurs at a slower pace due to the heat sink effect of tablet bed. In inlet temperature control, there is a slight drop in exhaust temperature after the spray is started. The drop in temperature occurs as a result of evaporative cooling. All the product, exhaust and inlet temperatures are important as the drying of moisture content from the spray droplets occurs by both conduction (due to product temperature) and convection (due to process air). Several factors have a control on the desired exhaust temperature, for instance:

(a) Product temperature limits: The product must be kept under temperature boundaries if it displays instability issues at higher temperatures. It is very crucial to maintain this temperature limit during preheating of tablet bed as at that time evaporative cooling will not occur and if the pan is not constantly rotated, then the product may not achieve uniform heat. Also, after stopping the spray, the temperature of the product might increase immediately owing to the loss of the evaporative cooling effect. Thus, after the spray cycle gets completed, there might be a need to start a cool-down cycle immediately.
(b) Coating solution characteristics: If the coating gets tackier on drying, then the product or exhaust temperature must be increased to prevent overwetting defects.

Volume

The coating pans employ airflow along with elevated temperatures for evaporating the coating solvent on the tablets into vapour and transfer it away from the coated tablets. Usually, the quantity of water vapour that can be withdrawn is proportionate to the volume of air that passes via the coating pan. Thus, it would be beneficial to utilize high airflow to achieve maximum evaporative capacity. Ideally, the process air volume must be accustomed to the highest volume that can yield a nonturbulent laminar flow. A nonturbulent flow is desired as a turbulent airflow leads to distortion of the air pattern. The manufacturers generally mention the maximum airflow which produces an acceptable turbulence level. The capacity of the process air to hold water vapour increases by heating the air stream. Compared to exhaust air volume, the inlet air volume is a better marker of the evaporative capacity. This is because the inlet air is the air that passes via the tablet bed and then evaporates the coating solution from the tablets. Moreover, the exhaust air volume will usually be somewhat higher than that of inlet air volume owing to adding up of water vapour and atomizing air by the spray guns. The inlet air temperature must be as high as possible if the rate-limiting factor is maximum evaporative capacity. However, the spray rate is constrained by the spray zone size available and the number of spray guns, rather than evaporative capacities. Thus, between different-sized pans, the airflow capacity must be proportional directly to the spray zone. For instance, if a coating pan with two spray guns with 20-cm spray pattern airflow of 100 CMH (cubic metres per hour) is used, then in scale-up to a pan comprising of four spray guns, the airflow of 2000 CMH should be ideally employed.

Humidity

The process air utilized during the coating process is either unconditioned or conditioned. Day-to-day variations in moisture content exist in either type of air utilized in the air stream. The spray drying is highly affected by the moisture content present in the air stream. Thus, there is an emerging trend towards using the dehumidified air stream. Employing a dehumidified air stream not only provides steady coating conditions but also offers higher evaporative capacity. This provides an advantage of achieving higher moisture evaporation at a given temperature and airflow than a more humid airflow. The dew point temperature is a measure representing the moisture content of the air stream. A chilled mirror-type sensor and capacitance are used to measure the dew point temperatures. To maintain proper drying rate, the dew point should be maintained in a controlled range. Pandey et al. utilized PyroButton (data logging device) that records temperature and humidity of the tablets throughout the coating process via relating the end product quality characteristics such as chemical stability, bilayer tablet delamination when kept for stability and logo bridging. Pyrobuttons (16-mm-diameter tablet-sized devices) were allowed to tumble in the tablet bed along with the tablets. On comparing with the conventional monitoring, the relative humidity measured by Pyrobuttons was found to be more sensitive. It provides real-time detailed information regarding the coating process thermodynamics [16]. Some of the case studies are published that demonstrates the utilization of Pyrobuttons for evaluating coating thermodynamics. A study was conducted for establishing the film coating spray rate, exhaust temperature and tablet hardness on delamination of bilayer tablets when kept for stability. It was observed that high tablet bed relative humidity led to greater delamination of bilayer tablets [17]. Another case study was done to establish the effect of various processing parameters on tablet bed microenvironment by employing logo-bridging defect as the coating quality attribute. It was observed that the relative humidity of the tablet bed significantly affected the logo bridging, and suspension solid percentage and gun-to-bed distance that influenced the tablet bed microenvironment significantly [14].

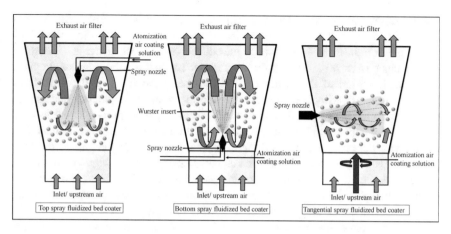

Fig. 4 Coating mechanism in top, bottom and tangential spray-fluidized bed coater

3.2 Fluidized Bed Coating

The fluidized bed technology has been employed in the pharmaceutical industry since a long duration. The process involves placing the feed material into the processing chamber (a cylindrical column) where it is held in the fluidized state with the help of carrier gas, usually air. The fluidization of the feed occurs in a columnar pattern in which the feed raises in the centre of the column because of the maximum entry of air in the centre. The feed falls in a downward direction towards the outer wall from where it re-enters the air stream again from the bottom region. The coating solution is sprayed on the feed via spraying nozzles that are placed in the top, bottom or side of the chamber. A schematic diagram of the top, bottom and tangential spray-fluidized bed coating is represented in Fig. 4. Compared to coating pans, the fluidized bed coating equipment is more efficient of water removal due to high airflow. The top spray technique is majorly used for odour- and taste-masking purposes as this technique results in highly porous coating, and it is difficult to achieve uniform film thickness by top spraying.

In the bottom spray technique, an inner cylindrical chamber (Wurster insert) is used. Dr. Dale Wurster, in 1959, introduced Wurster system at the University of Wisconsin. The Wurster technique is widely used for applying rate-controlling polymers because highly uniform film thickness can be achieved. It is compatible for delayed coating, enteric coating as well as controlled release coating of tablets. It is used commercially to coat particles from size less than 100-μm tablets. In Wurster coating, the atomized polymer droplets are sprayed from the bottom direction in the inner column with the product concurrently moving through it. Thereafter, due to product deceleration and gravitational forces, the particles fall outside the Wurster insert towards the bottom of the equipment. The recirculation of the feed occurs continuously which makes multiple passes of the feed via the spray zone. An orifice plate is there at the bottom of the chamber that is separated into two regions. A high volume of air with a high velocity transports the feed vertically inside the Wurster column. A spray nozzle is placed at the centre of the up-bed orifice plate from which the atomized coating liquid is introduced on the feed material. The spray angle ranges from 30° to 50° with a spray pattern like a solid cone of droplets. The outside region of the Wurster insert is usually identified as the down bed. The orifice plate in this area is configured on the basis of the density and size of the substrate to be processed. The down-bed region also requires airflow to keep the feed in a near-weightless suspension and to make it travel down rapidly (for minimizing the cycling time) and thereafter be dragged into the gap of the base partition. Usually, the larger feed such as tablets necessitates a high amount of air to create this condition compared to fine particles or pellets. Thus, the selection of the orifice plate is done accordingly for different substrates. Another processing variable in Wurster coating is the height at which the partition (Wurster insert) sits on the orifice plate that manages the feed flow in the horizontal direction into the coating zone. A relatively lesser gap is convenient for smaller particle coating. The expansion area height above the Wurster insert should be less for tablets as too high expansion height may lead to attrition of tablets. The partition height and the orifice plate need to be optimized as such tablets travel to a very little distance upwards outside the partition [18].

A Wurster coating equipment is usually recommended only when the film quality is very significant which is the case most probably in modified-release tablets. The film coating achieved by Wurster coater is of high quality because of high drying efficiency. Some of the modifications are done in the Wurster coating process for tablet coating such as modification in partition geometry, spray nozzle surrounds and airflow [19]. The processing variables affecting the tablet coating in Wurster coater are batch size, fluidization pattern, the impact of fluidized bed on spray pattern, evaporation rate and product temperature [20].

Batch Size

For Wurster coater, the working capacity is the volume outside the Wurster insert/partition and the partition at rest on the orifice plate. At the beginning of the process, the product is loaded only in the outer volume of the Wurster insert. However, this is done only for pellets or fine particle coating. For tablet coating usually up to one-half of the volume within the Wurster insert is also utilized. Around 20–25% of the working capacity is the minimum batch size. For accumulation of maximum of the coating solution/suspension being sprayed, it is important that sufficient feed is present in the up-bed region. However, sometimes in a small volume batch, the coating of partitions' inner wall may be experienced. Thus, small volume batch is only recommended when the final volume of the batch will be significantly higher than the starting volume (e.g. in the case of layering). When a batch size of approximately half of the working capacity of down bed is used, nearly maximum efficiency of the coater can be achieved.

Fluidization Pattern

The fluidization pattern is regulated by the partition height, fluidization air volume and orifice plate conformation. The aim is to keep the down bed smooth; however, that depends on the particle size. Moreover, some of the coating materials are tacky inherently, or due to temperature sensitivity, they move sluggishly. In such cases, it is inevitable to keep the whole bed moving; also, rather than getting a smooth flow, it is more desirable to achieve marginally over fluidized pattern. To achieve this either a more permeable down-bed plate is utilized or the partition is raised somewhat for allowing more air to percolate via the descending product. For tablets, a larger air volume is required in the down bed compared to pellets or granules to hold it well aerated. In the partition region, lesser airflow is desirable to minimize the distance travelled by the tablets outside the partition (to avoid tablet attrition). Furthermore, the partition height is a critical parameter for fluidization pattern in a Wurster coating. For tablets, large partition height is convenient so that a satisfactory number of tablets would pass via the gap per unit time and the highest quantity of coating could be sprayed on them.

Impact of Fluidized Bed on Spray Pattern

In the bottom spray technique owing to the close distance between the spray nozzle and the circulating bed, the substrate might arrive in the spray pattern before its full development. This may lead to decreased effectiveness of the system and uncontrolled droplet formation. Modification in the design of the spray nozzle has been done by various inventors to overcome this issue. Jones et al. developed a means to shield spray nozzle intended to keep the particles away from coating liquid until full development of spray pattern. It was achieved by surrounding the tip of the nozzle with an impermeable cylindrical shield. This modification helped to allow the full development of spray pattern before coming in contact with the substrate material. Furthermore, Bender modified the development of Jones to attain a more uniform product. The modification involved a permeable cylindrical shield intended to allow smaller particles to penetrate in the developing spray zone.

Evaporation Rate

The evaporation rate is controlled by the temperature, absolute humidity (dew point) and fluidization air volume. To sustain a persistent product temperature, an adjustment in temperature of fluidization air is done. The spray rate and incoming air humidity influence the product temperature. The drying condition will not be reproducible if the dew point of the incoming air is not regulated. There is an impact on the dew point due to weather changes which in turn affects the processing. In summer high humidity will affect the drying capacity, while in winter the static electricity generated during fluidization could be problematic. For thermosensitive coating materials or substrates, the effect of variation in dew point is more pronounced. Variation in dew point can lead to change in residual moisture of the film applied which can, in turn, affect the glass transition temperature for some coatings. Also, for latex materials, changes in dissolution with time may occur owing to variation in residual moisture. To minimize this effect of weather, a dew point range of 10–20 °C is recommended throughout the year.

Product Temperature

A varied range of product temperatures can be utilized for the Wurster coating process. For heat-sensitive substrates, the temperature below 30 °C is usually employed, while high product temperatures are used for aqueous-based spray liquids. Psychrometry is employed for ascertaining the limit at which the applied moisture at the substrate surface starts to remain on its layer instead of evaporating with the process air. It is the point at which the agglomeration usually begins. This exit humidity threshold is dependent on the product temperature, for example, the water elimination rate of a product temperature of 40 °C having an exit humidity 60% will be 100% higher compared to the product temperature of 30 °C [21].

4 Novel Techniques for Tablet Coating

Several novel coating techniques have been employed for tablet coating which are developed to overcome the challenges associated with conventional coating techniques. These techniques are mostly solventless techniques. For example, injection moulding technique, mechanical dry coating, compression coating, atomic layer deposition, in situ coating technology, magnetically assisted impaction coating, vacuum film coating, electrostatic coating and supercell coating technology are novel coating techniques. Some of the novel techniques employed in tablet coating are described along with their advantages and challenges associated in Table 2.

5 Modelling and Process Analytical Technology (PAT) for Tablet Coating Optimization

Irrespective of the category of coating method employed, superior coating properties can only be established if the formulation technique is completely comprehended and controlled. The main aim of PAT is to understand and control the manufacturing process. PAT can be defined as 'a system to design, analyze and control the manufacturing process by timely measuring the CQAs of raw materials and CPPs intended to ensure final product quality'. Thus, to obtain a predefined quality of the

Technique	Description	Benefits	Challenges associated	References
Injection moulding technique	In injection moulding technique, the molten polymers are injected under high pressure at raised temperatures into the mould, and on cooling of the polymer, a solid product is obtained. For tablet coating employing this technique, the tablet core is kept inside the mould, and then melted polymer is injected which forms a thin coat on tablet after solidification. Two surfaces of the tablets (upper and lower) are coated by employing an injection moulding unit. It is essential to select appropriate polymer as the final quality largely depends on the polymer properties	• It is a promising method offering product functionality and differentiation because precision coat moulds have the ability to modulate coat features and shape • It is a solvent-free technique with lesser processing time (no drying or curing required) • It can be scaled out and it is a continuous process	• Requirement of understanding the robustness of core tablet for selecting the processing conditions • Identification of coating materials having optimal melt processing properties • Necessity of investing in the equipment and precise dedicated coat moulds according to the tablet type	Puri et al. [22], Desai et al. [23], Desai et al. [24]
Electrostatic dry coating	The electrostatic dry coating technique was initially developed by electrostatic dry powder coating performed in a pan coater. The technique involves spraying of polymer and particle mixture on tablet surface without using solvent and further heating it until the mixture forms a film and fuses onto the tablet core. Two charging mechanisms are involved, namely, corona charging and tribo charging. The spraying of charged powder is done from a region of robust electric area and unfastened ion concentration. Within the area of corona discharge, for governing the charging of powdered particles, Pauthenier's equation is used	• Shorter coating process compared to other dry coating techniques • The method utilizes lesser energy and offers overall reduced processing costs • It enhances the coating powder adhesion and also offers uniform surface morphology and coating thickness • Beneficial for moisture-sensitive product	• The tablet core and the coating material should hold some conductive properties; otherwise, modification is required for satisfying the necessities of electrostatic powder coating • The resistivity of tablet core should be less than 10^9 Ωm so that the core can be properly earthed while in contact of grounded material (bose)	Qiao et al. [25], Bose and Bogner [26]

(continued)

Table 2 (continued)

Technique	Description	Benefits	Challenges associated	References
Atomic layer deposition	It is a surface-controlled technique of layer-by-layer coating process. It is widely employed in microelectronics and nanotechnology; however, for larger substrates also it has been successfully developed. By utilizing self-limiting chemical reactions amongst surface of solid substrate and gaseous precursors chemisorbed, the atomic layer deposition films are fabricated. For instance, for depositing metal oxide films, aluminium and titanium can be employed as metal precursors. Mostly, the initiation of atomic layer deposition takes place by initiation by metal precursor molecules that chemisorbs on -OH groups of the substrate surface	• Ultra-thin, high-quality slender films with high aspect-ratio structures are obtained • Smooth, continuous, attractive, dense coating is obtained • Also, substrates having low gas and moisture permeability can be coated with excellent diffusion barriers	• The surface modification, protection and functionalization are critical aspects of this process • The metal precursors increase the cost associated • For heat-sensitive substrates, the coating with this method is challenging because at reduced temperatures, the precursors do not exhibit sufficient activity which leads to failure of deposition	Hautala et al. [27], Kapoor et al. [2]
Compression coating	The compression-coated tablets have an inner core and a surrounding coat. The core tablet is the inner portion of compression-coated tablet. It is compressed with the small-diameter punch compared to the outer coated layer. The coating tablet is the outer portion of the compression-coated tablet. The coated tablet is prepared by transferring the core tablet in a die cavity of larger diameter and preliminarily filled with 70% coating material in such a way that it is placed exactly in the centre. The remaining coating material is placed above the core tablet and again	• Two incompatible materials can be compressed in a single tablet • Can be used for delivering more than one API • Simple and less expensive technique • Very less quantity of organic solvents is utilized • Requires shorter manufacturing time compared to liquid coating techniques	• Specially designed compression machines are necessary for formulating compression-coated tablets • During second compression, the core tablet may get eroded • Mixing of polymer while compression might modify the release pattern of API	Gaikwad and Kshirsagar [28], Himaja et al. [29]

product at the end by designing and developing the process is the main objective of the PAT framework. According to QBD principles, for ensuring consistent product quality, measurements are necessary on particular time intervals during the coating process or at the end of the process to enable identification of CPPs, CMAs and CQAs. These measurements are intended to monitor or control the coating process, estimate coating endpoint and assess coating quality. Sahni and Chaudhari have recently summarized various commonly employed modelling approaches and techniques to characterize and analyse the coating process [30]. The process analysis measurement can be performed through four ways: (a) in-line (sample is not removed), (b) on-line (sample is diverted, analysed and redirected into the process), (c) at-line (the removal and analysis of the sample is done close to the process), and (d) off-line (removal and analysis of the sample is done away from the process). In-line and on-line measurements can provide fast results, while at-line and off-line results are often time-consuming. Various techniques have been employed for studying different aspects of film coating quality such as confocal laser scanning microscopy [31], magnetic resonance imaging [32], light and electron microscopy [33], near-infrared spectroscopy (NIR) [34], positron emission tomography [35] and Raman spectroscopy [36–38]. Novel non-destructive techniques such as NIR chemical imaging [39], attenuated total reflection-infrared imaging [40], optical coherence tomography [41, 42], terahertz pulsed imaging [43, 44] and X-ray microcomputed tomography [45] are nowadays widely used. Many of the in-process parameters of the coating process such as temperature, spray rate, airflow, etc. can be measured directly. However, information regarding some critical factors such as atomized droplet distribution in the spray zone, coating thickness uniformity around each tablet, air velocity at various locations in the pan, droplet viscosity at the contact point with tablet surface, etc. cannot be measured directly. For such factors, various modelling techniques such as computational fluid dynamics (CFD), discrete element modelling (DEM) and Monte Carlo modelling are employed. These widely employed techniques for process analysis can be categorized into numerical and probabilistic methods. The DEM and CFD are numerical methods, while Monte Carlo modelling is a type of probabilistic models. In a study done by Christodoulou et al., modelling of spreading and drying on aqueous polymer film coating was done. A mathematical model simulating film formation, drying and spray impact was developed. For predicting the film drying, mixture modelling theory was employed, while for simplifying the liquid-particle system equations, lubrication approximation theory was employed. Variance-based sensitivity analysis was performed to evaluate the impact of spray parameters on liquid film thickness, and coating spreading, and for investigating the effect of film properties and tablets on drying [46].

5.1   Modelling Approaches

Discrete Element Modelling (DEM) and Computational Fluid Dynamics (CFD) Modelling

For employing CFD and DEM simulations, it is not necessary to preadjust the modelling parameters. These simulation models are utilized for investigating gas-solid interactions and flow patterns in fluidized beds. The continuum media method and trajectory method are the types of calculation options. DEM is a type of trajectory model in which the particle-gas and particle-particle interactions are simulated by individually tracking them. In DEM, individual particles are treated as a discrete entity that is traced individually by using the Newtonian equation, whereas CFD modelling simulates the gas and solid flow using Navier-Stokes equations in a continuum manner. The DEM has the capability of tracking the information of the dynamic individual particle and thus is utilized for understanding the tablet moving mechanics in the coating process. Toschkoff et al. investigated three spraying techniques and further combined them into a tablet-coating process DEM simulation. The outcomes demonstrated that the discrete drop method was reliable and adaptable for assessing the effect of spray intervals, number of drops and spray area uniformity. The entire process thermodynamics (e.g. airflow pattern) cannot be modelled with DEM approach. Combining DEM with CFD can be beneficial to evaluate spray-related factors, pan-related factors and thermodynamics more efficiently [47]. Limited data such as tablet velocity and position can be simulated by DEM approach. Various approaches to overcome this have been proposed in some research studies. Freireich et al. integrated the DEM simulations in a compartment model with population balance method. The detection of the spray zone was done by projecting parallel rays onto the tablets in a rectangular region and detection of collisions [48]. For industry-relevant simulations, the computational cost for keeping the typical tablet shape is relatively high. These simpler shapes like spheres are approximated to decrease the associated cost. However, after such simplifications also, simulation is difficult as it takes months to complete. Recently, graphical processor unit (GPU) has made large-scale simulations for millions of shaped particles or spheres easier using XPS code. Kureck et al. developed a novel algorithm for contact detection between biconvex tablets by GPU. The algorithm was validated and implemented for many experiments. Thereafter, simulation of 20 million tablets was done in a drum coater for illustrating the benefit of GPU computing for coating applications at industrial scale [49]. Suzzi et al. developed a DEM simulation model for tablet coating intended to examine the effects of tablet fill level and shape on tablet coating variability. DEM was utilized for numerically reproducing the tablet motion in a coating pan. Three different tablet shapes (round, oval and biconvex) were modelled by employing the 'glued spheres' technique. Thereafter, the analysis of three different fill volumes and the rotational, as well as translational tablet velocities, was done [50].

Monte Carlo Modelling

The Monte Carlo modelling technique is a quantitative method used for prediction of outputs anticipated from both theory and experiments. It is done by random sampling from factors influencing process such as rotation speed of the drum, core bed temperature, physical properties of the material, etc. The average of outputs of several probability distribution samples provides an accurate estimation of the real process outputs. Numerous investigators have employed Monte Carlo modelling for understanding the effect of coating parameters such as air velocity, coating period, spray pattern, mixing rate of particles, etc. By using this modelling method, spray dynamics and particle movement have been simulated in both pan coaters and fluidized bed coaters. Pandey et al. investigated processing variables affecting weight variability (weight gain mass coating variability) in pan coater by employing Monte Carlo simulations and video imaging techniques. Effects of pan loading, pan speed, coating time, tablet size, spray shape and area and spray flux distribution were investigated. The results demonstrated that the weight gain mass coating variability was inversely proportional to the square root of coating time. It was also found that spray shape did not affect the weight variability. However, an increase in spray area led to lower weight gain mass coating variability. For verification of predictions established by Monte Carlo simulation, coating experiments were done, and the results represented that the trend predicted by modelling were in good agreement with the experimental results [51]. Choi patented the evaluation of weight uniformity and coating uniformity of tablets coated using the pan coating process by employing Monte Carlo modelling. However, as per the expert opinion, a priori prediction cannot be obtained using Monte Carlo modelling, and there is a need to experimentally measure some of the model parameters first.

5.2 Spectroscopic and Imaging Techniques

Near-Infrared Spectroscopy (NIR)

Various research studies have been performed by researchers for employing NIR spectroscopy for analysis of tablet coating optimization. NIR spectroscopy is a non-destructive and rapid method with minimum sample preparation requirement. NIR spectroscopy can be employed at-line, in-line and off-line in a pan coater. Kim et al. developed an in-line NIR spectroscopy method to allow real-time analysis of the weight gain during coating. A diffuse reflectance probe was designed that was inserted into the coating pan, and by utilizing DOE, the optimal measurement conditions were identified. The weight gain predicted using NIR spectroscopy was confirmed by correlating with the thickness measured by employing micro-CT [52]. Hattori et al. evaluated the effect of the concentration of coating polymer on the tablet properties by employing NIR spectroscopy. Tablet properties such as tablet hardness, coating amount, coating thickness and tablet dissolution parameters were evaluated. While performing tablet coating, an in-line NIR spectroscopy was done. The predicted values and the measured values for each tablet property represented linear relationships [53]. Perez-Ramos et al. developed an in-line NIR spectroscopy method for analysing film coating thickness on tablet manufactured in a laboratory-scale pan coater. The off-line measurement done to analyse volumetric growth in tablets and the values estimated via NIR data showed a good correlation [54]. NIR chemical imaging is a novel indirect technique that helps to determine the coating layer by using changes in absorbance values. The ability of NIR chemical imaging to penetrate to a greater depth allows obtaining simultaneous information from both the core and coat. Also, a greater field of view of NIR chemical imaging allows the visualization of large samples up to 40×32 mm^2. Moltgen et al. applied in-line Fourier transform NIR spectroscopy for monitoring industrial-scale tablet coating process of heart-shaped tablets. Five experimental runs were conducted to study the influence of processing variables such as pan load, spray rate, pan rotation and exhaust air temperature. Based on Karl Fischer reference, a PLS calibration model helped to determine tablet moisture trajectory throughout the coating process. In amalgamation with PLS discriminant analysis, at-line NIR chemical imaging tested the HPMC coating and the changes occurring at the coat-core interface during the coating process. The study depicted that the at-line NIR chemical imaging and in-line NIR spectroscopy can be implemented as a combined PAT tool for monitoring the pan coating process [34].

Raman Spectroscopy

As compared to NIR spectroscopy, the utilization of Raman spectroscopy as a PAT tool is quite constrained due to the higher cost of equipment and sensitivity towards interfering light background scattering. However, owing to its flexibility and constant progress in efficiency, it is considered to develop an effective PAT tool. Romero-Torres et al. utilized Raman spectroscopy for evaluating tablet coating thickness [55]. In other study done by the same authors, they investigated varied calibration techniques for employing Raman spectroscopy as a PAT tool for investigating coating comprised of fluorescent ingredients [55]. For Raman spectroscopy, the remote fibre-optic probes simplify in-line monitoring of the process. Schwab and McCreery reported the first remote fibre-optic probe that can be employed for Raman spectroscopy. The probe was comprised of two single optical fibres, one intended to deliver laser light to the sample (known as excitation fibre) and another for collection of the scattered light by the sample and further transmitting to the detector (known as collection fibre). However, the efficiency for excitation and collection of Raman photons from the sample was poor [56]. Thus, further development has been done for improving the intensity of Raman signals and, in turn, enhances its efficiency. Examples include altering the overlap amongst collection cone of collection fibres and emission cone of excitation fibre to increase collection efficiency. Also, employing multiple fibres rather than one collection fibre is an approach to enhance the Raman signal. Moreover, amendments in the design of collection and excitation fibres have been commenced to enhance light coupling efficiency and subsequently enhance the signal intensity. El Hagrasy et al. utilized Raman fibre-optic probes for monitoring coating done in a pan coater. Employing Raman spectroscopy, the influence of pan rotation speed was evaluated by interpreting the acquired signal. Also, for the determination of coating endpoint and coating kinetics, a quantitative calibration technique was developed [36].

Terahertz Pulsed Imaging

In the electromagnetic spectrum, terahertz radiation is in the far-IR region (2–120 cm^{-1}). The key advantage of terahertz radiation (due to longer wavelength than NIR) is that it penetrates deeper (around 3 mm) into the solid dosage form. Other advantages of this method are that it is non-destructive and no chemometric calculation model is necessary for calculating the film thickness. The imaging method can be utilized only for single-point measurement (within milliseconds) or for mapping the entire surface of the tablet (requires 20–50 min). It is sensitive to the chemical as well as physical properties and can be utilized to examine coating thickness, uniformity, density, roughness, internal structures and integrity. Also, this method can be combined with additional analytical methods like drug release studies to correlate density measurements and coating thickness with release kinetics and thus allow deeper understanding and proper control of the coating process. Terahertz pulsed imaging can be employed for measuring film thickness in-line during pan coating which allows it to be used as an endpoint determination tool. A terahertz sensor was mounted on a perforated coating pan of production scale coater by May et al. During the coating process, the film thickness on the coated tablet was determined in-line in real time via the pan's perforation. It was possible to evaluate the coating thickness of 80 tablets per minute with this technique [57]. Spencer et al. employed this method for mapping the coating thickness of Asacol tablets. A map was generated of the internal structures utilizing the time delays of reflected pulses [58]. Maurer and Leuenberger utilized NIR imaging and terahertz pulsed imaging for monitoring the coating technique of film-coated tablets. NIR imaging provided the inter- and intra-tablet differences via different absorbance values, while the terahertz imaging technique provided the coating thickness. They concluded that terahertz pulsed imaging provided the advantage of giving the direct thickness values while the NIR imaging provided a better output for thinner coating layers [59].

X-ray Microcomputed Tomography

X-ray microcomputed tomography allows 3-D visualization of object's internal structure. It is an off-line measurement technique. The technique has high penetration capability and has a good resolution level. The technique has been employed to characterize the microstructures of the coated product and reveal the characteristic details of the coating layer. Compared to other classic visualization techniques, this technique has better applicability as it allows both two-dimensional and three-dimensional examination of the internal structures. It is an exceptional technique for visualizing the damages on the surface or inside the coated products and identification and quantification of cracks. The calculation of factors such as surface porosity, density and thickness of coating is possible with this technique. However, the current technique does not facilitate at-line and/or in-line monitoring of the coating process. Another limitation of this technique is that it cannot provide information regarding the chemical nature of the sample. However, to overcome this shortcoming an innovative approach of combining conventional spectroscopic techniques as X-ray microcomputed tomography within a single integrated instrument is being developed.

6 Summary

The pharmaceutical coating on solid dosage forms has been performed since several years for achieving stable and elegant product, modify the release profiles of the drug, mask the unpleasant taste or odour and protect from environmental factors. Pan coating and fluidized bed technique are widely used techniques for coating the solid dosage forms. The coating process includes numerous formulation and processing factors affecting various parameters of the coated end product. The factors affecting pan coating process are coating formulation influences such as the type of excipients used, solid content and the viscosity of coating solution; substrate factors like porosity, hardness, density and stability; pan coater parameters like pan load and pan speed; spray-linked factors such as spray gun design, gun-to-bed distance and rate of spray; and thermodynamic considerations like volume, temperature and humidity. While employing fluidized bed coater, factors such as batch size, fluidization pattern, evaporation rate, product temperature and impact of fluidized bed on spray pattern affect the final coated product quality. At the beginning of the twenty-first century, QBD, risk management and product quality research institute (PQRI) initiatives were introduced for designing, monitoring and controlling the product quality in the USA, Japan, Europe and other countries. It is inevitable to understand the interdependent factors and to optimize the coating process based on QBD principles. In recent years, for better understanding of factors affecting the coating process, the researchers are more focusing on applying appropriate modelling techniques and PAT. Modelling techniques utilized for evaluating various factors affecting coating are DEM, CFD and Monte Carlo modelling. Using combined modelling techniques with the novel theoretical models can be advantageous to researchers to attain a deeper knowledge of the process and streamline the process based on principles of QBD. Applying PAT tools helps to identify suitable process control strategy, assess coating quality and estimate coating endpoint by monitoring the coating process.

Acknowledgements The authors are grateful to Nirma University for providing the necessary facilities.

References

1. Behzadi S, Toegel S, Viernstein H (2008) Innovations in coating technology. Recent Pat Drug Deliv Formul 2:209–230.
2. Kapoor D, Maheshwari R, Verma K, et al (2020) Coating technologies in pharmaceutical product development. In: Drug Delivery Systems. Elsevier, pp 665–719
3. Cahyadi C, Chan LW, Heng PWS (2013) The reality of in-line tablet coating. Pharm Dev Technol 18:2–16.
4. Felton LA, Porter SC (2013) An update on pharmaceutical film coating for drug delivery. Expert Opin. Drug Deliv. 10:421–435
5. Basu A, De A, Dey S (2013) Techniques of tablet coating: concepts and advancements: a comprehensive review. J Pharm Pharm Sci 2:1–6
6. Seo K, Bajracharya R, Lee SH, Han H (2020) Pharmaceutical application of tablet film coating. Pharmaceutics 12:853.
7. Agrawal AM, Pandey P (2015) Scale up of pan coating process using quality by design principles. J Pharm Sci 104:3589–3611.
8. Porter SC, Verseput RP, Cunningham CR (1997) Process optimization using design of experiments. Pharm Technol 21:60–70
9. Porter S, Sackett G, Liu L (2009) Development, optimization, and scale-up of process parameters. In: Qiu Y, Zhang G, Porter W; Chen Y; Liu L (ed) Developing Solid Oral Dosage Forms. Academic Press, pp 761–805
10. Wilson KE, Crossman E (1997) The influence of tablet shape and pan speed on intra-tablet film coating uniformity. Drug Dev Ind Pharm 23:1239–1243.
11. Porter S, Sackett G, Liu L (2017) Development, Optimization, and Scale-up of Process Parameters. In: Qiu Y, Zhang G, Mantri R, Chen Y, Yu L (ed) Developing Solid Oral Dosage Forms. Academic press, pp 953–996
12. Mueller R, Kleinebudde P (2007) Comparison of a laboratory and a production coating spray gun with respect to scale-up. AAPS PharmSciTech 8:E21–E31.
13. Chen W, Chang S-Y, Kiang S, et al (2008) The measurement of spray quality for pan coating processes. J Pharm Innov 3:3–14.
14. Pandey P, Bindra DS, Felton LA (2014a) Influence of process parameters on tablet bed microenvironmental factors during pan coating. AAPS PharmSciTech 15:296–305.
15. Am Ende MT, Berchielli A (2005) A thermodynamic model for organic and aqueous tablet film coating. Pharm Dev Technol 10:47–58.
16. Pandey P, Ji J, Subramanian G, et al (2014b) Understanding the thermodynamic micro-environment inside a pan coater using a data logging device. Drug Dev Ind Pharm 40:542–548.
17. Zacour BM, Pandey P, Subramanian G, et al (2014) Correlating bilayer tablet delamination tendencies to micro-environmental thermodynamic conditions during pan coating. Drug Dev Ind Pharm 40:829–837.
18. Sonar GS, Rawat SS (2015) Wurster technology: Process variables involved and Scale up science. Innov Pharm Pharm Technol 1:100–109
19. Shelukar S, Ho J, Zega J, et al (2000) Identification and characterization of factors controlling tablet coating uniformity in a Wurster coating process. Powder Technol 110:29–36.
20. Jones D (2009) Development, Optimization, and Scale-up of Process Parameters: Wurster Coating. In: Qiu Y, Zhang G, Porter W, Chen Y, Liu L (ed) Developing Solid Oral Dosage Forms. Academic press, pp 807–825

21. Jones D, Godek E (2017) Development, optimization, and scale-up of process parameters: Wurster coating. In: Qiu Y, Zhang G, Mantri R, Chen Y, Yu L (ed) Developing Solid Oral Dosage Forms: Pharmaceutical Theory and Practice: Second Edition. Academic Press., pp 997–1014

22. Puri V, Brancazio D, Harinath E, et al (2018) Demonstration of pharmaceutical tablet coating process by injection molding technology. Int J Pharm 535:106–112.

23. Desai PM, Puri V, Brancazio D, et al (2018a) European Journal of Pharmaceutics and Biopharmaceutics Tablet coating by injection molding technology – Optimization of coating formulation attributes and coating process parameters. Eur J Pharm Biopharm 122:25–36.

24. Desai PM, Puri V, Brancazio D, et al (2018b) Tablet coating by injection molding technology – Optimization of coating formulation attributes and coating process parameters. Eur J Pharm Biopharm 122:25–36.

25. Qiao M, Zhang L, Ma Y, et al (2010) A novel electrostatic dry powder coating process for pharmaceutical dosage forms: Immediate release coatings for tablets. Eur J Pharm Biopharm 76:304–310.

26. Bose S, Bogner RH (2007) Solventless pharmaceutical coating processes: A review. Pharm. Dev. Technol. 12:115–131

27. Hautala J, Kääriäinen T, Hoppu P, et al (2017) Atomic layer deposition—A novel method for the ultrathin coating of minitablets. Int J Pharm 531:47–58.

28. Gaikwad SS, Kshirsagar SJ (2020) Review on Tablet in Tablet techniques. Beni-Suef Univ J Basic Appl Sci 9:1–7.

29. Himaja V, Sai Koushik O, Karthikeyan R and Srinivasa Babu P (2016) A comprehensive review on tablet coating. Austin Pharmacol Pharm 1:1–8

30. Sahni E, Chaudhuri B (2012) Experimental and modeling approaches in characterizing coating uniformity in a pan coater: A literature review. Pharm Dev Technol 17:134–147.

31. Depypere F, Van Oostveldt P, Pieters JG, Dewettinck K (2009) Quantification of microparticle coating quality by confocal laser scanning microscopy (CLSM). Eur J Pharm Biopharm 73:179–186.

32. Dorożyński P, Jamróz W, Niwiński K, et al (2013) Novel method for screening of enteric film coatings properties with magnetic resonance imaging. Int J Pharm 456:569–571.

33. Bikiaris D, Koutri I, Alexiadis D, et al (2012) Real time and non-destructive analysis of tablet coating thickness using acoustic microscopy and infrared diffuse reflectance spectroscopy. Int J Pharm 438:33–44.

34. Möltgen C-V, Puchert T, Menezes JC, et al (2012) A novel in-line NIR spectroscopy application for the monitoring of tablet film coating in an industrial scale process. Talanta 92:26–37.

35. Parker DJ, Dijkstra AE, Martin TW, Seville JPK (1997) Positron emission particle tracking studies of spherical particle motion in rotating drums. Chem Eng Sci 52:2011–2022.

36. El Hagrasy AS, Chang S-Y, Desai D, Kiang S (2006) Raman spectroscopy for the determination of coating uniformity of tablets: assessment of product quality and coating pan mixing efficiency during scale-up. J Pharm Innov 1:37–42.

37. Kauffman JF, Dellibovi M, Cunningham CR (2007) Raman spectroscopy of coated pharmaceutical tablets and physical models for multivariate calibration to tablet coating thickness. J Pharm Biomed Anal 43:39–48.

38. Radtke J, Rehbaum H, Kleinebudde P (2020) Raman spectroscopy as a PAT-Tool for film-coating processes: In-Line Predictions Using one PLS Model for Different Cores. Pharmaceutics 12:796.

39. Palou A, Cruz J, Blanco M, et al (2012) Determination of drug, excipients and coating distribution in pharmaceutical tablets using NIR-CI. J Pharm Anal 2:90–97.

40. Chan KLA, Hammond S V., Kazarian SG (2003) Applications of attenuated total reflection infrared spectroscopic imaging to pharmaceutical formulations. Anal Chem 75:2140–2146.

41. Lin H, Dong Y, Markl D, et al (2017) Pharmaceutical film coating catalog for spectral domain optical coherence tomography. J Pharm Sci 106:3171–3176.

42. Markl D, Hannesschläger G, Sacher S, et al (2014) Optical coherence tomography as a novel tool for in-line monitoring of a pharmaceutical film-coating process. Eur J Pharm Sci 55:58–67.
43. Alves-Lima D, Song J, Li X, et al (2020) Review of terahertz pulsed imaging for pharmaceutical film coating analysis. Sensors 20:1–16
44. Ho L, Müller R, Gordon KC, et al (2009) Terahertz pulsed imaging as an analytical tool for sustained-release tablet film coating. Eur J Pharm Biopharm 71:117–123.
45. Perfetti G, Van De Casteele E, Rieger B, et al (2010) X-ray micro tomography and image analysis as complementary methods for morphological characterization and coating thickness measurement of coated particles. Adv Powder Technol 21:663–675. https://doi.org/10.1016/j.apt.2010.08.002
46. Christodoulou C, Mazzei L, Garcia-Muñoz S, Sorensen E (2018) Modeling of spreading and drying of aqueous polymer coatings on pharmaceutical tablets during film coating. In: Eden M, Lerapetritou M, Towler G (ed) Computer Aided Chemical Engineering. Vol. 44. Elsevier, pp 2095–2100
47. Toschkoff G, Just S, Funke A, et al (2013) Spray models for discrete element simulations of particle coating processes. Chem Eng Sci 101:603–614.
48. Freireich B, Li J, Litster J, Wassgren C (2011) Incorporating particle flow information from discrete element simulations in population balance models of mixer-coaters. Chem Eng Sci 66:3592–3604.
49. Kureck H, Govender N, Siegmann E, et al (2019) Industrial scale simulations of tablet coating using GPU based DEM: A validation study. Chem Eng Sci 202:462–480.
50. Suzzi D, Toschkoff G, Radl S, et al (2012) DEM simulation of continuous tablet coating: Effects of tablet shape and fill level on inter-tablet coating variability. Chem Eng Sci 69:107–121.
51. Pandey P, Katakdaunde M, Turton R (2006) Modeling weight variability in a pan coating process using Monte Carlo simulations. AAPS PharmSciTech 7:E2–E11.
52. Kim B, Woo YA (2020) Optimization of in-line near-infrared measurement for practical real time monitoring of coating weight gain using design of experiments. Drug Development and Industrial Pharmacy pp 1-11
53. Hattori Y, Sugata M, Kamata H, et al (2018) Real-time monitoring of the tablet-coating process by near-infrared spectroscopy - Effects of coating polymer concentrations on pharmaceutical properties of tablets. J Drug Deliv Sci Technol 46:111–121.
54. Pérez-Ramos JD, Findlay WP, Peck G, Morris KR (2005) Quantitative analysis of film coating in a pan coater based on in-line sensor measurements. AAPS PharmSciTech 6:E127–E136.
55. Romero-Torres S, Pérez-Ramos JD, Morris KR, Grant ER (2005) Raman spectroscopic measurement of tablet-to-tablet coating variability. J Pharm Biomed Anal 38:270–274.
56. Schwab SD, McCreery RL (1984) Versatile, efficient Raman sampling with fiber optics. Anal Chem 56:2199–2204.
57. May RK, Evans MJ, Zhong S, et al (2011) Terahertz in-line sensor for direct coating thickness measurement of individual tablets during film coating in real-time. J Pharm Sci 100:1535–1544.
58. Spencer JA, Gao Z, Moore T, et al (2008) Delayed release tablet dissolution related to coating thickness by terahertz pulsed image mapping. J Pharm Sci 97:1543–1550.
59. Maurer L, Leuenberger H (2009) Terahertz pulsed imaging and near infrared imaging to monitor the coating process of pharmaceutical tablets. Int J Pharm 370:8–16.

Continuous Twin-Screw Granulation Processing

Uttom Nandi, Tumpa Dey, and Dennis Douroumis

1 Granulation

Granulation is a well-known powder processing technique, used in the pharmaceutical industry for the manufacturing of solid dosage forms [1]. This term is used to describe the processing of powders for particle enhancement with the aim to improve a range of properties such as flowability, compressibility, tabletability and homogeneous distribution of active ingredients, etc. [2, 3]. A deep understanding of the technology may aid in the prediction and preparation of good-quality granules along with tablet manufacturing. The transformation of powders to agglomerated particles is usually performed prior to tableting to ensure minimal aggregation and a uniform flow of the powder through the hopper to the die [2]. Typically, granulation is a particle size enlargement process where particles are processed to form larger multi-unit entities with a distribution in between 0.2 and 0.4 mm [4]. Even larger size granules (around 1–4 mm) are also prepared for the capsule manufacturing [5]. Depending on the final particle size, granules are further processed with other excipients and used as an intermediate before compression to form tablets, or for filling of hard gelatin capsules. Furthermore, granulation technology is used to reduce the generation of toxic dust during powder handling [6]. A good-quality granule exhibits a less non-friable behaviour and also produces less amount of fines during processing. Pharmaceutical powders have often uneven particle size distribution leading to segregation during storage which can be minimised and improve content uniformity via granulation. The bulk powders present several practical implications such as higher packaging, storage and transportation which can be tackled through

U. Nandi (✉) · T. Dey · D. Douroumis
Faculty of Engineering and Science, School of Science, University of Greenwich, Kent, UK

CIPER Centre for Innovation and Process Engineering Research, Kent, UK
e-mail: D.Douroumis@greenwich.ac.uk

the manufacturing of granules with higher densities. Traditionally, granulation of powders can be achieved by two different methods, classified as (a) dry granulation and (b) wet granulation.

In general, pharmaceutical manufacturing can be divided into two distinct stages: primary manufacturing (i.e. upstream operations) which involves the production of the active ingredient from the starting reagents and secondary manufacturing (i.e. downstream operations) which involves the conversion of the active drugs into products suitable for administration such as granules, capsules or tablets [7]. The secondary manufacturing involves integration of multiple processing units; thus, this stage requires a fundamental understanding of processing parameters to optimise a formulation [8–10].

The manufacturing of granules can be conducted via three different ways: dry, wet and melt granulation. The dry granulation involves aggregation of primary powders in the absence of any liquids under high pressure to facilitate bonding of the particles by direct contact and subsequent milling to attain the desired size [1]. This method is suitable for processing moisture-sensitive active pharmaceutical ingredients (APIs), while it is cost-effective due to the less processing steps, little or no material waste and low dust exposure. A common approach for dry granulation is roller compaction where powder is fed into two counterrotating rolls producing flat-shaped ribbons of compacted material. The use of a dry binder, such as cellulose, starch or povidone, in the powder blend is essential to achieve a stronger ribbon [11]. Subsequently, the ribbons can be milled to obtain the desired granule size. In many cases the use of roller compaction/dry granulation has been described as a 'continuous production line' [12]. The technique has been frequently used over the past two decades as it improves drug dosage weight control, content uniformity and powder flow while it is easy to scale up and facilitates continuous manufacturing [13]. In some cases the generation of fines makes the technology unfavourable or even unwanted for further processing and might disqualify or complicate the process for highly potent drugs [14].

A wide range of powder processing methods are employed in the pharmaceutical industry to produce granules with particular characteristics in terms of their physical and pharmaceutical properties (e.g. bioavailability) [15]. According to several studies, wet granulation provides better control of drug uniformity, improves flowability and increases bulk density and porosity [16–18]. Wet granulation requires volatile and non-toxic solvent (e.g. ethanol, isopropanol) for the processing of powder blends which are an alternative for moisture-sensitive APIs, and they tend to dry quickly. The use of aqueous solution is a common approach to create strong bonds between the particles that lock them together. However, when the water dries, the powders might break, and thus it is a prerequisite to form a dense mass. Following the production of granules, further processing is carried out by sieving, milling or mixing with additional components to manufacture a finished dosage form. Wet

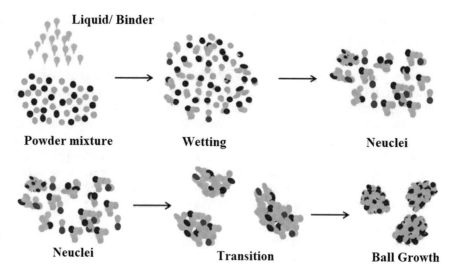

Fig. 1 Diagram of granule formation [19]

granulation technologies usually involve the use of high shear mixers and fluidised bed that produce dense and uniform granules.

Theoretically, granule mechanism requires the adhesion of particles for the formation of agglomerates and comprises of three key steps. The particle adhesion takes in various steps; as shown in Fig. 1, this involves wetting and nucleation, transition and ball growth [6]. Initially adhesion or cohesion forces take place through the formation of an immobile thin layer which results in the decrease of the interparticulate distance while increasing the contact area through van der Waals forces. This is the pendular state where water is distributed as mobile thin layer around the particles holding them together through lens-shaped rings. The transition state is entered by further addition of granulating liquid leading to the formation of stronger liquid bridges (funicular state) by filling up the interparticulate void space. This is usually the end of the wet granulation process, but further liquid saturation (80%) and air displacement lead to the capillary state where large snowballs are built up which are not suitable for pharmaceutical purposes.

Melt granulation is similar to dry granulation process where binder solution is replaced by a meltable binder. Fluidised bed melt and melt extrusion or even high shear granulations are processing technologies that can be effectively used where the binder is melted/soften near or above its melting point or glass transition temperature in order to obtain agglomerated granules [20–23]. Usually the melting point of binders varies between 30 and 100 °C, and they either melt or become tacky followed by solidification upon cooling.

2 Instrumentation of a Twin-Screw Granulation (TSG) (Extruder)

Extrusion granulation equipment is almost identical to that used for typical hot melt extrusion (HME) and consists of the extruder, auxiliary equipment, downstream processing equipment and some other monitoring tools for performance and evaluation of product [24]. The extruder typically composed of hopper, single or twin screw, barrels, die and driving unit for screw. The auxiliary equipment equipped with a cooling and heating device is connected to the barrels, the conveyer belt to cool down the extrudates and the solvent delivery pump. The monitoring screen displays screw speed, temperature scales, torque monitor and pressure scales.

Overall extrusion process is divided into four sections [25]:

- Feeding of the materials
- Conveying of materials (mixing and particle size reduction)
- Out flow from the extruder (no die)
- Downstream processing

During processing, temperature is controlled by electrical heating bands and monitored by thermocouples displayed on monitoring screen. Usually, the extruder comprises of single or twin rotating screws placed inside the barrel. The barrel is composed of sections which is bolted and clamped together and described as zones in the extruder. A die plate is attached to the end of barrel, which determines the shape of the final extruded product (Fig. 2).

Currently the most common extruder types are (a) the single-screw and (b) the twin-screw extruders. The single-screw extruder consists of only single screw placed in the extruder barrel, while more advanced twin-screw extrusion system consists of either in a same direction (co-rotating) or opposite direction (counterrotating).

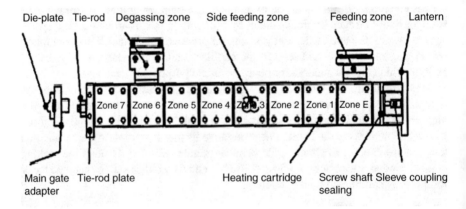

Fig. 2 Schematic diagram of an extruder [26]

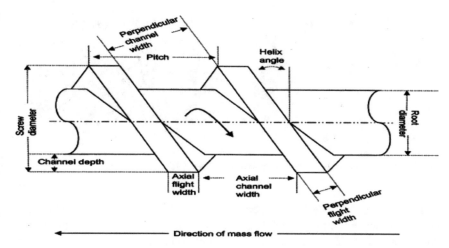

Fig. 3 Geometry of extruder screw [28]

Usually, the extruder screw is characterised by length/diameter (L/D) ratio of screw which typically ranges from 20 to 40:1.

The heat required (melt granulation) for the melting or fusing of the material is provided by the combination of electric or liquid clams on the barrels and friction of the materials produced by shear force between rotating screw and barrel wall [27].

The extrusion granulation process is fully controlled by applying the optimal temperature, screw speed and feed rate. The technique has a potential to control and process material at a specific requirement such as high shear extrusion or addition of solvent at solvent evaporation stage during processing. Screw configuration allows extruder to perform mixing and particle size rearrangement which performs a vital role for the dispersion of API into carrier matrices.

The material is fed from the hopper directly into the deeper flight or greater flight pitch. The geometry of flights (shown in Fig. 3) allows feeding materials to fall easily into rotating screw for conveying alongside the barrel. The helix angle and pitch of the screw control the constant rotation speed of screws. The materials fed as a solid into the transition zone where it is mixed, compressed, melted and plasticised. The compression process of materials into the barrel is regulated either by decreasing thread pitch but maintaining constant flight depth or maintaining constant thread pitch with decreasing flight depth [29]. This process creates pressure as the material moves into the barrel to the exit. The material moves in helical path as a result of some mechanisms such as transverse flow, pressure flow, drag flow and leakage, while movement of material in barrel is affected by two reverse mechanisms (a) screw diameter space and (b) width of the barrel. The material reaches the metering zones with uniform thickness and flowability which drag out the granulated material as uniform delivery of granules. The downstream processing is equipped with conveyer which permits extrudates to cool down at room temperature by applied air pressure.

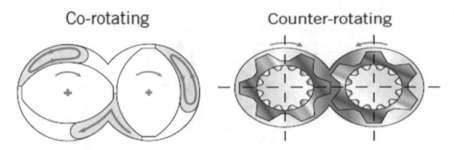

Fig. 4 Twin-screw co-rotating and counterrotating screw [31]

In twin-screw extruders, screws can be rotated either in the same (co-rotating) or opposite (counterrotating) direction as shown in Fig. 4. Two screws are placed into the barrel side by side, and it is designed to control operating parameters such as the filling level of material, the screw speed, the feed time and the residence time [30]. In counterrotating extruder, twin screw rotates in opposite direction in barrel. This type of extruder is usually applied for high shear materials as material squeezed through the gaps between screws. Counterrotating screw provides an excellent dispersion of blended particles, while it also exhibits some disadvantages of air entrapment, high pressure and low output as a result of low maximum screw speed. This type of extruder does not produce pushing effect of materials into the barrel due to opposite direction of screw rotation.

On the other hand, a co-rotating screw rotates at the same directions, and it states the advantage of self-wiping and intermeshing design [25]. This type of extruder is mainly used in the industry which has competency to operate at high screw speed and provide excellent high output with intensive mixing and conveying of materials during the process. Co-rotating is subclassified as non-intermeshing and intermeshing.

Intermeshing twin-screw extruders are very popular as they provide self-wiping to minimise the non-motion of materials and prevent overheating of materials and superior mixing in respect over single-screw extruder. Intermeshing extruders operate on the principle of first in, first out where the material does not rotate along with screw to barrel [32]. Non-intermeshing extruders are used to extrude a highly viscous material which is not liable to produce high torque during processing [33].

3 TSG Processing Parameters

3.1 Temperature

Each of the barrels can have a unique set point; therefore, the process can be run using a single temperature value or a temperature profile, depending on specific requirements of the process. Temperature has an effect on processability of the formulation as viscosity is temperature dependent, as well as on the quality of the final product. The bed temperature for lubricated powders varies from 5 to 15 °C and depends on the flow rate, screw speed, L/S ratio and the amount of polymer in the binding solution [34, 35]. The temperature variations within the barrel can easily reach 70 °C, while the presence of long mixing zones increases the temperature of the formed granules. The temperature can be also influenced by the different wetting behaviour of the processed powders [36].

3.2 Screw Design

Screw configuration is designed based on the type, number and sequence of phases of which the extrusion comprises. At the entrance of the extruder, conveying screw elements of high-pitch sizes are placed to ensure proper powder feeding since bulk density of the inlet materials is much smaller than extrudate density. A standard configuration presents conveying elements up to two thirds of the screw length, followed by high shear mixing zone. Venting during extrusion process is sometimes needed to remove entrapped air or residue moisture from the final product. Vent requires a drop in pressure in that part of the extruder to prevent the exiting of the material through the opening. This is achieved by positioning of high-pitch conveying elements are positioned. For extrusion through the die and shaping of the product, the pressure should be increased so the pitch is reduced.

The elements on the screw shaft are interchangeable so a customised screw configuration can be assembled to match the specific requirements of each process. Elements differ in design to suit the various steps of processing, such as transporting, mixing, melting and shaping. Conveying elements have self-wiping geometry needed for transportation of the material along the screw, whereas the free volume of the screw and speed is modulated by pitch size (Fig. 5). Mixing (kneading) elements are used for mixing, melting and homogenisation, while they comprised of disc, which are staggered under certain angle. The angle determines the conveying and mixing properties; conveying properties decrease, whereas mixing properties increase with increasing offset angle. Additionally, longer discs impart more shear, while shorter improve dispersive mixing. Therefore, kneading elements can be classified as:

- Forwarding
- Neutral
- Reversing

Screw configuration has a critical impact on the product properties where insufficient mixing results in non-homogenous blends or leads to incomplete product conversion or reaction. On the contrary, if the mixing zone is too long and imparting too much shear, residence time can increase as well as product temperature both resulting in API degradation.

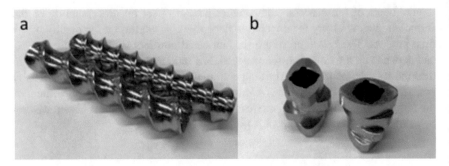

Fig. 5 Conveying elements (**a**) and mixing elements (**b**)

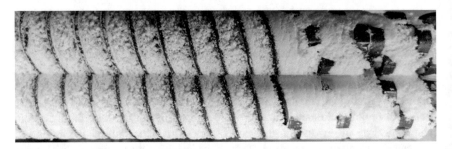

Fig. 6 Photo showing a wet TSG of microcrystalline cellulose/lactose monohydrate mixture with a kneading block (right most side of the image). Direction of flow is to the right

The use of conveying elements with different flight pitches can have a significant effect on the extruded granules. By increasing the flight pitch of the screws, the granule output is increased, while the fines are reduced due to the larger volume which is available for the wetted mass [37, 38]. The use of higher flight pitch facilitates the formation of porous granules, while the increased number of conveying elements results in increase of the granule strength. The presence of conveying elements right after a kneading zone plays a key role as it minimises the formation of large clumps and results in their breakage.

Furthermore, the kneading elements play a key role due to their capability to produce stronger compressive granules. Figure 6 shows a TSG process illustrating the granule development and compaction. When using high offset angles of kneading elements, granules appear larger and denser, while longer mixing zones produced less friable and breakable particles with narrow and controllable size.

On the contrary the usage of multiple kneading zones has a negligible effect on the granule particle size and distribution. Kneading elements control the morphology of extruded granules and usually produce elongated shapes compared to spherical-shaped granules obtained when only conveying screws are implemented [39, 40].

3.3 Feeding Rate and Screw Speed

The feeding rate is one of the most important process variables, and it has been found to influence the particle size and granule density/strength. High feeding rates are related to increased compressive forces which correspond to larger and dense granules. In the absence of kneading zones, high feed rates increase the formation of fines which are friable and easily break while the liquid distribution in the powder blend is non-uniform. Screw speed is related to the shear rate in a TSG, but it has low impact on the particle size of the granules and the residence time. By increasing the screw speed, only a minor size reduction has been observed only when high adhesive polymers are used in the granulation blend [41].

3.4 Mixing in a TSG

The powder mixing in a TSG is directly related to the screw configuration and the resulted shear rate as a function of the process settings and is classified as radial or axial based on the direction of spread. During the TSG process, radial mixing is a prerequisite for a homogeneous granule distribution at constant powder feeding, while axial mixing can also help to avoid inhomogeneities. The selection of feeding rate, screw speed and screw configuration determine the degree of mixing. The axial mixing is directly affected by the residence time distribution (RTD), screw speed and geometry. When suing high screw speeds, the axial mixing increases as estimated by the rise of the normalised variance ($\sigma 2\theta$) and the lowering of the Peclet number (Pe). However, there are contradictory studies suggesting that axial mixing is not affected by the processing parameters [42].

The most favourable feature of a TSG process is the capacity to processed high powder throughput in a short residence time (0–20s). Despite the possible gains of TSG over batch manufacturing, this is not always straightforward because there is a limited time frame to achieve homogeneous granule distribution, granule formation and breakage to obtain the final product. Hence, in order to achieve high TSG yield, the process should be designed carefully with longer residence time than the mixing time across the extruder barrel. The process is more complicated when mixing powders with the granulating liquid which requires homogeneous liquid distribution within the powder. Sayin et al. observed that the site of liquid addition and the periodicity of the peristaltic pump have a strong impact on the moisture content and distribution [43]. The use of more kneading zones can help to improve the distribution of granulation liquid, but further improvements required the addition of screw elements with modified geometries that can induce distributive mixing.

The addition of granulating liquid results in the formation of liquid bridges between the powder particles, and subsequently aggregation takes place to produce larger granules. The evolution of particle size and the primary shaping mechanism in the TSG is limited due to the capacity of the extruder. Extensive studies have shown that granule size increases not only after the kneading zones but also upstream (before) suggesting there are not only two granule formation mechanisms such as the dispersive and distributive mixing. In the third mechanism, the built-up material before the kneading zone (flow restriction) is forced-mixed with the inbound powder due to the throughput force. As a result, the increase in the throughput (feeding) leads to the increase of granule size assuming there is enough granulating liquid to form large agglomerates.

Kumar et al. investigated the interrelations of the residence time and mixing settings over the quality of extruded granules [44]. The study demonstrated that the increase of kneading elements had no influence on the yield fraction despite the improvement of powder mixing and residence time. The same was observed by increasing the L/S ratio which resulted only in the formation of larger granules.

4 Twin-Screw Granulation

TSG is an advanced processing technology that has been extensively used for granule production over the last couple of decades [4]. Several studies have been reported related to TSG optimisation by investigating the effect of the formulation composition and operational variables such as screw configuration, pitch and length of conveying element, thickness and angle of kneading element, and influence of kneading blocks. A schematic diagram of a TSG line is illustrated in Fig. 7.

The first study for the development of pharmaceutical granules at a laboratory scale using a single-screw extruder was reported by Goodhart et al. [46]. The investigation was undertaken to evaluate various factors related to wet granulation such as the effect of granulating fluid, type of end plate, number of mixing anvils and screw speed. The studies were conducted to also understand the level of content uniformity during granulation. The use of water isopropanol as granulating fluid reduced the sugar solubility in the granulating fluid, creating increased torque

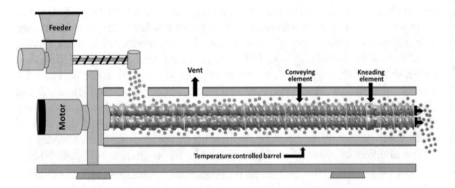

Fig. 7 Schematic representation of a continuous twin-screw granulation [45]

during high-speed processing. The granules prepared by using this granulating fluid resulted in the compression of less gritty and smoother tablets compared to water. It was concluded that the water isopropanol granulating fluid created processing interruption but produced granules with low bulk densities.

Later on, in 1986 Gamlen and Eardley introduced the twin-screw extruder in pharmaceutical research, to produce paracetamol extrudates with a combination of excipients, i.e. Avicel, lactose and/or hydroxypropyl methylcellulose (HPMC), and using water as a granulating fluid [47]. The results revealed that addition of HPMC in the formulation influenced significantly on the extrusion properties. HPMC helped to retain water in its interstitial spaces, reducing frictional forces between extruder and the plate. Micrographs of both extruded formulations with or without HPMC showed similar appearances. Hence, the addition of HPMC improved the extrudability without affecting the extrudate quality. A year later, Lundeberg and later Kleinebudde (1988) also employed twin-screw extruders for the formation of effervescent granules [48–52]. Furthermore, TSG has been implemented to perform dry, wet and melt granulation process [53] including scaling up of continuous granulation coupled with process analytical technologies (PAT) by applying quality by design (QbD) approaches [54].

Dhenge et al. conducted an empirical study on a TSE with model pharmaceutical formulations focused on the physical properties of the final granules [42]. The authors investigated the effect of screw speed, powder feed rate and liquid-to-solid (L/S) ratio on the residence time and torque which was found to affect the particle size, strength, shape and structure of the granules. The most pronounced effect on granule properties was observed with a liquid-to-solid (L/S) ratio of 0.4, showing a monomodal distribution of granule sizes with a peak around the 1000 μm mark. At higher L/S, the extra liquid caused an increase in the residence time of material in the granulator, resulting in a reduction of undersized and oversized granules. The granule's shape and hence the flow were improved due to the increased amount of granulating fluid which helped to achieve stronger liquid bridges between the particles. The powder feed rate influenced the transition and final state of granule properties such as size, shape, structure, porosity, strength and dissolution time. At low feed rate, the residence time became long, resulted in strong granules with an increased average granule size, whereas higher feed rate reduced the granule size. At a powder feed rate of 3.5 and 5 kg/h, the sphericity of the granules was found to be increased. The improved sphericity of granule was related to the increased filling at high powder feed rate which led to increase in shearing forces within the barrel and turned the processed powder to spherical agglomerates. The surface morphology of the granules became smooth by increasing the length of the screw while porosity was decreased. A high feed rate not only increased the granules' morphological strength and stability but also affected the dissolution rates. It was concluded that TSG optimisation is a complex process and is affected significantly by the critical processing parameters.

Vercruysse et al. investigated the operational parameters related to TSG and their effect on the manufacturing process using theophylline as model API [34]. There was no significant relationship of screw configuration and screw speed to the granules' morphology, but a high number of kneading elements and increased throughput resulted in higher torque during granulation. The high torque resulted in temperature rise in the barrel which led to reduced amount of fines and less friable granules. The binder was found to be more effective when it was dissolved in the granulating fluid. Increasing the number of kneading elements yielded denser granules with a longer disintegration time and dissolution rate. The findings of this work suggested that the granule and tablet quality can be optimised by adjusting specific process variables. Khorsheed et al. also investigated the effect of TSG processing parameters on the powder and granule and tablet properties [55] using microcrystalline cellulose (MCC) or mannitol C160. Their study showed increasing MCC granule size and strength can reduce tabletability and vice versa. Although mannitol C160 granules did not affect tabletability, particle size reduction has shown significant compactibility improvement. They found a correlation between the yield pressure, plastic and elastic work of the initial powders and changes in tabletability performance as a result of the granulation process. Authors mentioned that increasing the strength and size of granules may cause their reduction of the tabletability.

The granule structure is closely related to tablet's quality attributes, and it can be controlled by the selection of appropriate excipients as it was recently reported by Megarry et al. [56]. Allopurinol-granulated formulations were prepared by wet granulation using twin-screw and high shear processing. By using different mannitol grades (200SD and C160), it was found to present a polymorphic transition during processing, containing mostly β-mannitol. The 200SD granules presented needle-shaped morphology with high porosity and specific surface area, which led to poorer flow properties but higher tablet tensile strength. The study suggested that the understanding of specific excipient grade and their effect during processing is crucial to optimise tablet manufacturability.

Lute et al. investigated the influence of varying barrel fill levels on the mean residence time, granule properties and tensile strength of tables using MCC and lactose [57]. They reported that specific feed load or powder feed volume directly affects the granule size and shape. Increasing fill levels of MCC inside the extruder barrel caused shorter residence time along with decreased granule size. On the other hand, lactose maintained its granule size at all fill levels. Again, usage of specific pharma excipients and their processing parameters are crucial parts of the granulation optimisation process.

Twin-screw dry granulation is considered more effective for granule manufacturing as it limits heat exposure to only one-barrel zone, much shorter than melt granulation. Lui Y. et al. (2017) studied formulations containing different polymeric binders (AF15, Kollidon VA64, Soluplus, Kollidon SR), with glass transition temperature less than 130 °C [58]. Granulation of the primary powders with some degree of moisture was found to be beneficial for processed polymers with high glass transition temperatures. Selected polymer particles are more prone to soften and flow under frictional forces if their T_g was closer to the barrel zone temperature in the kneading section. A higher zone temperature highly increases the opportunities for successful granulations. Screw speed was a major cause for friction heating, while the kneading block offset was only minor in its influence on the granulation process. According to their results, higher screw speed tended to increase the particles size, producing bigger chunks (> 3350 μm). Conversely, an increase of moisture content in the excipient resulted in smaller particle size distribution. So, successful granulation can be achieved by varying the processing parameters, and preformulation studies will aid to quickly optimise the process.

Ye et al. (2019) used twin-screw dry granulation to improve the flow property of moisture-sensitive materials [59]. They produced dry granule formulations using four different APIs processed with Klucel, Ethocel and magnesium stearate for sustained release. A DoE was employed to determine the effect of different processing parameters, i.e. screw speed, feeding rate, barrel temperature and screw configuration on the product properties (flow properties, particle size distribution and dissolution time). It was revealed that an increased screw speed is related to a higher percentage of medium size granules while a negative correlation was found between the amount of large size granules and screw speed. This was attributed to the decrease of the mean residence time due to the high screw speeds and the subsequent reduction of the kneading effect on primary powders and the formation of smaller granules. Higher feeding rates improve the flow properties of the powders, and decreased angles of repose were obtained. The morphology of granules was affected by the powder flow where long stripe shape exhibited poor flowability compared to round-shaped particles. Finally, drug release was affected by the binder content in the granule and presented significant variations, i.e. large stronger granules with more binder showed relatively slow release. On the other hand, small amount soft binder provided less particle adhesion which resulted in faster disintegration and hence faster dissolution rates. The continuous processing and simplicity of operation, in the absence of milling, suggest that TSDG is more effective compared to other conventional dry granulation approaches.

Kallakunta et al. applied heat-assisted dry granulation using a twin-screw extruder to formulate sustained-release granules [60]. Granulation feasibility was studied with different binders (e.g. Klucel EF, Kollidon VA64), sustained-release agents (e.g. Klucel MF, Eudragit RSPO) and diluents at various drug loads. The processing conditions were below the melting point or glass transition temperature of the formulation ingredients. They have found a size correlation to the binding capacity of the excipient. Formulations with Klucel produced granules with a size of around 250 μm, whereas Kollidon VA64F promoted finer granules related to its own particle size (20 μm). Hence, the good binding properties of the ingredients in the formulation facilitated easier granule formation and larger granule size. On the other hand, formulations consisting of only Klucel MF showed very minimal erosion (approximately 5%) over 24 h. The drug release was found to be incomplete in these formulations, as the high viscosity of Klucel MF might be the reason for the low drug release profiles. The excellent binding properties and viscosity of Klucel MF resulted in dosage forms with good matrix integrity, which then became one of the controlling factors for drug release. Conversely, formulations with Kollidon are reported to undergo greater erosion which destabilised the tablet matrix and led to fast drug release. In summary, heat-assisted dry granulation could be applied for continuous twin-screw granulation, which may ameliorate the process constraints and stability problems in conventional granulation techniques.

Unlike wet and dry granulation, melt granulation offers several advantages for processing pharmaceutical actives. Twin-screw melt granulation is carried out at higher temperatures than traditional batch melt granulation, and thermoplastic polymers can be used as binders. This is a clear benefit, considering the limited number of traditional binders that are suitable for use in conventional granulation processes. The process of twin-screw melt granulation is also advantageous as it eliminates the need for organic solvents and water, while it is cost-effective and environmentally friendly. As a totally water-free process, twin-screw melt granulation is suitable for drugs that undergo hydrolysis or degradation in the presence of water.

Van Melkebeke et al. studied twin-screw melt granulation for the manufacturing of immediate release formulation using two grades of polyethylene glycol (PEG 400 and 4000) as a binder [20]. Authors described the importance of granulation temperature on its dissolution properties. A high yield and fast dissolution rate were obtained only at a processing temperature near the melting point of PEG. Post-granulation characterisations showed a homogeneous dispersion of the BCS class II drug within the polymeric matrix created a micro-environment around the drug particles enhancing the dissolution rate. Addition of small surfactant amounts (polysorbate 80 or Cremophor) helped to achieve a complete drug release within 10 min. A high drug content required more PEG content and surfactant to obtain 100% drug release.

Batra A. et al. investigated polymeric binders with high melting points (180 °C) for improving tabletability of pharmaceutical APIs using twin-screw melt granulation [61]. For the purposes of the study, metformin hydrochloride and acetaminophen were used as active ingredients and several polymers, i.e. hydroxypropyl cellulose, hydroxypropyl methylcellulose, polyvinylpyrrolidone and methacrylate-based polymers, including Klucel EXF, Eudragit EPO and Soluplus, as binders. The prepared granules demonstrated good tablet tensile strength with even as low as 10% w/w polymer concentrations. As the melting temperature of acetaminophen is below 180 °C, its TSG temperature was achieved at 130 °C, and even at that temperature, extruded granules provided acceptable compatibility of >2 MPa, suggesting that compressed tablets could withstand manufacturing and end-use stresses during coating, packaging, transportation and handling. The work demonstrated that a pool of polymeric binders can be successfully used for twin-screw melt granulation and further exploited in the future.

Unlike wet or dry granulation, in melt granulation the growth mechanism involves an additional nucleation mechanism known as immersion or distribution as shown in Fig. 8.

The mechanism was studied by Monteyne et al. for the development of immiscible drug-binder formulations [63]. They implemented thermal analysis, rheological characterisation and microscopic images to reach an in-depth understanding of material behaviour during agglomeration. They reported that the distribution of the binder in the immiscible blends caused a double T_g and a clear loss peak

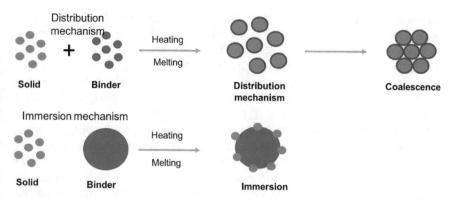

Fig. 8 Nucleation mechanism of melt granulation [62]

in the thermogram. The binder was found to act as a separate phase favouring efficient binder distribution where a thin binder layer with restricted mobility is formed on the surface of the primary drug particles during granulation. Then it is covered by a second layer with improved mobility when the binder concentration is sufficiently high. The granules manufactured with 20% (w/w) Soluplus or higher became smaller and more spherical as a function of temperature, whereas a lower binder concentration resulted in larger and more needle-shaped granules. The study showed strong evidence of the binder distribution during TSG strongly affected the granule characteristics.

In another study, the same group carried out TSG studies with Soluplus and metoprolol or caffeine [64]. In this case, thermal analysis showed only one T_g, indicating a highly miscible system. A high barrel temperature was used to process granules larger than 500 μm which also showed minimum torque fluctuation during granulation. Surprisingly, granules prepared with 20% or more binder concentration resulted in large aggregates at processing temperatures <90 °C. Prepared granules with caffeine-Soluplus blends remained broad size distribution over the different binder concentrations and were not affected by the process temperatures, whereas the granule size distribution of the MPT/SLP blends appeared narrower and shifted towards lower particle sizes with an elevated granulation temperature.

5 Twin-Screw Granulation and Continuous Manufacturing

Traditional manufacturing of medicinal products in the pharmaceutical industry uses batch processing, where every single unit operation is conducted separately. The adoption of continuous manufacturing (CM) from pharmaceutical industry is relatively new, and it takes place in a stepwise manner. On the other hand, food, petrochemical, polymer and oil refining industries have been undertaking continuous manufacturing operations for decades [13, 14, 65, 66] and produce large volume production at a cost-effective manner. The term 'continuous' means a required process may run for an extended period, with raw material constantly fed into the process. The pharmaceutical industry has faced many obstacles in attempting such a continuous production method on a day-to-day basis. The main perceived issue is the industry's rigid structure, because of the strict supervision of regulatory agencies such as the FDA in the USA or the European Medicines Agency (EMA) in Europe [67, 68]. Despite the fact that there are no regulatory hurdles for implementing continuous processes, pharmaceutical industry needs to reform regulatory framework, pharmaceutical equipment design and operation.

Some pharmaceutical companies plan to convert 70% of their production lines to continuous manufacturing to allow a more efficient product and process development as part of the product operation. Nevertheless, twin-screw granulation is an ideal example of such a process that has successfully been introduced for CM production. Recently, GEA introduced a continuous platform for oral solid dosage forms which integrates multiple operation units comprising of granulation, drying and tablet compression. As shown in Fig. 9, the process involves the dosing and mixing of raw materials using multiple feeders, followed by the high shear granulator for mixing, wetting and granulation through the coupling with a highly accurate dosing system (e.g. water, solvents, binder solutions). Subsequently the granules are continuously transferred (e.g. vacuum or gravity) to a fluidised bed dryer for drying and milled to achieve the desired particle size and content uniformity. The drying process is monitored with an on-line moisture LightHouse probe. Prior to tablet compression in a rotary tablet press, the dried powders are blended with the external phase (e.g. lubricants, disintegrants, fillers). The tablet press comprises of six compression modes such as compression to equal porosity, exchangeable compression module with a wash-off-line capability which are coupled with advanced in-line PAT sensors and a control system. The technology is versatile, and processed amounts vary from 500 g for R&D purposes up to 100 kg/h.

A similar processing technology known as MODCOS has been developed by Glatt for the conversion of the batch mode to a continuous fluid bed system. As shown in Fig. 10, loss in weight feeders is used for the dosing of the active drug substance and excipients through vacuum conveyor in a twin-screw extruder to produce medium- to high-density granules. The wet granules are pneumatically conveyed into the process insert of the fluid bed via a specially designed transfer line, where they are continuously dried to the required moisture level. Before the granules are compressed in tablets with other ingredients, a dry mixer is used to achieve homogeneous mixing. A key advantage of the MODCOS line is the narrow retention time distribution during drying, while a sophisticated discharge system facilitates complete emptying of the process chambers and thus prevents any cross-contamination with consistent product quality. The continuous line is coupled with a range of PAT tools including two NIR probes to determine content uniformity at the end of the extruder or the discharge system. A moisture probe is used at the fluid bed dryer discharge point and particle size probe at the powder discharge (feeders).

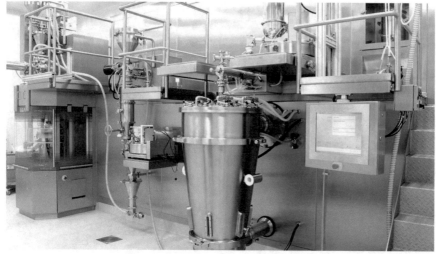

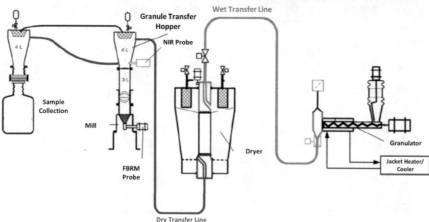

Fig. 9 ConsiGma continuous high shear granulation process by GEA

A unique feature of the continuous line is the intelligent control system where all the process parameters are controlled together and continuously monitored to provide the basis for automatic process control. The manufacturing process is controlled by recipes which include the distribution of residence times, while the data for all process units can be displayed as tables of graphs.

In batch manufacturing of solid dosage form, there is a limited process under-standing and control which requires the application of more intensive and advanced manufacturing processes. Continuous granulation processing is fully automated, and thus scale-up issues related to batch manufacturing are no longer encountered. Often in batch granulation the active substances tend to agglomerate especially when they present highly cohesive properties. This problem can be easily mitigated in

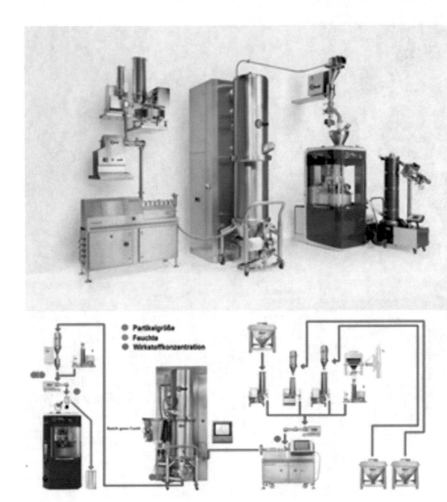

Fig. 10 MODCOS continuous high shear granulation process by Glatt

continuous granulation by combining high shear co-milling of the drug substances and excipients followed by low-shear blending. The powder blends are immediately compressed to produce tablets and unlike batch processing do not allow time for particles to re-agglomerate. CM lines can be built in a flexible way for the processing of multiple formulations (products) through careful consideration and optimal design. Continuous granulation lines can be easily adopted for both dry and wet processing which eventually results in a good return on the initial investment. Other advantages of continuous granulation processing include the following:

- Enhanced development approach by implementing QbD approaches and incorporating PAT tools.
- Reduce risk of manufacturing failure and prevent drug shortages.

- Decrease the risk of out-of-specification failures both for intermediates and finished products.
- Flexibility by using the same system to develop a manufacturing process.
- Effect on supply chain by increasing supply speed and reacting to market demands.
- Agility and reduced scale-up efforts.
- Real-time quality assurance-secure quality attributes and measure critical quality parameters.
- Reduction of capital and operational costs and environmentally friendly.
- Cost reductions in R&D, product transfer and productivity.
- Reduced system's footprint.

5.1 Regulatory Aspects

The business of pharmaceutical industry and its regulatory environments are constantly evolving. Regulatory authorities are continuously reviewing their guidelines for the pharmaceuticals to achieve a continuous manufacturing process to understand the processing parameters and better monitoring of the production line. All these guidelines suggest continuous processing will be a key manufacturing approach for pharmaceuticals in the near future. This should allow a greater degree of control over the processing parameters during production.

Advances are also accompanied by worldwide regulatory initiatives, such as the FDA (Food and Drug Administration) and the ICH (International Conference on Harmonization). According to ICH Q8, quality is defined as 'The suitability of either a drug substance or drug product for its intended use and this term includes such attributes as the identity, strength and purity' [69]. The ICH Q8 provides an idea of the documentation process of the shear knowledge acquired during product and process development which can be used to analyse the product quality. It suggests that quality cannot be tested into a product; instead quality should be present due to the design of the product and process and testing is merely a method to confirm this.

The pharmaceutical industry relies on innovation and manufacturing development, where a quality by test (QbT) system is applied to maintain product quality using the following steps: raw material tests, fixed drug manufacturing processes and finished product tests. However, the development of the quality by design (QbD) concept, implemented by regulatory agencies, introduces higher level of product and process understanding but also potential regulatory flexibility. Hence, it can lead to increased successes rate in the development of finished products, process robustness, less manufacturing deviations and failed/reworked batches. In addition, it promotes easy of post-approval changes and real-time release testing with lower costs and cycle times. The QbD concept was first introduced by the quality pioneer Joseph M. Juran who introduced asset of universal processing steps to establish quality goals in order to avoid the loss of market share, failure of finished products and waste as a result of poor product quality planning [70].

Over the years, pharmaceutical QbD has been developed with the issuance of a series of guidelines such as ICH Q8 (pharmaceutical development), ICH Q9 (quality risk management), ICH Q10 (pharmaceutical quality system) and ICH Q11 (development and manufacture of drug substances) [69, 71–73]. Also, the FDA took notice of developments in other industries that are using continuous manufacturing to increase processing efficiency. Application of QbD approach into the pharmaceutical industry will certainly ensure improved pharmaceutical drug quality and safety and to achieve a desired pharmaceutical manufacturing process on the basis of scientific and engineering knowledge [74].

5.2   Quality by Design (QbD)

Quality by design (QbD) is defined in ICH Q8 guidelines as 'A systemic approach to development that begins with predefined objectives and emphasizes product and process understanding and process control, based on sound science and quality risk management' [69]. Widely accepted elements of the foregoing QbD are as follows: quality target product profile (QTPP), critical quality attributes (CQAs), critical material attributes (CMAs) and critical process parameters (CPPs). The definitions of theses parameters are described below [69, 75].

Quality target product profile (QTPP). This is a prospective summary of the quality characteristics of a drug product such as dosage form, delivery systems, dosage strength, etc. The dosage strength and container closure system of the drug product have to be taken into account because these directly involve pharmacokinetics properties (e.g. dissolution) of the drug and drug product quality criteria (e.g. sterility, purity, stability).

Critical quality attributes (CQAs). Critical quality attributes are included with physical, chemical, biological or microbiological properties or characteristics of an output material including finished product. A potential CQA stipulation for a drug product derived from QTPP involves guidance relating to product and process development within an appropriate limit, range or distribution to ensure the desired product quality.

Critical material attributes (CMAs). This is included with the physical, chemical, biological or microbiological properties or characteristics of an input material. To ensure the desired quality of the drug substances, excipients or in-process materials, CMAs should be within an appropriate limit, range or distribution.

Critical process parameters (CPPs). This parameter helps to monitor before or in-process quality that influences the appearance, impurity and yield of the final product.

Steps for QbD implementation:

- Define the desired performances of the product and identity the QTPPS.
- Identify the CQAs.
- Identify possible CMAs and CPPs.

- Set up and execute the design of space, which is linked to CMAs, CPPs and also CQAs and to obtain enough information of how these parameters impact on QTPP. Hence, a process design space should be defined and lead to an end product with the desired QTPP.
- Identify and control the sources of variability from the raw materials and the manufacturing process.
- Continually monitor and improve the manufacturing process to assure consistent product quality.

Upon understanding the elements and the steps for QbD implementation, it is important to be familiar with the commonly used tools in QbD which is based on the science underlying the design and the science of manufacturing. This includes design of experiment (DoE), process analytical technology (PAT) and risk assessment [69].

5.3   Design of Experiment (DoE)

A design of experiment is an excellent tool, which allows pharmaceutical scientists to determine the relationship among factors that influence the output of a process. This methodology was first reported by Fisher in his book *The Design of Experiment* [76]. The application of DoE in QbD helps to gain the maximum information about a pharmaceutical process, factors affecting the raw material attributes (e.g. particle size) and process parameters (e.g. screw speed, time) which helps to reduce the number of experiments required involved in quality attributes such as blend uniformity, tablet hardness, thickness and friability. It is almost impossible to assess each operation individually because each unit operation has many different input and output variables as well as process parameters. Thus, the results are investigated by DoE and help to identify optimal conditions, the critical factors that influence most CQAs and those which do not as well as the existence of interactions and synergies between factors [77].

5.4   QbD Approaches in Twin-Screw Granulation

The benefits of using QbD approaches in pharmaceutical manufacturing have been recognised and promoted by regulatory bodies such as the Food and Drug Administration (FDA) combined with PAT principles and closed loop quality assurance. Continuous manufacturing lines have been implemented in pharmaceutical industry such as the drug product Orkambi by Vertex for the treatment of cystic fibrosis in 2015. There are only a few studies in literature related to QbD approaches coupled with PAT tools related to twin-screw granulation.

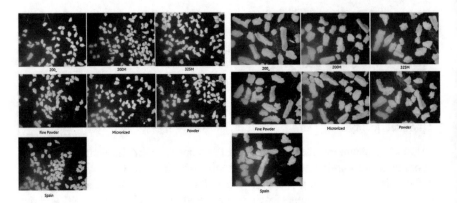

Fig. 11 Pictures of two sieve fractions of the seven granule loads (500–710 μm and 1000–1400 μm)

The first report was conducted by Fonteyene et al. (2014) who investigated the effects of variation in raw material properties on the CQAs of granules produced by wet granulation followed by tableting [78]. By using a powder-to-tablet wet granulation line, a model formulation of theophylline–lactose–PVP (30%–67.5%–2.5%) was investigated while the process parameters are kept steady. For the purposes of the study, seven grades of theophylline were processed, and the features of granules/tablets were evaluated. The granule particle size for all experiments showed a bimodal distribution with granules being in-spec containing either large amounts of fines (>150 μm) or large amounts of oversized particles (>1400 μm). The differences were directly correlated to the initial particle size of the theophylline grade. The granules obtained with fine powders presented higher bulk density and lower tapped density compared to the initial powder blend suggesting that no tapped volume reduction can be produced when granule powders have high tapped densities.

As shown in Fig. 11, the granule morphology showed needle-shaped, while for the small size fractions, more spherical particles were observed without however having been able to identify any differences for the granules of the various theophylline grades.

PCA applied for the content uniformity showed that smaller granules present more lactose monohydrate while larger granules more theophylline. The investigations on the processability showed that theophylline powders play a key role in feeding with large powders pushing the injectors out of the granulator barrel. Regarding the tableting process, a direct relation between the granule size and compression forces was observed with small size fractions (<150 μm) require higher compaction forces.

Maniruzzaman et al. applied a QbD approach by introducing for the first time a design of experiment to investigate the effect of formulation composition in a wet extrusion granulation process [79]. Twin-screw granulation was conducted by using blends of polymer/inorganic excipients (hydroxypropyl methylcellulose and magnesium aluminometasilicate–MAS) as carriers and PEG as the binder to produce ibuprofen granules. The MAS/polymer ratio, PEG amount (binder) and liquid-to-solid (L/S) ratios were set as the independent variables and the dissolution rates, mean particle size, the dissolution rates, mean particle size and the loss on drying (LoD) of the extruded granules (D_{50}) and the loss on drying (LoD) of the extruded granules as the dependent variables. The morphology of the obtained granules appeared spherical for all processed batches compared to the needle-shaped IBU with the D_{50} particle size varying from 100 to 300 µm. Dynamic vapour sorption analysis showed a reversible water uptake of all batches and provided evidence that the inorganic excipient prevents significant water uptake. The content uniformity was assessed using confocal Raman mapping and demonstrated excellent ibuprofen distribution within the granules which was partially amorphous as a result of the processing during twin-screw granulation. The DoE analysis revealed that the PEG amounts and the L/S ratio had a significant effect on both the ibuprofen release and the LOD. The granule particle size distribution was found to be affected significantly by the MAS/polymer ratios but also the binder amounts.

The same group conducted an identical study by using a DoE to investigate the effect of the excipient composition, binder amount and liquid-to-solid (L/S) ratio (independent variables) on drug dissolution rates, median particle size diameter and specific surface area (dependent variables), shown in Fig. 12 [80]. This time ethanol was used as granulating liquid instead of water.

The use of a different liquid resulted in the formation of larger granules with D_{50} varying from 200 to 583 µm. For most of the batches, a monomodal particle size distribution was obtained, while the granule morphology appeared spherical as before. This time all independent variables were found to have a significant effect on the drug dissolution rates and particle size distribution, while the two-way interactions identified after the data integration suggested a complex granulation process.

The granule's specific surface area was only affected by the MAS/polymer ratios and the PEG amounts at a significant level. Interestingly the water-insoluble ibuprofen demonstrated relatively fast release rates with 2 h (pH 1.2) due to the increased amorphous content which resulted due to the solubilisation effect of ethanol and the drug absorption within the porous network of the inorganic magnesium aluminometasilicate excipient.

Another comprehensive study was conducted by Grymonpre et al., who investigated the impact of critical process parameters (CPPs) and critical material parameters (CMPs) on the CQAs in twin-screw melt granulation process followed by milling and tableting of the formed granules [81]. Two active substances, acetaminophen (APAP) and hydrochlorothiazide (HCT), were co-processed with a range of hydrophilic polymers such as Kollidon VA64, Soluplus (SOL), Eudragit EPO and Affinisol grades (15 LV, 4 M). The processing temperatures were affected by the glass transition of the binders, and for the HPMC grades, higher temperatures were used due to their complex viscosities.

The milled granules presented lower moisture content (<1%) with regular shape and good flowability. More fines were received when EPO and Affinisol were used

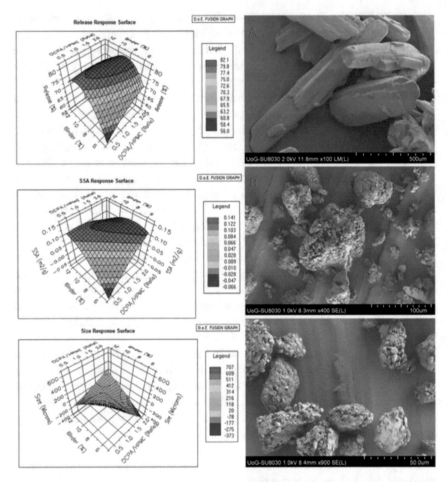

Fig. 12 Response surface plots of IBU release, specific surface area and particle size distribution dependent variables (left). SEM images of (**a**) bulk IBU, (**b**) F2 granules (DCPA/Polymer 1.0, Binder 8.0%, L/S ratio 0.30) and (**c**) F10 granules (DCPA/Polymer 1.0, Binder 8.0%, L/S ratio 0.30) (right)

as binders, but overall, all polymers were suitable for melt granulation processing. SOL and VA64 outperform the rest of the binders due to their high milling efficiency and resistance to form fines. Compatibility studies showed identical performance for both drugs irrespective of the polymeric binder. The tabletability studies (Fig. 13) showed significant improvement of melt granulated products compared to physical mixtures. The T_g of the polymer was found to affect the extrusion processing especially for VA64 which resulted in increased torque, while binders with low T_g (e.g. SOL, EPO) facilitated a smoother granulation process. Similarly, the tableting process was also affected by the binder grade where EPO showed less fragmentation and higher elastic deformation during tablet compaction in comparison with SOL

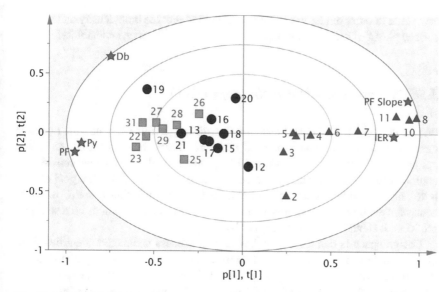

Fig. 13 PC1 vs. PC2 bi-plot of the determined compaction properties (loadings) for the experimental runs of the DoE (scores). The numbers represent corresponding experimental run of HCT-EPO formulations (*blue triangles*), HCTSOL formulations (*dark red circles*) and HCT-VA64 formulations (*orange boxes*), plotted against loadings (*star shaped*) for which PF represents the plasticity factor, IER the anti-correlated in-die elastic recovery, PF slope the slope of the plasticity factor over four compaction pressures, Py the Heckel value and Db the fragmentation factor

and VA64. Overall, the study demonstrated that twin-screw melt granulation was robust for both low and high drug loading processes and CQAs were well identified.

In another study the same group applied a QbD methodology by using the continuous ConsiGma extrusion line to investigate the formulation optimisation of twin-screw granulated composition of various binary filler/binder grades and ratios. By using multiple linear regression models, the authors were able to understand the impact of the filler/binder properties on the granule and tablet CQAs. A DoE with 27 batches was combined with PCA plot to reduced large data sets and used to identify similarities or differences of materials with different chemical characteristics. The overall scope of the study was to identify the impact of materials on CQAs and consequently develop predicting formulation models with suitable characteristics for the processing of APIs with unfavourable properties. For example, the study demonstrated that the granule particle size was not affected by the original particle size or the water uptake of the filler. The granule flowability was found to be affected by the binder higher concentration amounts but not of the filler properties. The granule friability was decreased when PVP was used at higher concentrations. Finally, the tabletability was not affected by the grade of the filler which showed no impact at all. On the contrary the binder grade and the use of higher PVP concentrations demonstrated a significant effect on the improved tabletability. When compared to other binder grades, it was identified that the bulk density and specific surface play a role on the deformation mechanisms and hence tabletability.

5.5   Process Analytical Technology (PAT)

PAT is defined as 'Tools and systems that utilize, analyze and control real-time measurements of raw and processed materials during manufacturing, to ensure optimal processing condition are used to produce final product that consistently conforms to established quality and performance standards' [71]. The goal of PAT is to enhance understanding of and control the manufacturing process, which is consistent with our current drug quality system. So, quality cannot be tested into products; it should either be built-in or by design.

Design space is defined by the key critical process parameters identified from process characterisation studies and their acceptable ranges. These parameters are the primary focus of on-, in- or at-line PAT applications [74]. In most cases, spectroscopic techniques, such as Raman spectroscopy, UV-Vis spectroscopy and NMR (nuclear magnetic resonance), are commonly used. Besides the foregoing, near-infrared spectroscopy (NIR) [82], nano metric temperature measurement (MTM) [83] and tunable diode laser absorption spectroscopy (TDLAS) are widely applied tools in the pharmaceutical manufacturing field and play important roles in real-time monitoring of the processes used. Among these, NIR has drawn great attention in industry because it is a rapid, non-invasive analytical technique, and there is no need for extensive sample preparation [84–87]. In most research, it is used for the identification and characterisation of raw materials and intermediates, analysis of dosage forms, manufacturing and prediction of one or more variables in the process line or the final product stream(s) on the basis of on-line, in-line or at-line spectroscopic measurement [88]. The fast growth of interest in QbD and its tools DoE, PAT and risk assessment approaches makes the QbD available and feasible to the pharmaceutical field to achieve a better understanding of the material and process parameters used.

5.6   Process Analytical Technology (PAT) in Extrusion Granulation

The framework of PAT is intended to support innovation and efficiency in pharmaceutical processes, manufacturing and quality assurance [89]. This includes systems that can be employed to design, analyse and control manufacturing by measuring critical quality and performance attributes in a timely manner. This involves measurements of raw and in-process materials aiming to ensure the quality of the finished products. PAT is not only away to implement real-time release testing but also to effectively detect failures and help understand the manufacturing processes. Due to the versatility of PAT tools, relevant information can be obtained by monitoring a range of physical, chemical and biological attributes. This can be achieved mainly by four key components which include:

- Multivariate tools for design, data acquisition and analysis which helps to build scientific understanding and identify CPPs and CMAs which eventually leads to process understanding while the generated information is integrated into the process control.
- Process analytical chemistry tools can effectively provide real-time and in situ data for the processed materials and process. The process measurements can also be near real time (e.g. on-, in- and at-line) in an invasive or non-invasive manner.
- Process monitoring and control involves the design of process controls and development of mathematical relations that provide adjustments to achieve control of all critical attributes.
- Continuous process optimisation and knowledge management relate to data collection and analysis from generated databases over the life cycle of the finished product.

PAT tools have been successfully implemented in continuous wet granulation production line, namely, ConsiGma developed by GAE Pharma [90]. The process consists of five locations where the critical quality attributes are measured. The first and the third measure the blend uniformity of the processed powders and the moisture content of the dried granules, while the second monitors the moisture distribution of the formed granules. A NIR sensor is coupled to the first location to allow accurate control of the powder feeding and blending and if possible to provide feedback for controlling blending operations [91–94]. Similarly, NIR probes were used to measure the moisture content and distribution.

Fonteyne et al. introduced a combination of PAT tools by using Raman, NIR and photometric imaging technique for the evaluation of the powder-to-tablet ConsiGma production line [95]. The aim of the study was to acquire solid-state information and granule size distribution data and in turn use them to predict a range of granule properties such as moisture content, bulk/tapped density and flowability. As shown in Fig. 14, the Raman and NIR spectra were collected to apply principal component analysis (PCA) and determine whether the formed granules contained theophylline monohydrate. Similarly, a PC plot was used to analyse all data collected through 11 DoE experiments when using the FlashSizer 3D process for the estimation of granule size and particle distribution.

The same group conducted a separate study in order to obtain an in-depth understanding of the twin-screw extrusion granulation and fluidised bed drying processes by using Batch Statistical Process Monitoring (BSPM) principles [96]. For the purposes of the study, the group implemented multivariate data analysis in terms of PCA, partial least squares regression and its various extensions such as multiblock PCA/PLS and orthogonal PLS. The work demonstrated how multivariate data analysis can be routinely used to generate data from the variable monitored by

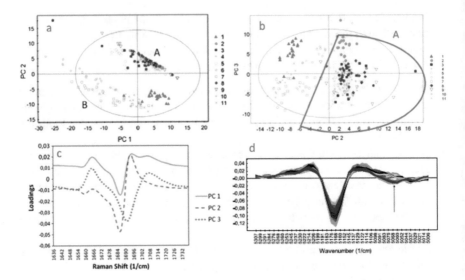

Fig. 14 (**a**) Raman spectra, PC 1 (47.12%) versus PC 2 (26.95%) scores plot; (**b**) Raman spectra, PC 2 (26.95%) versus PC 3 (16.24%) scores plot; (**c**) Raman spectroscopy, PC A loadings plots of PC 1, PC 2 and PC 3; (**d**) NIR spectroscopy, second derivative of NIR spectra. Coloured applied as above for Cluster A (*dashed line*) and Cluster B (*full line*)

the univariate sensors for a continuous granulation process and also how the BSMP concepts are used to monitor variables in order to identify operational variations.

Madarász et al. studied real-time feedback control of twin-screw wet granulation by using dynamic image analysis [97]. In a typical granulation process of lactose and starch blends, a process camera was coupled with image analysis to monitor the particle size distribution of the obtained granules. The real-time feedback control was implemented by controlling the feeding rate of the granulating liquid (peristaltic pump) through a PC.

As shown in Fig. 15, the image analysis software consisted of three main stages:

(a) Preprocessing: Greyscale filter and binarisation.
(b) Post-processing: Excluding particles on the edges of the image, edge detection and removing noise.
(c) Analysing and classification: Particle count, determining particle characteristics (minimum and maximum calliper diameter, aspect ratio), classification and summarisation.

The peristaltic pump is controlled through the image analysis software by using a manual RPM or an auto mode (Fig. 16) where the software controls the pump's rotation speed via a P controller. By setting the desired granule particle size (e.g. D_{50}: 1200 μm), the granulation process was tested by simulating different

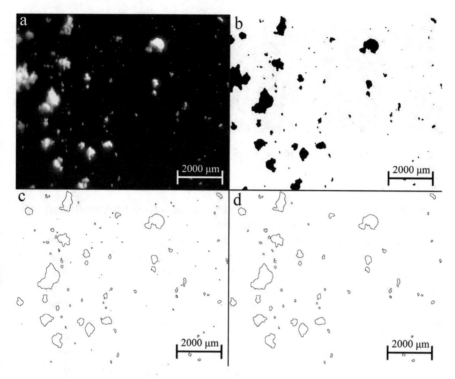

Fig. 15 Stages of image processing: (**a**) raw image; (**b**) preprocessing; (**c**), (**d**) post-processing

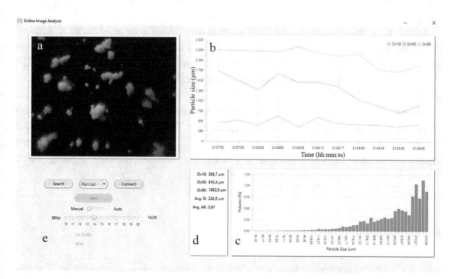

Fig. 16 User interface of the developed online image analysis software. (**a**) Current picture being analysed (**b**) Dv10, Dv50 and Dv90 over time (**c**) Particle size distribution (**d**) Current particle size and average diameter (**e**) Control panel for the peristaltic pump

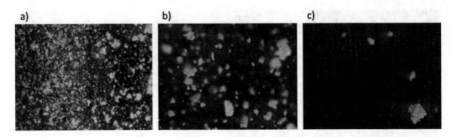

Fig. 17 Representative images captured during experiments using 7KE90 configuration at L/S ratio of 0.15 (**a**), 0.25 (**b**), 0.30 (**c**)

events including system startup and pump malfunction. Eventually the system could automatically adjust the granule particle size at the set value.

In-line monitoring via image analysis was carried out by Sayun et al., who used a twin-screw granulator with two different screw configurations and various liquid-to-solid (L/S) ratios [98]. The real-time high-speed imaging system features a red–green–blue light that targets the sample creating 3D images and can record particles with size distributions from 50 to 3000 μm. The work revealed that the fraction of fines increased with increasing L/S ratio suing both screw configurations.

It was also found that the screw configuration imparts a strong effect on the granule porosity while increases in L/S ratio result in decreasing porosity. The authors observed that the small window of imaging (Fig. 17 for capturing granule particles) resulted in measurement fluctuations originated from powder and liquid feeding methods. The recorded d10 values presented less variations compared to d50 and d90 but were prone to L/S variations.

Rehrl et al. introduced the concept of using soft PAT sensor in order to control the three different continuous processing lines such as hot melt extrusion, direct compression and wet granulation [99]. By measuring the concentration of the API at specific locations using NIR probes, for example, directly after granulation, it was able to predict the concentration of the drug in the feeder. The concentration prediction from on-line spectral measurements (at specific regions) can be done by constructing calibration curves at various w/w % and combined PLS regression models. The developed PLS model had a R^2 of 98.3% and validation experiments carried out at flow rates of 20–20 kg/h. The experiments revealed the dependence of the wet granulation process on the feeder excitation.

6 Conclusions

Despite the fact that twin-screw granulation is a relatively new process in pharmaceutical industry, it represents an excellent paradigm of pharmaceutical processing that combines principles of QbD and PAT monitoring for process control and quality while translating the existing batch processing to continuous manufacturing.

However, there is still a lack of adequate association between the experimental findings and theoretical prediction regarding material transport and kinetics in twin-screw granulation. Nevertheless, TSG is one of the few pharmaceutical processes that has proved its potential and applicability for the commercialisation of finished products through the implementation of continuous manufacturing.

References

1. D.M. Parikh, Handbook of pharmaceutical granulation technology, CRC Press, 2016.
2. G.M. Walker, Chapter 4 Drum Granulation Processes, in: A.D. Salman, M.J. Hounslow, J.P.K.B.T.-H. of P.T. Seville (Eds.), Granulation, Elsevier Science B.V., 2007: pp. 219–254.
3. G.K. Bolhuis, H. de Waard, Compaction properties of directly compressible materials, Pharm. Powder Compact. Technol. 2 (2011) 154.
4. T.C. Seem, N.A. Rowson, A. Ingram, Z. Huang, S. Yu, M. de Matas, I. Gabbott, G.K. Reynolds, Twin screw granulation—A literature review, Powder Technol. 276 (2015) 89–102.
5. M.E. Aulton, K. Taylor, Pharmaceutical preformulation, Aulton's Pharm. Des. Manuf. Med. Elsevie r Heal. Sci. Edinburgh. (2013).
6. M.E. Aulton, Pharmaceutics. The Science of Dosage Form Design. 2nd edn. Churchill Livingstone, (2005).
7. J. Rantanen, J. Khinast, The future of pharmaceutical manufacturing sciences, J. Pharm. Sci. 104 (2015) 3612–3638.
8. S. Mascia, P.L. Heider, H. Zhang, R. Lakerveld, B. Benyahia, P.I. Barton, R.D. Braatz, C.L. Cooney, J.M.B. Evans, T.F. Jamison, End-to-end continuous manufacturing of pharmaceuticals: integrated synthesis, purification, and final dosage formation, Angew. Chemie Int. Ed. 52 (2013) 12359–12363.
9. R. Lakerveld, B. Benyahia, P.L. Heider, H. Zhang, A. Wolfe, C.J. Testa, S. Ogden, D.R. Hersey, S. Mascia, J.M.B. Evans, The application of an automated control strategy for an integrated continuous pharmaceutical pilot plant, Org. Process Res. Dev. 19 (2015) 1088–1100.
10. R. Lakerveld, B. Benyahia, R.D. Braatz, P.I. Barton, Model-based design of a plant-wide control strategy for a continuous pharmaceutical plant, AIChE J. 59 (2013) 3671–3685.
11. H. Mangal, M. Kirsolak, P. Kleinebudde, Roll compaction/dry granulation: Suitability of different binders, Int. J. Pharm. 503 (2016) 213–219.
12. R. Singh, M. Ierapetritou, R. Ramachandran, An engineering study on the enhanced control and operation of continuous manufacturing of pharmaceutical tablets via roller compaction, Int. J. Pharm. 438 (2012) 307–326.
13. P. Kleinebudde, Roll compaction/dry granulation: pharmaceutical applications, Eur. J. Pharm. Biopharm. 58 (2004) 317–326.
14. Y. Funakoshi, T. Asogawa, E. Satake, The use of a novel roller compactor with a concavo-convex roller pair to obtain uniform compacting pressure, Drug Dev. Ind. Pharm. 3 (1977) 555–573.
15. S.M. Iveson, J.D. Litster, K. Hapgood, B.J. Ennis, Nucleation, growth and breakage phenomena in agitated wet granulation processes: a review, Powder Technol. 117 (2001) 3–39.
16. C. Wang, S. Hu, C.C. Sun, Expedited development of a high dose orally disintegrating metformin tablet enabled by sweet salt formation with acesulfame, Int. J. Pharm. 532 (2017) 435–443.
17. L. Cai, L. Farber, D. Zhang, F. Li, J. Farabaugh, A new methodology for high drug loading wet granulation formulation development, Int. J. Pharm. 441 (2013) 790–800.
18. S.-H. Kim, K.-M. Hwang, C.-H. Cho, T.-T. Nguyen, S.H. Seok, K.-M. Hwang, J.-Y. Kim, C.-W. Park, Y.-S. Rhee, E.-S. Park, Application of continuous twin screw granulation for the metformin hydrochloride extended release formulation, Int. J. Pharm. 529 (2017) 410–422.

19. P. Thapa, J. Tripathi, S.H. Jeong, Recent trends and future perspective of pharmaceutical wet granulation for better process understanding and product development, Powder Technol. 344 (2019) 864–882.

20. B. Van Melkebeke, B. Vermeulen, C. Vervaet, J.P. Remon, Melt granulation using a twin-screw extruder: a case study, Int. J. Pharm. 326 (2006) 89–93.

21. B. Mu, M.R. Thompson, Examining the mechanics of granulation with a hot melt binder in a twin-screw extruder, Chem. Eng. Sci. 81 (2012) 46–56.

22. J.M. Keen, C.J. Foley, J.R. Hughey, R.C. Bennett, V. Jannin, Y. Rosiaux, D. Marchaud, J.W. McGinity, Continuous twin screw melt granulation of glyceryl behenate: development of controlled release tramadol hydrochloride tablets for improved safety, Int. J. Pharm. 487 (2015) 72–80.

23. T. Monteyne, J. Vancoillie, J.-P. Remon, C. Vervaet, T. De Beer, Continuous melt granulation: Influence of process and formulation parameters upon granule and tablet properties, Eur. J. Pharm. Biopharm. 107 (2016) 249–262.

24. H.F. Mark, J.I. Kroschwitz, Encyclopedia of polymer science and engineering, 1985.

25. J. Breitenbach, Melt extrusion: from process to drug delivery technology, Eur. J. Pharm. Biopharm. 54 (2002) 107–117.

26. D. Ridhurkar, A. Vajdai, Z. Zsigmond, Hot-melt extrusion (HME) and its application for pharmacokinetic improvement of poorly water soluble drugs., Pharmacol. Toxicol. Biomed. Reports. 2 (2016).

27. C. Martin, Guidelines for Operation of Leistritz Twinscrew Extruder, Am. Leistritz Corp. Somerv. (2001) 21–25.

28. M. Maniruzzaman, D. Douroumis, S.J. Boateng, J.M. Snowden, Hot-melt extrusion (HME): from process to pharmaceutical applications, Recent Adv. Nov. Drug Carr. Syst. (2012).

29. P.S. Johnson, Developments in extrusion science and technology, Rubber Chem. Technol. 56 (1983) 575–593.

30. M. Mollan, Historical overview, DRUGS Pharm. Sci. 133 (2003) 1–18.

31. P. Pitayachaval, P. Watcharamaisakul, A review of a machine design of chocolate extrusion based co-rotating twin screw extruder, in: IOP Conf. Ser. Mater. Sci. Eng., IOP Publishing, 2019: p. 12012.

32. W. Thiele, Twin-screw extrusion and screw design, DRUGS Pharm. Sci. 133 (2003) 69–98.

33. I. Ghebre-Sellassie, I. Ghebre-Selassie, C.E. Martin, F. Zhang, J. DiNunzio, C. Martin, Melt-Extruded Molecular Dispersions, in: Pharm. Extrus. Technol., CRC Press, 2003: pp. 264–279.

34. J. Vercruysse, D.C. Díaz, E. Peeters, M. Fonteyne, U. Delaet, I. Van Assche, T. De Beer, J.P. Remon, C. Vervaet, Continuous twin screw granulation: influence of process variables on granule and tablet quality, Eur. J. Pharm. Biopharm. 82 (2012) 205–211.

35. M.R. Thompson, S. Weatherley, R.N. Pukadyil, P.J. Sheskey, Foam granulation: new developments in pharmaceutical solid oral dosage forms using twin screw extrusion machinery, Drug Dev. Ind. Pharm. 38 (2012) 771–784.

36. K.E. Rocca, S. Weatherley, P.J. Sheskey, M.R. Thompson, Influence of filler selection on twin screw foam granulation, Drug Dev. Ind. Pharm. 41 (2015) 35–42.

37. U. Shah, Use of a modified twin-screw extruder to develop a high-strength tablet dosage form, Pharm. Technol. 29 (2005) 52–66.

38. D. Djuric, P. Kleinebudde, Impact of screw elements on continuous granulation with a twin-screw extruder, J. Pharm. Sci. 97 (2008) 4934–4942.

39. R.M. Dhenge, J.J. Cartwright, M.J. Hounslow, A.D. Salman, Twin screw granulation: Steps in granule growth, Int. J. Pharm. 438 (2012) 20–32.

40. M.R. Thompson, J. Sun, Wet granulation in a twin-screw extruder: Implications of screw design, J. Pharm. Sci. 99 (2010) 2090–2103.

41. M.R. Thompson, K.P. O'Donnell, "Rolling" phenomenon in twin screw granulation with controlled-release excipients, Drug Dev. Ind. Pharm. 41 (2015) 482–492.

42. R.M. Dhenge, R.S. Fyles, J.J. Cartwright, D.G. Doughty, M.J. Hounslow, A.D. Salman, Twin screw wet granulation: Granule properties, Chem. Eng. J. 164 (2010) 322–329.

43. R. Sayin, A.S. El Hagrasy, J.D. Litster, Distributive mixing elements: towards improved granule attributes from a twin screw granulation process, Chem. Eng. Sci. 125 (2015) 165–175.
44. A. Kumar, M. Alakarjula, V. Vanhoorne, M. Toiviainen, F. De Leersnyder, J. Vercruysse, M. Juuti, J. Ketolainen, C. Vervaet, J.P. Remon, Linking granulation performance with residence time and granulation liquid distributions in twin-screw granulation: An experimental investigation, Eur. J. Pharm. Sci. 90 (2016) 25–37.
45. N. Kittikunakorn, T. Liu, F. Zhang, Twin-screw melt granulation: Current progress and challenges, Int. J. Pharm. 588 (2020) 119670.
46. F.W. Goodhart, J.R. Draper, F.C. Ninger, Design and use of a laboratory extruder for pharmaceutical granulations, J. Pharm. Sci. 62 (1973) 133–136.
47. M.J. Gamlen, C. Eardley, Continuous extrusion using a raker perkins MP50 (multipurpose) extruder, Drug Dev. Ind. Pharm. 12 (1986) 1701–1713.
48. P. Kleinebudde, H. Lindner, Experiments with an instrumented twin-screw extruder using a single-step granulation/extrusion process, Int. J. Pharm. 94 (1993) 49–58.
49. P. Kleinebudde, A.J. Sølvberg, H. Lindner, The power-consumption-controlled extruder: A tool for pellet production, J. Pharm. Pharmacol. 46 (1994) 542–546.
50. N.-O. Lindberg, C. Tufvesson, L. Olbjer, Extrusion of an effervescent granulation with a twin screw extruder, Baker Perkins MPF 50 D, Drug Dev. Ind. Pharm. 13 (1987) 1891–1913.
51. N.-O. Lindberg, M. Myrenas, C. Tufvesson, L. Olbjer, Extrusion of an effervescent granulation with a twin screw extruder, Baker Perkins MPF 50D. Determination of mean residence time, Drug Dev. Ind. Pharm. 14 (1988) 649–655.
52. N.-O. Lindberg, C. Tufvesson, P. Holm, L. Olbjer, Extrusion of an effervescent granulation with a twin screw extruder, Baker Perkins MPF 50 D. Influence on intragranular porosity and liquid saturation, Drug Dev. Ind. Pharm. 14 (1988) 1791–1798.
53. M.R. Thompson, Twin screw granulation-review of current progress, Drug Dev. Ind. Pharm. 41 (2015) 1223–1231.
54. F.R. Parker, Department of Health and Human Services, US Food and Drug Administration: Authority and Responsibility, in: FDA Adm. Enforc. Man., CRC Press, 2005: pp. 21–60.
55. B. Khorsheed, I. Gabbott, G.K. Reynolds, S.C. Taylor, R.J. Roberts, A.D. Salman, Twin-screw granulation: Understanding the mechanical properties from powder to tablets, Powder Technol. 341 (2018) 104–115.
56. A. Megarry, A. Taylor, A. Gholami, H. Wikström, P. Tajarobi, Twin-screw granulation and high-shear granulation: The influence of mannitol grade on granule and tablet properties, Int. J. Pharm. 590 (2020).
57. S. V. Lute, R.M. Dhenge, A.D. Salman, Twin screw granulation: An investigation of the effect of barrel fill level, Pharmaceutics. 10 (2018) 1–21.
58. A.S. Liu Y, Thompson MR, O'Donnell KP, Heat Assisted Twin Screw Dry Granulation, AIChE J. 63 (2017) 4748–4760.
59. X. Ye, V. Kallakunta, D.W. Kim, H. Patil, R. V. Tiwari, S.B. Upadhye, R.S. Vladyka, M.A. Repka, Effects of Processing on a Sustained Release Formulation Prepared by Twin-Screw Dry Granulation, J. Pharm. Sci. 108 (2019) 2895–2904.
60. V.R. Kallakunta, H. Patil, R. Tiwari, X. Ye, R.S. Vladyka, S. Sarabu, D.W. Kim, S. Bandari, M.A. Repka, Exploratory studies in heat-assisted continuous twin-screw dry granulation: A novel alternative technique to conventional dry granulation, HHS Public Access. 555 (2019) 380–393.
61. A. Batra, D. Desai, A.T.M. Serajuddin, Investigating the Use of Polymeric Binders in Twin Screw Melt Granulation Process for Improving Compactibility of Drugs, J. Pharm. Sci. 106 (2017) 140–150.
62. T. Schfer, C. Mathiesen, Melt pelletization in a high shear mixer, VIII Eff. Bind. Viscosity. Int. J. Pharm. 139 (1996) 125–138.

63. T. Monteyne, L. Heeze, S.T.F.C. Mortier, K. Oldörp, R. Cardinaels, I. Nopens, C. Vervaet, J.P. Remon, T. De Beer, The use of Rheology Combined with Differential Scanning Calorimetry to Elucidate the Granulation Mechanism of an Immiscible Formulation During Continuous Twin-Screw Melt Granulation, Pharm. Res. 33 (2016) 2481–2494.

64. T. Monteyne, L. Heeze, S.T.F.C. Mortier, K. Oldörp, I. Nopens, J.P. Remon, C. Vervaet, T. De Beer, The use of rheology to elucidate the granulation mechanisms of a miscible and immiscible system during continuous twin-screw melt granulation, Int. J. Pharm. 510 (2016) 271–284.

65. L.D. Bruce, N.H. Shah, A.W. Malick, M.H. Infeld, J.W. McGinity, Properties of hot-melt extruded tablet formulations for the colonic delivery of 5-aminosalicylic acid, Eur. J. Pharm. Biopharm. 59 (2005) 85–97.

66. C. Martin, Twin screw extrusion for pharmaceutical processes, in: Melt Extrus., Springer, 2013: pp. 47–79.

67. S. Byrn, M. Futran, H. Thomas, E. Jayjock, N. Maron, R.F. Meyer, A.S. Myerson, M.P. Thien, B.L. Trout, Achieving continuous manufacturing for final dosage formation: challenges and how to meet them. May 20–21, 2014 continuous manufacturing symposium, J. Pharm. Sci. 104 (2015) 792–802.

68. S.L. Lee, T.F. O'Connor, X. Yang, C.N. Cruz, S. Chatterjee, R.D. Madurawe, C.M. V Moore, X.Y. Lawrence, J. Woodcock, Modernizing pharmaceutical manufacturing: from batch to continuous production, J. Pharm. Innov. 10 (2015) 191–199.

69. Q. ICH, Pharmaceutical development, Q8, Curr. Step. 4 (2009).

70. J.M. Juran, Juran on quality by design: the new steps for planning quality into goods and services, Simon and Schuster, 1992.

71. I.C.H. ICH, Q9 Quality Risk Management, in: Proc. Int. Conf. Harmon. Tech. Requir. Regist. Pharm. Hum. Use, 2005.

72. I.C.H.H.T. Guideline, Pharmaceutical quality system q10, Curr. Step. 4 (2008).

73. R. Ogilvie, ICH Q11: Development and manufacture of drug substance, ICH Qual. Guidel. An Implement. Guid. (2017) 639–665.

74. Food and Drug Administration, Guidance for industry, PAT-A Framework for Innovative Pharmaceutical Development, Manufacturing and Quality Assurance, http://http//www.fda.gov/cder/guidance/published.html (2004).

75. X.Y. Lawrence, G. Amidon, M.A. Khan, S.W. Hoag, J. Polli, G.K. Raju, J. Woodcock, Understanding pharmaceutical quality by design, AAPS J. 16 (2014) 771–783.

76. T. Seidenfeld, RA Fisher on the design of experiments and statistical estimation, in: Founders Evol. Genet., Springer, 1992: pp. 23–36.

77. A. Gawade, S. Chemate, A. Kuchekar, Pharmaceutical Quality by Design: A new approach in product development, Res. Rev. J. Pharm. Pharm. Sci. 2 (2013) 5–12.

78. M. Fonteyne, H. Wickström, E. Peeters, J. Vercruysse, H. Ehlers, B.-H. Peters, J.P. Remon, C. Vervaet, J. Ketolainen, N. Sandler, J. Rantanen, K. Naelapää, T. De Beer, Influence of raw material properties upon critical quality attributes of continuously produced granules and tablets, Eur. J. Pharm. Biopharm. 87 (2014) 252–263.

79. M. Maniruzzaman, A. Nair, M. Renault, U. Nandi, N. Scoutaris, R. Farnish, M.S.A. Bradley, M.J. Snowden, D. Douroumis, Continuous twin-screw granulation for enhancing the dissolution of poorly water soluble drug, Int. J. Pharm. 496 (2015).

80. M. Maniruzzaman, S.A. Ross, T. Dey, A. Nair, M.J. Snowden, D. Douroumis, A quality by design (QbD) twin—Screw extrusion wet granulation approach for processing water insoluble drugs, Int. J. Pharm. 526 (2017) 496–505.

81. W. Grymonpré, G. Verstraete, V. Vanhoorne, J.P. Remon, T. De Beer, C. Vervaet, Downstream processing from melt granulation towards tablets: In-depth analysis of a continuous twin-screw melt granulation process using polymeric binders, Eur. J. Pharm. Biopharm. 124 (2018) 43–54.

82. M.T. Islam, M. Maniruzzaman, S.A. Halsey, B.Z. Chowdhry, D. Douroumis, Development of sustained-release formulations processed by hot-melt extrusion by using a quality-by-design approach, Drug Deliv. Transl. Res. 4 (2014) 377–387.

83. V. Lourenço, D. Lochmann, G. Reich, J.C. Menezes, T. Herdling, J. Schewitz, A quality by design study applied to an industrial pharmaceutical fluid bed granulation, Eur. J. Pharm. Biopharm. 81 (2012) 438–447.

84. T.R.M. De Beer, P. Vercruysse, A. Burggraeve, T. Quinten, J. Ouyang, X. Zhang, C. Vervaet, J.P. Remon, W.R.G. Baeyens, In-line and real-time process monitoring of a freeze drying process using Raman and NIR spectroscopy as complementary process analytical technology (PAT) tools, J. Pharm. Sci. 98 (2009) 3430–3446.

85. L. Saerens, L. Dierickx, T. Quinten, P. Adriaensens, R. Carleer, C. Vervaet, J.P. Remon, T. De Beer, In-line NIR spectroscopy for the understanding of polymer–drug interaction during pharmaceutical hot-melt extrusion, Eur. J. Pharm. Biopharm. 81 (2012) 230–237.

86. F. De Leersnyder, E. Peeters, H. Djalabi, V. Vanhoorne, B. Van Snick, K. Hong, S. Hammond, A.Y. Liu, E. Ziemons, C. Vervaet, Development and validation of an in-line NIR spectroscopic method for continuous blend potency determination in the feed frame of a tablet press, J. Pharm. Biomed. Anal. 151 (2018) 274–283.

87. M.T. Islam, N. Scoutaris, M. Maniruzzaman, H.G. Moradiya, S.A. Halsey, M.S.A. Bradley, B.Z. Chowdhry, M.J. Snowden, D. Douroumis, Implementation of transmission NIR as a PAT tool for monitoring drug transformation during HME processing, Eur. J. Pharm. Biopharm. 96 (2015) 106–116.

88. R. Singh, A.D. Román-Ospino, R.J. Romañach, M. Ierapetritou, R. Ramachandran, Real time monitoring of powder blend bulk density for coupled feed-forward/feed-back control of a continuous direct compaction tablet manufacturing process, Int. J. Pharm. 495 (2015) 612–625.

89. P.A.T. FDA, A Framework for Innovative Pharmaceutical Development, Manufacturing and Quality Assurance. Guidance for Industry (2004), (n.d.).

90. S. Laske, A. Paudel, O. Scheibelhofer, S. Sacher, T. Hoermann, J. Khinast, A. Kelly, J. Rantannen, O. Korhonen, F. Stauffer, A review of PAT strategies in secondary solid oral dosage manufacturing of small molecules, J. Pharm. Sci. 106 (2017) 667–712.

91. A.U. Vanarase, M. Alcalà, J.I.J. Rozo, F.J. Muzzio, R.J. Romañach, Real-time monitoring of drug concentration in a continuous powder mixing process using NIR spectroscopy, Chem. Eng. Sci. 65 (2010) 5728–5733.

92. A.U. Vanarase, M. Järvinen, J. Paaso, F.J. Muzzio, Development of a methodology to estimate error in the on-line measurements of blend uniformity in a continuous powder mixing process, Powder Technol. 241 (2013) 263–271.

93. L. Martínez, A. Peinado, L. Liesum, G. Betz, Use of near-infrared spectroscopy to quantify drug content on a continuous blending process: influence of mass flow and rotation speed variations, Eur. J. Pharm. Biopharm. 84 (2013) 606–615.

94. V. Kehlenbeck, Use of near infrared spectroscopy for in-and off-line performance determination of continuous and batch powder mixers: opportunities & challenges, Procedia Food Sci. 1 (2011) 2015–2022.

95. M. Fonteyne, S. Soares, J. Vercruysse, E. Peeters, A. Burggraeve, C. Vervaet, J.P. Remon, N. Sandler, T. De Beer, Prediction of quality attributes of continuously produced granules using complementary pat tools, Eur. J. Pharm. Biopharm. 82 (2012) 429–436.

96. A.F. Silva, J. Vercruysse, C. Vervaet, J.P. Remon, J.A. Lopes, T. De Beer, M.C. Sarraguça, European Journal of Pharmaceutics and Biopharmaceutics Process monitoring and evaluation of a continuous pharmaceutical twin-screw granulation and drying process using multivariate data analysis, (n.d.).

97. L. Madarász, Z.K. Nagy, I. Hoffer, B. Szabó, I. Csontos, H. Pataki, B. Démuth, B. Szabó, K. Csorba, G. Marosi, Real-time feedback control of twin-screw wet granulation based on image analysis, Int. J. Pharm. 547 (2018) 360–367.

98. R. Sayin, L. Martinez-Marcos, J.G. Osorio, P. Cruise, I. Jones, G.W. Halbert, D.A. Lamprou, J.D. Litster, Investigation of an 11 mm diameter twin screw granulator: screw element performance and in-line monitoring via image analysis, Int. J. Pharm. 496 (2015) 24–32.

99. J. Rehrl, A.-P. Karttunen, N. Nicolaï, T. Hörmann, M. Horn, O. Korhonen, I. Nopens, T. De Beer, J.G. Khinast, Control of three different continuous pharmaceutical manufacturing processes: Use of soft sensors, Int. J. Pharm. 543 (2018) 60–72.

Continuous Powder Feeding: Equipment Design and Material Considerations

Brian M. Kerins and Abina M. Crean

1 Introduction

Continuous feeding of raw materials is a critical step of all continuous manufacturing (CM) processes. The function of the feeder is to transfer material into the following operation using an accurate and reliable feed rate. In the case of solid oral dosage forms, the predominant materials fed are active pharmaceutical ingredients (APIs) and excipient powders. If there is variability in the feeding process, there is a risk that downstream processes will be impacted, leading to the material critical quality attributes (CQAs) being outside the specified limits [1]. All feeders share this primary function to control the rate of powder flow; however, the underlying feeding mechanism varies depending on the equipment design. The most common feeder types employed in the pharmaceutical industry are based on one of the following moving elements: screw, vibratory channel, belt or rotary valve [2–4]. Feeder selection is carried out by assessing the compatibility with several key aspects of the CM process.

The material properties of fed API and excipients can vary significantly [5, 6]. Therefore, it is important to employ a suitable feeder design to minimise unwanted powder flow patterns. Table 1 outlines some of the main points for feeder-material compatibility. Feeder design also impacts the degree of feed rate control. For example, twin-screw feeders can better regulate powder flow in comparison with single-screw configurations. This is because twin screws tend to dispense material in smaller pulses [7]. Closed-loop feedback control is often incorporated into pharmaceutical feeders to further reduce feed rate variability and is used in loss-in-weight (LIW) systems which are discussed in more detail in Sect. 2.2. The

B. M. Kerins · A. M. Crean (✉)
University College Cork, Cork, Ireland
e-mail: a.crean@ucc.ie

© The Author(s), under exclusive license to Springer Nature Switzerland AG 2022
A. Fytopoulos et al. (eds.), *Optimization of Pharmaceutical Processes*, Springer
Optimization and Its Applications 189, https://doi.org/10.1007/978-3-030-90924-6_7

Table 1 Overview of material compatibility with feeder types [7, 8]

Feeder design		
Screw	Vibratory channel	Belt
• Various screw types available which allow the feeder to handle a wide range of materials • Available in single-screw or twin-screw setups • Single-screw feeders may encounter issues when dispensing fine/cohesive powders as they can build up on the screw and decrease feeder efficiency. Certain twin-screw designs can overcome this by using screws which intermesh, providing a self-cleaning function	• Gently handles powders • The vibrations may generate dust for low-density materials • The vibrations may promote powder segregation. This is particularly relevant if feeding blends • Adhesive powders can build up on the feeder tube or on the tray	• Gently handles powders • Ideally want the powder to form a stable bed on the belt, which may make it suitable for low-density materials that aerate and form dust • Adhesive material may stick to the belt which can produce feed rate variability and affect the belt tracking

maximum volumetric capacity of a feeder is dependent on the moving element used. To ensure a feeder is compatible with the CM process, the feed rate required in the next unit operation must be comfortably within the operational limits of the chosen feeder.

2   Overview of Feeding Fundamentals

Pharmaceutical feeders may vary in design; however, the core elements of the feeding process remain the same. This section will discuss these shared fundamentals and outline how they impact feeding control.

2.1   Volumetric Feeding

Conventional volumetric feeders operate using open-loop control where there is no feedback signal integrated into the process. In relation to screw feeders, this means the screws will rotate at a constant speed unless the operator manually intervenes. While running in this fixed manner, there is often variability in the produced feed rate. Investigations into the volumetric feeding process have highlighted physical mechanisms behind these mass flow deviations, with several examples being discussed in the chapter.

If fluctuations are present, it suggests that the mass of powder being conveyed by the screws is inconsistent. Screw design will be discussed in more detail in

Sect. 2.4, but in brief, the screws transport material within channels between the screw flights. The first source of variability may be identified here as the volume of material contained within these pockets may not be consistent. There are several root causes that could contribute to this. Cohesive material may adhere to the screws, form stagnant zones and limit the volumetric transport capacity [9]. Alternatively, with each screw rotation, a uniform volume of powder may struggle to flow into the screw flights from the hopper. This is called inconsistent flight filling which again is more commonly seen in poorly flowing and cohesive materials. Powder bridging is one form of flow obstruction which can cause this non-uniform filling [10].

Next it must be considered if the volume of material being transported remains constant (i.e. consistent flight filling). If the mass flow is still not stable, this suggests that the bulk density of the material is variable. One possible cause for fluctuating powder density is the hopper refilling process. Compressive forces generated by the incoming material can result in the densification of powder in the lower portions of the hopper. An increase in density would allow a greater mass of material to be transported within the screws resulting in higher feed rates [11].

For these reasons outlined, volumetric feeding has an increased risk of mass flow variability. Accordingly, this type of feeder is usually used if feed rate accuracy and precision is not critical which is seldom applicable for pharmaceutical manufacturing.

2.2 Gravimetric Feeding

Feeding complications which occur during volumetric feeding similarly occur when using gravimetric, loss-in-weight (LIW) feeders. However, in LIW feeders there is an in-built gravimetric system which enables minimisation of feed rate deviations. LIW feeders can consist of the same volumetric feeding component, but also require a weighing platform and a control module (Fig. 1). The control module is often a type of proportional-integral derivative (PID) controller and is the primary enabler for the closed-loop gravimetric system. During operation, the load cell within the platform continuously monitors the net weight of the material in the feeding unit. This sensory data is transferred back to the control module to calculate the instantaneous feed rate. If there is any disparity between the actual feed rate and the setpoint (i.e. the input feed rate target selected by the operator), the controller will determine a desired actuator output. This will signal the motor to adjust the screw speed and to minimise this deviation from the defined setpoint.

The main advantage of this gravimetric system is that the feeder can self-regulate the screw speed to compensate for feeding inconsistencies. For example, if the material density increases, the controller will detect the higher feed rate produced, and it will signal the motor to reduce the screw speed. Conversely, if screw flight filling worsens, the controller will detect a lower feed rate, and increase the screw speed.

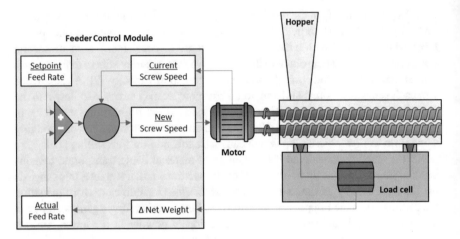

Fig. 1 Schematic of a LIW system for a twin-screw feeder

2.3 Hopper Refill Procedure

During the feeding operation, the hopper depletes, and when it reaches a predefined level, the feeder controller initiates a refill cycle to replenish the material back to a preset upper fill level. The fresh powder entering the hopper can create compressive forces, causing densification of the lower portion of material [12]. With a greater density, a higher mass of powder can enter the screw flights and cause a spike in the feed rate. Refilling also has the potential to aerate the powder, an unwanted effect, as the material may then behave more like a liquid and flush uncontrollably through the screws, again causing overfeeding [13].

As discussed above, gravimetric feeding uses a feedback signal (derived from the net weight changes in the hopper) to regulate the screw speed, thereby reducing feed rate deviations. This feedback system is compromised during hopper refill as the material is entering and leaving the feeder at the same time, obscuring the weight readings, and as a result the feed rate cannot be calculated. Without a feedback signal, the feeder temporarily switches from gravimetric to volumetric mode. Operating in volumetric mode, the process is essentially blind to the density changes that can occur which can result in temporary feed rate deviations. It will remain operating in this manner for the duration of the refill and for a short post-refill delay, after which it will return to gravimetric feeding. Once the feeder switches back to gravimetric mode, it can recognise the feed rate deviation and begin to regulate the screw speed. However, this can lead to an abrupt speed change which can further contribute to feeding variability [14]. Feed rate variability during refills can impact downstream processes as shown by Berthiaux et al. [1] where the refilling procedure produced feed rate deviations which negatively affected the following mixing operation.

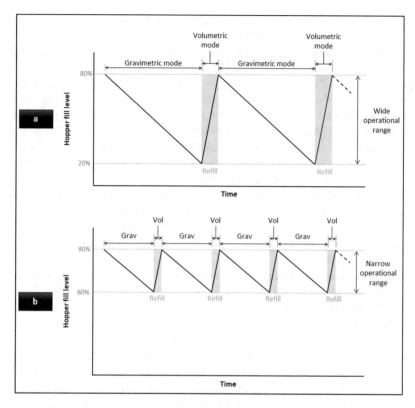

Fig. 2 Examples of a (**a**) low- and (**b**) high-frequency hopper refill schedule

While establishing a hopper refill procedure, several factors must be considered to optimise the process and minimise any unwanted effects. These factors include the frequency/size of refills; the material properties; the post-refill delay duration; and the refilling device. All these factors cannot be decided in isolation as they are highly interlinked. Two refill procedures which differ in the frequency/size of refills are shown in Fig. 2. Larger, low-frequency refills (a) mean that less refills are needed in total and that the feeder doesn't have to revert to volumetric mode as often. The downside is that a greater mass of refill material is added to a shallower bed of bulk powder. This can accentuate the alteration to the powder properties. In contrast, smaller, high-frequency refills (b) minimise this effect, although as more refills are required, the gravimetric system is more regularly disengaged.

Engisch and Muzzio [13] investigated the impact of refill scheduling for a zinc oxide powder and a acetaminophen/silica blend. In both cases the feed rate deviation was highest using the larger, less frequent refills, and improved as the refills became smaller. Although the same trend was observed for each material, the mechanism behind the deviation was different. The overfeeding for the zinc oxide was primarily caused by powder densification due to compressive effects. In contrast, the deviations for the acetaminophen/silica blend were due to fluidisation and flushing of materials through the feeder screws.

During the refill process, there are vibrational disturbances created which distort the net weight readings of the load cell. Accordingly, in LIW feeders there is often a post-refill delay function which designates a waiting period once the refill has completed before switching back to gravimetric mode. The post-refill delay function allows time for the vibrational disturbances to dissipate before the weight readings are utilised for the feedback loop. Engisch and Muzzio [13] compared a 5- and 10-s post-refill delay. No improvement was observed using the longer delay which indicated that the majority of the deviation occurred while the hopper was physically being refilled, rather than the period directly after.

The refilling device is another important factor as it controls how the new material is transferred into the hopper. Various options are available such as gate vales, rotary valves, pneumatic receivers and volumetric screw feeders. Ideally the rate of the refilling should be quick to reduce the time spent in volumetric mode, although adding material too quick and with too much force can result in greater feed rate deviations by altering the powder density [13]. Therefore, the selection of a suitable refill device should be tailored to the properties of the fed material and the acceptable level of feed rate deviation of the feeding process.

As discussed, the overall problem with the hopper refill process is that the feeder switches to volumetric mode, and the screw speed is fixed for the duration of the refill. To directly address this issue, more advanced approaches are being developed to improve control during this period. One example of this is the 'refill array' function [14]. In brief, this method allows the screw speed to change during the refill based on previously stored feeding data which can reduce feed rate deviations and lead to a smoother transition back to gravimetric feeding.

2.4   Volumetric Capacity and Feed Factor

The screws in pharmaceutical feeders are often flood fed from the hopper [15]. Flood feeding the screws means material flows directly into the screw conveyor by gravity without assistance from additional pneumatic or conveyor systems. The volume of powder that the screws can transport is dependent on the screw design and its dimensions. Several of the primary screw design features are illustrated in Fig. 3. Material entering from the hopper flows into the channels between the screw flights. As the screws rotate, the material is then conveyed through the barrel. The pitch (distance between adjacent screw flights) and the flight depth are among the key factors that dictate the size of these pockets, which then controls the volumetric transport capacity [16]. Selection of an appropriate screw configuration is essential during process design as the feed rate required by the next unit operation must be within the screws' volumetric range.

An important parameter used to describe the transport efficiency of screws is the feed factor. Feed factor represents the mass of powder delivered per revolution

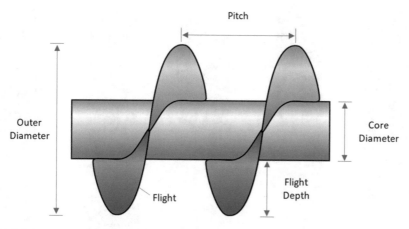

Fig. 3 Diagram of the typical screw geometries

of the feeder screw (g/rev) [17]. Feed factor can be affected by several equipment and process variables which involve the physical design of the screw, the screw speed and the hopper fill level, and by the bulk properties of the fed material. In regard to screw design, a study by Yadav et al. [18] highlighted that screws with a larger pitch produced higher feed factors due to larger channels within the flights to accommodate material. Moreover, the magnitude of difference in feed factor due to the pitch sizes was dependent on the material being fed. Using a multivariate approach, Bostijn et al. [11] correlated the maximum feed factor for 15 pharmaceutical powders with the raw material properties. The resulting analysis highlighted that the feed factor was linked to the bulk density and flowability of the materials. Additionally, this study demonstrated how the feed factor decreases as the hopper gradually depletes. The feed factor can also be used to help detect feeding complications as fluctuations may be indicative of inconsistent flight filling and material density changes.

3   Twin-Screw Feeders: Equipment Considerations

Twin-screw feeders are commonly used during pharmaceutical continuous manufacturing and offer a range of designs and tooling configuration options. Therefore, a specific feeder can be tailored to the process and material requirements to improve feeding performance. In this section, several of these equipment options will be discussed such as screw type, discharge screen type and hopper/agitators.

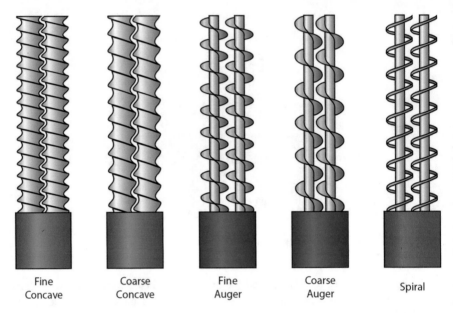

| Fine | Coarse | Fine | Coarse | Spiral |
| Concave | Concave | Auger | Auger | |

Fig. 4 Example of twin-screw types

3.1 Screw Type

While selecting an appropriate screw type for a feeding process, there are two primary considerations: (a) the feed rate required to the next unit operation and (b) the properties of the powder being fed. As discussed in Sect. 2.4, the volumetric capacity of the screws is impacted by the screw design. Several twin-screw setups are displayed in Fig. 4. Note that the primary difference between the fine and coarse screws is the pitch size, with the coarse design having a greater capacity. To optimise the screw configuration to a specific material, a thorough characterisation of its physical properties is required. Feeding behaviour of material is linked to its flow, which in turn is related to powder properties such as particle size and shape, bulk and true density, electrostatic charge, moisture content and surface texture [19–22].

Cohesive, low-density and poorly flowing powders can be some of the most difficult to feed. Firstly, these powder particles have a greater tendency to adhere to available surfaces. If this occurs on the screws, it can lead to the formation of stagnant powder zones. Throughout the feeding process, this can cause the feeder efficiency to gradually decrease resulting in a reduced volumetric capacity [9]. Cartwright et al. [23] encountered a similar issue where a low-density API compacted within the barrel housing. To compensate, the LIW feeder progressively increased the motor torque to meet the feed rate setpoint. This eventually led to the feeder shutting down as the upper torque limit was reached. These unwanted flow patterns also raise concerns regarding material traceability and degradation [24]. Auger screw types have been shown to be particularly prone to these issues and therefore should be used with care if processing very cohesive materials [10]. Due to the design of concave screws, in a twin-screw setup, they are capable of a self-cleaning ability which helps to reduce material build-up [24]. An additional consideration if using concave screws with a cohesive material is the size of the screw pitch. A study by Engisch and Muzzio [24] found that colloidal silicon dioxide, which is a low-density and highly cohesive powder, had difficulty fully filling the flights of the fine concave screws. Therefore, the screw configuration was unable to reach the desired feed rate capacity. One method which was found to improve the flight filling was the use of a larger feeder with bigger screws.

In contrast to cohesive powders, the feeding performance of free-flowing materials is less dependent on screw type [25]. However, if powders are allowed to flow too freely through the screws, it can impact feed rate control and lead to increased variability. In this scenario auger screw types offer less control in comparison with concave screws. Concave screws have smaller pockets to convey the material and as a result can dispense powder in smaller pulses which reduces the tendency of material to flush through the screws, thereby improving the performance [24].

3.2 Screen Type

In some twin-screw feeder models, there is an option to place a discharge screen at the outlet directly after the screws. Like the screws, by providing tooling choices, it grants the operator more flexibility to optimise the process based on the fed material. There are two primary functions of the screen component: to help regulate flow and to break up powder aggregates [24]. An example of two screens which can be placed at the outlet of a K-Tron MT12 twin-screw feeder is shown in Fig. 5. The size and shape of the screen gratings impact its ability for flow regulation, with smaller gratings providing increased resistance. Feeders can also be operated without a screen in place.

Materials, particularly those with good flowability, may flush out of the screws too freely if the feeder configuration lacks control. This can result in increased feed rate variability. A good example of this was shown by Engisch and Muzzio [24]. In this study, a free-flowing excipient, Prosolv HD90, was gravimetrically fed using various tooling configurations. It was found that the feed rate variability could be reduced with the inclusion of a screen at the outlet. In a subsequent study, the additional flow control gained with the screen was shown to help reduce feed rate fluctuations caused by hopper refills [13].

Screens may be beneficial for some cohesive materials as they can help to break up powder clumps; however, they can also cause other issues. If the powder is prone to adhering to the equipment, the addition of a screen will provide extra available surface which could accentuate the problem of material adherence. Material may accumulate on the screen and then fall off periodically causing feed rate fluctuations [24]. The flow regulation of the screen occurs by forcing the powder to pass through the gratings. Poorly flowing material may struggle to get through finer screen

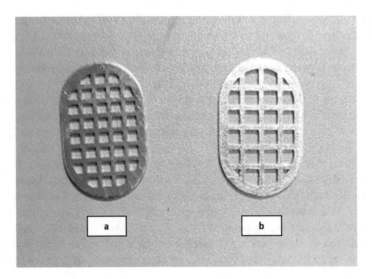

Fig. 5 Example of two discharge screens: (**a**) a fine square screen, and (**b**) a coarse square screen

gratings which can lead to the powder building up and compacting before the screen. The powder compaction causes the feed rate to drop, and due to the gravimetric feedback system, the controller then increases the screw speed to compensate for the drop-off in feed rate. As more and more powder compacts, the torque needed by the motor to rotate the screws increases. If an upper torque threshold is met, the motor can shut down, halting the feeding process [10].

3.3 Hopper and Agitator

Flow patterns in the hopper are an important aspect of continuous feeding as it controls how the material transitions into the screws. There are two primary modes of flow seen within the hopper: mass flow and funnel flow. Mass flow is the desired behaviour and works under the principle of first in, first out (Fig. 6). In this mode, all particles in the hopper are in a uniform motion which provides a steady discharge. Funnel flow, which is often described as first in, last out, occurs when a preferential flow channel develops directly over the hopper outlet [26]. During funnel flow the material in the centre flows faster versus the material at the edges, which can also lead to the formation of stagnant zones. Ratholing is a term used to describe extreme cases of funnel flow where the material nearer the walls is completely stationary and only the central material is discharged [27]. Ratholing was observed by Santos et al. [28] which resulted in a feed rate reduction for a poorly flowing material. Funnel flow can also have other negative effects on the bulk powder. It has the potential to

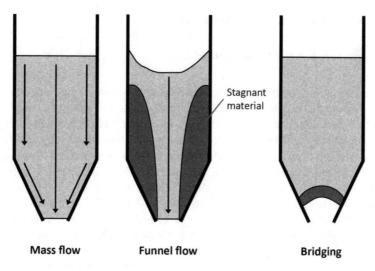

Mass flow   **Funnel flow**   **Bridging**

Fig. 6 Flow patterns in the hopper

induce powder segregation into non-uniform fractions [29]. Additionally, it raises concerns regarding material residence times.

Aside from funnel flow, powder bridging is another undesirable flow issue which can occur in the hopper (Fig. 6). Obstruction to flow due to bridging arises when a stable arch forms over the hopper outlet, which prevents material from being discharged [27]. The obstruction to flow would have a significant impact on the overall CM process as it would starve the feeder screws, and the continuous stream of material into the next unit operation would cease.

Similar to screw and screen selection, thorough material characterisation is recommended prior to selecting a hopper design. Choosing a suitable design can help mitigate the flow issues of troublesome materials. The shape of the hopper, including the wall slope and outlet width, can have a significant impact on powder flow behaviour [30]. A rotating agitator can be installed inside the hopper which can facilitate improved flow and screw flight filling. However, these agitators may not be compatible in all processes. Cartwright et al. [23] observed significant ratholing during a feeding study and noted it was partly due to the agitator. The rotating blade aided the compaction of the low-density API which required repeated operator intervention to resolve. The solution used in this study was to select a feeder with a flexible hopper design. These specialised hoppers allow the bulk powder to be gently massaged from the outside via external agitators, thereby improving flow behaviour [7].

4   Additional Process Considerations

4.1   Time to Reach Steady State

The start-up procedure of a CM process must be given careful consideration as the unit operation must be allowed to achieve a steady state. The time required is heavily dependent on factors such as the feed rate employed and the material being fed. While steady state can be achieved in a relatively short time frame during the feeding process, it is important to understand this time frame as large fluctuations may occur prior to reaching steady state which can produce significant feed rate variability. Simonaho et al. [31] investigated this by monitoring the individual feeding of microcrystalline cellulose and acetylsalicylic acid at 17.14 kg/h and 2.86 kg/h, respectively. In both cases it was shown that a steady-state mass flow was achieved after 3 min from start-up. Blackshields and Crean [32] also studied the feeding of microcrystalline cellulose, although a much lower feed rate of 0.25 kg/h was used. Additionally, the definition of the time to reach steady state employed was the time taken until the feed rate remained within ±3 standard deviations of the gravimetric setpoint. In this study, approximately 12 min was needed for the mass flow to remain within these limits. Ervasti et al. [33] investigated a continuous process for manufacturing extended release ibuprofen tablets. Within the experimental design, the API was fed at 3 different mass flow rates: 0.070, 0.525 and 0.770 kg/h. A settling time of under 5 min was seen for both the higher feed rates. In contrast, the 0.070 kg/h feed rate required approximately 10 min to stay within the ±3 standard deviations limits.

4.2   Powder Triboelectrification

Triboelectrification or tribo-charging is a charge transfer process which can occur when particle contact involves frictional forces generated by rubbing, sliding, rolling or impaction [22]. Triboelectrification can apply to anywhere in the manufacturing process where particles frequently collide with other powder particles, or with the surfaces of equipment. Pharmaceutical powders are often dielectric materials, giving them a greater tendency to tribo-charge [34]. These insulating properties additionally mean the accumulated charge will decay slowly, which may be of particular concern to CM processes where each unit operation connects directly to the next [35]. The electrostatic charge generated can be quite problematic during manufacturing as it can:

- Increase the risk of powder handling hazards such as creating an electrical spark or causing a dust explosion [36].
- Lead to powder agglomeration and segregation.
- Reduce powder flow.

- Increase particle adhesion.

Due to the influence of electrostatic charges, there have been many studies investigating its impact on unit operations such as feeding [11, 35, 37, 38] and blending [34, 39, 40]. There has also been several reviews discussing tribo-charging in a pharmaceutical setting [22, 41, 42].

Engisch and Muzzio [24] encountered electrostatic issues when feeding colloidal silicon dioxide which lead to significant powder build-up at the feeder outlet. Using an electrostatic eliminator, the tendency for powder adhesion was reduced although not completely resolved.

A study by Beretta et al. [35] investigated the tribo-charging of various pharmaceutical powders and found the magnitude of the charge generated was highly material dependent. Additionally, the particle charge density was compared after (a) allowing the powder to flow through a GranuCharge instrument and (b) feeding using a twin-screw feeder. There was a good correlation between these results which suggests that the tribo-charging may be mainly due to frictional interparticle forces rather than interaction with equipment surfaces.

While feeding controlled release grades of hypromellose, Allenspach et al. [37] reported significant electrostatic material build-up on the feeder barrel. The accumulated material occasionally fell and caused feed rate fluctuations, which was reflected in the higher feed rate variability of those samples. Another finding of this study was that the location of the material build-up changed when the powder was fed directly from the feeder into another hopper. In this case, instead of accumulating on the feeder barrel, the powder adhered to the output of the following hopper which highlights the additional considerations when integrating the feeder into a continuous process.

5 Low-Dose Powder Feeding

Special consideration must be given to feeding processes which require very low feed rates. In relation to pharmaceutical manufacturing, this is most frequently seen with excipients, such as flow aids and lubricants, which are only required in small quantities proportional to the overall formulation. Low-dose feeding also applies for feeding highly potent active pharmaceutical ingredients. An increasing number of highly potent active pharmaceutical ingredients have emerged from development in recent years [43]. Fluctuations in the feed rate can occur with all feeders, although when using lower feed rate setpoints this can become particularly troublesome [28]. One solution is to pre-blend the API or excipient with another material in the formulation and then feed at a higher feed rate where there is greater control. The drawback of this approach is that it necessitates an additional processing step. Alternatively, the issue can be directly addressed by establishing a feeding process capable of dispensing a continuous and reliable powder stream at lower feed rates.

Bostijn et al. [11] investigated feed rates of 100 and 550 g/h using a twin-screw LIW feeder. The relative standard deviation (RSD) of the feed rate was significantly higher in the lower 100 g/h runs. Additionally, the powder properties were a critical factor which impacted the feed rate variability. A micro-pump feeder setup has been utilised in several studies where accurate feed rates were achieved at 1–25 g/h [44], 1–15 g/h [45] and 1–5 g/h [46]. In this design the feed rate is primarily controlled by the displacement of the powder from a cartridge via a pump/piston. Besenhard et al. [47] assembled a vibratory sieve and chute system which produced a stable flow from 4 to 90 g/h. However, the powder had to be preprocessed via sieving prior to feeding.

6 Modelling to Predict Feeder Performance

The APIs and excipients used in pharmaceutical formulations can differ significantly in relation to their material properties. These differences affect the material performance in all operations throughout the manufacturing process, including blending [48], tableting [49], granulating [50] and feeding [11, 24]. Therefore, research which aims to investigate and further our understanding of these interactions is an indispensable tool during process design. The key benefits of this modelling are:

- It can predict which tooling configurations would be most suitable.
- It can lead to a faster and more efficient drug development process.
- It can reduce the consumption of materials, which are often in limited supply during the early design phases.

The first step in the modelling process is to create a database of the material properties. To improve the quality and reliability of the data, standardised characterisation methods should be used [51]. From this material library, a model can be produced using multivariate analysis techniques such as principal component analysis (PCA). In technical terms, PCA is a mathematical algorithm which reduces the dimensionality of data while still retaining most of variation [52]. PCA can position the materials within a design space so the relationship between the properties can be assessed. During process design, this method can also be used to identify a surrogate material which shares the same critical material attributes.

Partial least squares (PLS) regression is another multivariate analysis technique which can be used. While PCA determines the relationship between the material properties, PLS correlates the independent variables (material properties) to output responses. In relation to continuous feeding, the responses studied include the feed rate RSD, and deviation from the feed rate setpoint. The established correlation can be used to predict feeder performance based on the material properties. Examples of studies using multivariate analysis methods are shown in Table 2.

Powder behaviour during the feeding process has also been investigated using discrete element modelling (DEM) [54–56]. The DEM approach determines the

Table 2 Examples of studies which used modelling to investigate the feeding process

Study	Brief outline
Polizzi et al. [27]	PLS was used to model the relationship between the material properties and the flow in conical hoppers
Wang et al. [25]	Both PCA and PLS were used to create predictive correlations between material flow properties and feeder performance
Escotet–Espinoza et al. [5]	PCA and hierarchical clustering were used to analyse a material library based on flow properties. The material clusters were linked to the performance in the characterised equipment
Van Snick et al. [6]	A material library was created using over 100 raw material descriptors. It was then analysed with PCA to identify the relationship between the properties
Bostijn et al. [11]	PLS was used to correlate several feeding responses to the material descriptors. Two volumetric (the maximum feed factor and its relative decay) and two gravimetric (the feed rate RSD and deviation from the setpoint) feeding responses were assessed
Wang et al. [53]	PCA and hierarchical clustering were used to analyse a material library. The feeding performance of several materials was assessed to determine if samples within the clusters exhibited similar feeding behaviour
Yadav et al. [18]	A PCA model was used to investigate the relationship between the material properties, the feeder tooling configuration and the feeding performance
Stauffer et al. [38]	PCA and PLS models were used to optimise the feeding performance of a blend and to identify the critical material properties
Tahir et al. [17]	First, material-specific PLS models were generated. Then, PCA was used to cluster the materials, and a generic PLS model was developed for each cluster to predict the feed factor profile

trajectory of individual particles using simulations which focus on particle-particle and particle-wall interactions. Important information regarding powder behaviour can be extracted using these simulations while not consuming any physical material.

7 Considerations for Feeder Integration into CM Lines

In a CM process, it is common for APIs and excipients to be fed using individual feeders, and then blended in the following operation. As previously discussed (Sect. 2.2), gravimetric feeders can improve feeding performance of materials. Further levels of control are also of interest when integrating multiple feeders into a continuous process. Three types of control systems have been described [57] (Fig. 7):

1. Local control – Each feeder independently controls its feed rate.

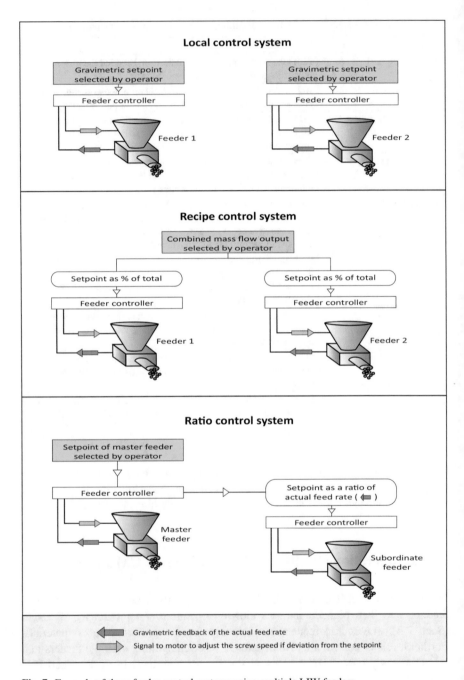

Fig. 7 Example of three feeder control systems using multiple LIW feeders

2. Recipe control – The feed rate of each feeder is determined as a percentage of the main recipe (i.e. overall combined feed rate).
3. Ratio control – One feeder is assigned as the master while the other feeders are assigned as subordinates. The subordinate feeders determine their feed rate targets as a percentage of the master feeder's output. This means they can react to the actual mass flow of the master feeder.

A study by Hanson [9] compared feeding performance while using local and ratio control. It was found that the variability of the fed concentrations of the API and excipients was lower while using ratio control.

While designing the feeding step, it is important to define the acceptable level of feed rate variability that the following unit operations can tolerate without compromising the quality of the final product. For example, variability in feed rate can result in subsequent blend variability and variability in the final dosage uniformity of content. The frequency of feed rate fluctuations should be assessed, as continuous blenders can only offset short-term (i.e. high-frequency) fluctuations [58]. Vanarase and Muzzio [59] were able to reduce feeding variability by using higher feed rates; however, this did not improve blend uniformity after the blending step. It was suggested that the variability due to the feeding process was almost completely filtered out by the continuous mixing step. In contrast, Berthiaux et al. [1] found that the feeding variability caused by the hopper refill process resulted in the post-mixer blend being outside the specified uniformity limits.

In contrast to batch processing, material traceability is a key requirement and challenge for integrated pharmaceutical CM processes. From patient safety and product quality perspectives, it is a regulatory requirement to identify the batches of raw materials' input at the feeding stage which composes a specific batch/lot of the final drug product. To trace materials through the CM process, measurement of residence time distribution (RTD) is proposed [60]. RTD is defined as a probability distribution that describes the amount of time a mass or fluid element remains in a process. Addition of a tracer compounds, the application of online measurements of a specific material attribute (e.g. near-infrared or Raman spectral properties) and process modelling can be used to measure RTD [61]. RTD profiles of materials in LIW feeders are influenced by material feed rate but also powder flow patterns (i.e. mass flow versus funnel flow and bridging) and feeder equipment design, configuration and settings.

A study by Van Snick et al. [62] established a PLS regression model which linked the properties of a range of pharmaceutical excipients and feeder process variables with RTD responses as outputs, for two twin-screw feeders. RTDs for both feeders could be represented by a combination of plug flow and mixed flow. Material flow rate, hopper level and density of the material were identified as critical factors for both feeders. Plug-flow and mixed-flow times were reduced to a similar extent by an increase in powder flow and decrease in material density. However, difference in RTD profiles was noted for both screw feeder types. Therefore, feeder type, configuration and processing parameters should be considered and investigated as critical process factors in relation to material traceability for a pharmaceutical continuous process.

8 Summary

Continuous feeding is an integral step in the continuous manufacturing of pharmaceutical products. As highlighted in this chapter, there is no one feeder setup suitable for all APIs and excipients. For this reason, many studies have been carried out to further our understanding of the underlying feeding mechanisms, and to correlate feeding behaviour with elements of the process design. Of the various considerations, the properties of the fed material have been identified as a highly influential factor. It has been repeatedly shown that the feeder type, the relative tooling and the process parameters must be tailored to the material properties to optimise feeding. High emphasis is put on this relationship in the pharmaceutical sector as highly accurate and precise feeding is required. A nonoptimal feeding process with high variability could cause failures of downstream processes, reducing the quality of the final drug product. As the industry follows its current trajectory towards an increased uptake of CM, it is essential that we continue to develop our understanding of the mechanisms behind the feeding process. Research to date has been primarily focused on how the equipment and process parameters affect feeder performance. An area which may warrant more research in future work is if the feeding process itself is affecting the physical properties of the fed material, as this could impact the following unit operations.

References

1. Berthiaux H, Marikh K, Gatumel C (2008) Continuous mixing of powder mixtures with pharmaceutical process constraints. Chem Eng Process Process Intensif 47:2315–2322. doi: https://doi.org/10.1016/j.cep.2008.01.009
2. Coperion (2021) Feeders - Coperion. https://www.coperion.com/en/products-services/process-equipment/feeders. Accessed 20 Jan 2021
3. Gericke (2021) Volumetric and gravimetric feeders. https://www.gerickegroup.com/feeding. Accessed 20 Jan 2021
4. Schenck Process (2021) Products for pharmaceuticals and feeding. https://www.schenckprocess.com/products?industry=pharmaceuticals&technology=industrial-feeding-technology. Accessed 20 Jan 2021
5. Escotet-Espinoza MS, Moghtadernejad S, Scicolone J, et al (2018) Using a material property library to find surrogate materials for pharmaceutical process development. Powder Technol 339:659–676. doi: https://doi.org/10.1016/j.powtec.2018.08.042
6. Van Snick B, Dhondt J, Pandelaere K, et al (2018a) A multivariate raw material property database to facilitate drug product development and enable in-silico design of pharmaceutical dry powder processes. Int J Pharm 549:415–435. doi: https://doi.org/10.1016/j.ijpharm.2018.08.014
7. Messmer T (2013) Technical article choosing a feeder. https://www.schenckprocess.com/brochures/technical-reports. Accessed 20 Jan 2021
8. Nowak S (2015) Optimizing feeding accuracy for your batch or continuous process. Powder Bulk Eng
9. Hanson J (2018) Control of a system of loss-in-weight feeders for drug product continuous manufacturing. Powder Technol 331:236–243. doi: https://doi.org/10.1016/j.powtec.2018.03.027

10. Engisch WE, Muzzio FJ (2012) Method for characterization of loss-in-weight feeder equipment. Powder Technol 228:395–403. doi: https://doi.org/10.1016/j.powtec.2012.05.058
11. Bostijn N, Dhondt J, Ryckaert A, et al (2019) A multivariate approach to predict the volumetric and gravimetric feeding behavior of a low feed rate feeder based on raw material properties. Int J Pharm 557:342–353. doi: https://doi.org/10.1016/j.ijpharm.2018.12.066
12. Hopkins M (2006) LOSS in weight feeder systems. Meas Control 39:237–240. doi: https://doi.org/10.1177/002029400603900801
13. Engisch WE, Muzzio FJ (2015) Feedrate deviations caused by hopper refill of loss-in-weight feeders. Powder Technol 283:389–400. doi: https://doi.org/10.1016/j.powtec.2015.06.001
14. Nowak S (2016) Three ways to improve continuous loss-in-weight feeding accuracy. Powder Bulk Eng
15. Bates L (2000) Guide to the design, selection, and application of screw feeders. Professional Engineering Pub, pp 19–37
16. Dai J, Cui H, Grace JR (2012) Biomass feeding for thermochemical reactors. Prog Energy Combust Sci 38:716–736. doi: https://doi.org/10.1016/j.pecs.2012.04.002
17. Tahir F, Palmer J, Khoo J, et al (2020) Development of feed factor prediction models for loss-in-weight powder feeders. Powder Technol 364:1025–1038. doi: https://doi.org/10.1016/j.powtec.2019.09.071
18. Yadav IK, Holman J, Meehan E, et al (2019) Influence of material properties and equipment configuration on loss-in- weight feeder performance for drug product continuous manufacture. Powder Technol 348:126–137. doi: https://doi.org/10.1016/j.powtec.2019.01.071
19. Faqih AMN, Alexander AW, Muzzio FJ, Tomassone MS (2007) A method for predicting hopper flow characteristics of pharmaceutical powders. Chem Eng Sci 62:1536–1542. doi: https://doi.org/10.1016/j.ces.2006.06.027
20. Garg V, Mallick SS, Garcia-Trinanes P, Berry RJ (2018) An investigation into the flowability of fine powders used in pharmaceutical industries. Powder Technol 336:375–382. doi: https://doi.org/10.1016/j.powtec.2018.06.014
21. Jager PD, Bramante T, Luner PE (2015) Assessment of pharmaceutical powder flowability using shear cell-based methods and application of Jenike's methodology. J Pharm Sci 104:3804–3813. doi: https://doi.org/10.1002/jps.24600
22. Wong J, Kwok PCL, Chan HK (2015) Electrostatics in pharmaceutical solids. Chem Eng Sci 125:225–237. doi: https://doi.org/10.1016/j.ces.2014.05.037
23. Cartwright JJ, Robertson J, D'Haene D, et al (2013) Twin screw wet granulation: Loss in weight feeding of a poorly flowing active pharmaceutical ingredient. Powder Technol 238:116–121. doi: https://doi.org/10.1016/j.powtec.2012.04.034
24. Engisch WE, Muzzio FJ (2014) Loss-in-weight feeding trials case study: Pharmaceutical formulation. J Pharm Innov 10:56–75. doi: https://doi.org/10.1007/s12247-014-9206-1
25. Wang Y, Li T, Muzzio FJ, Glasser BJ (2017) Predicting feeder performance based on material flow properties. Powder Technol 308:135–148. doi: https://doi.org/10.1016/j.powtec.2016.12.010
26. Søgaard SV, Olesen NE, Hirschberg C, et al (2017) An experimental evaluation of powder flow predictions in small-scale process equipment based on Jenike's hopper design methodology. Powder Technol 321:523–532. doi: https://doi.org/10.1016/j.powtec.2017.08.006
27. Polizzi MA, Franchville J, Hilden JL (2016) Assessment and predictive modeling of pharmaceutical powder flow behavior in small-scale hoppers. Powder Technol 294:30–42. doi: https://doi.org/10.1016/j.powtec.2016.02.011
28. Santos B, Carmo F, Schlindwein W, et al (2018) Pharmaceutical excipients properties and screw feeder performance in continuous processing lines: a Quality by Design (QbD) approach. Drug Dev Ind Pharm 44:2089–2097. doi: https://doi.org/10.1080/03639045.2018.1513024
29. Ketterhagen WR, Curtis JS, Wassgren CR, Hancock BC (2009) Predicting the flow mode from hoppers using the discrete element method. Powder Technol 195:1–10. doi: https://doi.org/10.1016/j.powtec.2009.05.002
30. Schulze D (2016) Storage and discharge of bulk solids. In: Merkus H., Meesters G. (eds) Production, handling and characterization of particulate materials, Particle Technology Series, vol 25. Springer, Cham, pp 425–478

31. Simonaho SP, Ketolainen J, Ervasti T, et al (2016) Continuous manufacturing of tablets with PROMIS-line - Introduction and case studies from continuous feeding, blending and tableting. Eur J Pharm Sci 90:38–46. doi: https://doi.org/10.1016/j.ejps.2016.02.006

32. Blackshields CA, Crean AM (2018) Continuous powder feeding for pharmaceutical solid dosage form manufacture: a short review. Pharm Dev Technol 23:554–560. doi: https://doi.org/10.1080/10837450.2017.1339197

33. Ervasti T, Simonaho SP, Ketolainen J, et al (2015) Continuous manufacturing of extended release tablets via powder mixing and direct compression. Int J Pharm 495:290–301. doi: https://doi.org/10.1016/j.ijpharm.2015.08.077

34. Pu Y, Mazumder M, Cooney C (2009) Effects of electrostatic charging on pharmaceutical powder blending homogeneity. J Pharm Sci 98:2412–2421. doi: https://doi.org/10.1002/jps.21595

35. Beretta M, Hörmann TR, Hainz P, et al (2020) Investigation into powder tribo-charging of pharmaceuticals. Part I: Process-induced charge via twin-screw feeding. Int J Pharm 591:120014. doi: https://doi.org/10.1016/j.ijpharm.2020.120014

36. Glor M (2003) Ignition hazard due to static electricity in particulate processes. Powder Technol 135–136:223–233. doi: https://doi.org/10.1016/j.powtec.2003.08.017

37. Allenspach C, Timmins P, Lumay G, et al (2021) Loss-in-weight feeding, powder flow and electrostatic evaluation for direct compression hydroxypropyl methylcellulose (HPMC) to support continuous manufacturing. Int J Pharm 596:120259. doi: https://doi.org/10.1016/j.ijpharm.2021.120259

38. Stauffer F, Vanhoorne V, Pilcer G, et al (2019) Managing active pharmaceutical ingredient raw material variability during twin-screw blend feeding. Eur J Pharm Biopharm 135:49–60. doi: https://doi.org/10.1016/j.ejpb.2018.12.012

39. Engers DA, Fricke MN, Storey RP, et al (2006) Triboelectrification of pharmaceutically relevant powders during low-shear tumble blending. J Electrostat 64:826–835. doi: https://doi.org/10.1016/j.elstat.2006.02.003

40. Karner S, Urbanetz NA (2012) Arising of electrostatic charge in the mixing process and its influencing factors. Powder Technol 226:261–268. doi: https://doi.org/10.1016/j.powtec.2012.04.062

41. Naik S, Mukherjee R, Chaudhuri B (2016) Triboelectrification: A review of experimental and mechanistic modeling approaches with a special focus on pharmaceutical powders. Int J Pharm 510:375–385. doi: https://doi.org/10.1016/j.ijpharm.2016.06.031

42. Sarkar S, Mukherjee R, Chaudhuri B (2017) On the role of forces governing particulate interactions in pharmaceutical systems: A review. Int J Pharm 526:516–537. doi: https://doi.org/10.1016/j.ijpharm.2017.05.003

43. Wollowitz S (2010) Managing high-potency active pharmaceutical ingredients-A drug sponsor's guide. Drug Dev Res 71:420–428. doi: https://doi.org/10.1002/ddr.20385

44. Besenhard MO, Fathollahi S, Siegmann E, et al (2017) Micro-feeding and dosing of powders via a small-scale powder pump. Int J Pharm 519:314–322. doi: https://doi.org/10.1016/j.ijpharm.2016.12.029

45. Fathollahi S, Sacher S, Escotet-Espinoza MS, et al (2020) Performance evaluation of a high-precision low-dose powder feeder. AAPS PharmSciTech 21:301. doi: https://doi.org/10.1208/s12249-020-01835-5

46. Sacher S, Heindl N, Afonso Urich JA, et al (2020) A solution for low-dose feeding in continuous pharmaceutical processes. Int J Pharm 591:119969. doi: https://doi.org/10.1016/j.ijpharm.2020.119969

47. Besenhard MO, Karkala SK, Faulhammer E, et al (2016) Continuous feeding of low-dose APIs via periodic micro dosing. Int J Pharm 509:123–134. doi: https://doi.org/10.1016/j.ijpharm.2016.05.033

48. Vanarase AU, Osorio JG, Muzzio FJ (2013) Effects of powder flow properties and shear environment on the performance of continuous mixing of pharmaceutical powders. Powder Technol 246:63–72. doi: https://doi.org/10.1016/j.powtec.2013.05.002

49. Van Snick B, Grymonpré W, Dhondt J, et al (2018b) Impact of blend properties on die filling during tableting. Int J Pharm 549:476–488. doi: https://doi.org/10.1016/j.ijpharm.2018.08.015
50. Willecke N, Szepes A, Wunderlich M, et al (2017) Identifying overarching excipient properties towards an in-depth understanding of process and product performance for continuous twin-screw wet granulation. Int J Pharm 522:234–247. doi: https://doi.org/10.1016/j.ijpharm.2017.02.028
51. Hlinak AJ, Kuriyan K, Morris KR, et al (2006) Understanding critical material properties for solid dosage form design. J Pharm Innov 1:12–17. doi: https://doi.org/10.1007/BF02784876
52. Ringnér M (2008) What is principal component analysis? Nat Biotechnol 26:303–304. doi: https://doi.org/10.1038/nbt0308-303
53. Wang Y, O'Connor T, Li T, et al (2019) Development and applications of a material library for pharmaceutical continuous manufacturing of solid dosage forms. Int J Pharm 569:118551. doi: https://doi.org/10.1016/j.ijpharm.2019.118551
54. Bhalode P, Ierapetritou M (2020) Discrete element modeling for continuous powder feeding operation: Calibration and system analysis. Int J Pharm 585:119427. doi: https://doi.org/10.1016/j.ijpharm.2020.119427
55. Hou QF, Dong KJ, Yu AB (2014) DEM study of the flow of cohesive particles in a screw feeder. Powder Technol 256:529–539. doi: https://doi.org/10.1016/j.powtec.2014.01.062
56. López A, Vivacqua V, Hammond R, Ghadiri M (2020) Analysis of screw feeding of faceted particles by discrete element method. Powder Technol 367:474–486. doi: https://doi.org/10.1016/j.powtec.2020.03.064
57. Weinekötter R, Gericke H (2000) Mixing of Solids. Springer Netherlands, pp 118–124
58. Pernenkil L, Cooney CL (2006) A review on the continuous blending of powders. Chem Eng Sci 61:720–742. doi: https://doi.org/10.1016/j.ces.2005.06.016
59. Vanarase AU, Muzzio FJ (2011) Effect of operating conditions and design parameters in a continuous powder mixer. Powder Technol 208:26–36. doi: https://doi.org/10.1016/j.powtec.2010.11.038
60. U.S. Food and Drug Administration (2019) Quality considerations for continuous manufacturing guidance for industry. Center for Drug Evaluation and Research.
61. Pedersen T, Karttunen AP, Korhonen O, et al (2021) Determination of residence time distribution in a continuous powder mixing process with supervised and unsupervised modeling of in-line near infrared (NIR) spectroscopic data. J Pharm Sci 110:1259–1269. doi: https://doi.org/10.1016/j.xphs.2020.10.067
62. Van Snick B, Kumar A, Verstraeten M, et al (2019) Impact of material properties and process variables on the residence time distribution in twin screw feeding equipment. Int J Pharm 556:200–216. doi: https://doi.org/10.1016/j.ijpharm.2018.11.076

Ultrasound for Improved Encapsulation and Crystallization with Focus on Pharmaceutical Applications

Chinmayee Sarode, Yashraj Jagtap, and Parag Gogate

1 Introduction

"Ultrasound" is waves that are similar to sound or light waves but have a frequency greater than 20 kHz. Like sound waves, they are pressure waves that can be transmitted through any medium like water or air. Similarly, they can be focused, reflected, refracted, and absorbed like light waves. The ultrasound frequencies are above human's hearing capacity. Ultrasound waves consist of alternating compression and rarefaction regions that can create pressure variations in the applied medium driving various applications ranging from medicine, engineering, to material science. Moreover, ultrasound can provide the user with flexibility in the sense that their frequencies and amplitudes can be tuned. Also, they can physically act upon cells or biomolecules, bringing about desired changes. The absorption capacity of ultrasound is very low in water, tissues, or flesh in the human body. So ultrasound offers advantages such as being noninvasive, safe, and painless. These characteristics make them very attractive for usage in the pharmaceutical industry including usage as a diagnostic tool to targeted drug delivery to synthesis of drugs of specific morphology and characteristics.

In the pharmaceutical industry, there is a growing trend to explore novel and robust technologies that can be used to prepare high-quality and safe products with an enhanced process efficiency and reduced energy consumption. Ultrasound is one such approach that can be employed in various applications including encapsulation and crystallization. Integration of ultrasound into the conventional processes can give added benefits in the synthesis of microspheres and microparticles. For example, in a normal spray-drying process where heterogeneous particle size distribution

C. Sarode · Y. Jagtap · P. Gogate (✉)
Chemical Engineering Department, Institute of Chemical Technology, Mumbai, India
e-mail: pr.gogate@ictmumbai.edu.in

© The Author(s), under exclusive license to Springer Nature Switzerland AG 2022
A. Fytopoulos et al. (eds.), *Optimization of Pharmaceutical Processes*, Springer Optimization and Its Applications 189, https://doi.org/10.1007/978-3-030-90924-6_8

is an issue, using ultrasound leads to formation of small and uniform particles with a greater control over their formation. Similarly, an ultrasonic spray freeze-drying process also leads to creation of uniform, spherical, and porous particles. Even in the case of ultrasound-assisted extrusion, by virtue of ultrasonic vibrations, a homogeneous dispersion of particles is created, resulting in better product. Crystallization is one of the most significant operations in the pharmaceutical industry as more than 90% of all active pharmaceutical ingredients (APIs) are crystals. The method of crystallization determines the final crystal properties including particle size distribution, form, and polymorphic composition, which also significantly affect downstream processing and bioavailability. Ultrasound application in crystallization provides advantages such as improved crystallization parameters like nucleation, crystal growth, and distribution. It is also important to note that the application is restricted to laboratories and the employment for industrial scale operations needs to be explored.

Ultrasonic processing is dependent on various process parameters like pressure, temperature, and viscosity as well as ultrasonic parameters such as frequency and intensity. Ultrasound effects are mainly based on the vibrations induced by passage of ultrasound and the generation of cavitating conditions. For example, in the case of encapsulation, the governing mechanism is based on either the capillary wave hypothesis or cavitation theory that eventually yields better quality product. The capillary wave hypothesis focuses on the formation of a capillary wave with crests and troughs on a vibrating surface, whereas cavitation hypothesis refers to the formation of cavities leading to droplet formation from the liquid film on the surface. The proper selection of the operating conditions usually allows tailoring a given controlling mechanism that also decides the expected product characteristics. This chapter offers such discussion on the governing mechanisms for the improvement, the information on the possible reactor configurations, as well as the selection of operating conditions for the specific applications of encapsulation and crystallization. Such application of ultrasound under the desired conditions can give advantages such as greater control over particle size, enhanced solubility of drugs, controlled crystallization, and production of nanomaterials.

2 Drug Encapsulation

The global biopharmaceutical market is valued at US$ 228 billion in 2016. A recent trend is to search for novel methods of drug development that will facilitate drug production with increased efficiency and safety. There are many challenges faced by the drug developers in the initial phases of which maintaining the chemical and physical stability of the biopharmaceuticals during the manufacturing, transportation, and storage phase is the main one. This is most relevant because the stability of these biomolecules is largely dependent on a diverse range of factors like temperature, pH, interface exposure, and mechanical stress faced [1]. Cell encapsulation is among the most well-known technology in the pharmaceutical industry that provides a solution to these issues faced by the developers.

2.1 Encapsulation in Pharmaceutical Industry

Encapsulation is one of the crucial processes that has been subjected to continuous innovation in order to guarantee the success of pharmacological therapies [2]. It is characterized as a process by which solid particles or liquid/gas droplets are enclosed in an inert shell. This helps to isolate the core material from the external environment [3]. Encapsulation results in the formation of particles that have diameters of a few nm to a few mm [4]. There are various physical, chemical, and mechanical processes that can be utilized for encapsulation of various materials. Process selection depends on a variety of parameters like the nature of polymer, desired particle morphology, and chemical characteristics of a drug like solubility [5]. Stirring, static mixing, spraying, extrusion, and dripping are all common methods for microsphere formation, but ultrasonic irradiation has recently become a popular technique due to better efficiency and productivity [2]. Synthesizing microspheres requires a great deal of knowledge about (1) core material, (2) encapsulant, (3) core-matrix-environment interaction, (4) stability, and (5) core release mechanism [6, 7].

Fundamental steps in encapsulation include incorporation of bioactive compounds, droplet formation, removal of solvent, microparticle harvesting, and drying treatments [5]. The process output is extremely reliant on processing parameters like solution conditions including temperature, concentration, pH, stirring rate, sonication conditions, etc. [8]. A key performance parameter indicating the efficacy of the encapsulation process is the extent of entrapment, characterized by encapsulation efficiency or adsorption capacity [9]. While designing a system of production for any product, there are four factors that attain higher importance: encapsulation materials, production process, final morphology, and ultimate application. Along with these, other factors like the stability and functional properties of the bioactive (core) component, process reproducibility, and targeted release profile should also be considered. Caution should also be exercised to overcome certain drawbacks of microsphere aggregation and adherence [10]. Increasing the encapsulation effectiveness of a drug in drug carrier particles would result in a more potent therapeutic effect with fewer side effects [8]. Thus, encapsulation offers advantages to improve the solubility of the drug, reduce toxicity, and protect the drug from external conditions such as pH, temperature, enzymes, and oxidation [8]. It also increases the mechanical stability and achieve long-lasting matrices. It is possible to use the encapsulating vehicle as a targeting platform, thus allowing the drug to be delivered to specific cells in the body. Control of sustained or sequential drug delivery by encapsulated cells in response to external stimuli or environmental changes can also be brought about by encapsulation [11]. Table 1 provides details about the commonly applied encapsulation techniques.

Table 1 Encapsulation techniques

Method	Core	Size (μm)	Active load (%)	Morphology	Principle	References
Spray drying	Liquid/solid	10–400	5–50	Matrix	Atomization of core material takes place in a hot chamber with concurrent evaporation of water	Zuidam and Shimoni [4], Roos and Livney [12], Đorđević et al. [13]
Spray cooling/chilling	Liquid/solid	20–200	10–20	Matrix	Solidification of molten core compound takes place in a cold chamber after spraying	Zuidam and Shimoni [4], Đorđević et al. [13]
Fluidized bed coating	Solid	5–5000	5–50	Reservoir	Coating material is sprayed onto solid particles fluidized by air	Zuidam and Shimoni [4], Roos and Livney [12], Đorđević et al. [13]
Lyophilization/freeze drying	Liquid	1–1000	1–95	Matrix	Mixing the core in a coating solution and freeze-drying under low pressure or vacuum	Đorđević et al. [13], Sanguansri and Augustin [7], Jyothi, et al. [3]
Melt extrusion	Liquid/solid	300–5000	5–40	Matrix	Extrusion of melt takes place along with active compounds after passage through orifices or extruder	Zuidam and Shimoni [4], Đorđević et al. [13]
Emulsification	Liquid	10–1000	20–50	Matrix	Gelling agent is added to emulsion of biopolymer-with-water in oil under conditions of shear	Zuidam and Shimoni [4], Roos and Livney [12], Đorđević et al. [13]
Co-extrusion	Liquid/solid	150–8000	70–90	Reservoir	Dissolve active in oil phase, prepare an aqueous coating and use concentric nozzles to press simultaneously water phase through outer nozzle and oil phase through inner nozzle	Zuidam and Shimoni [4], Roos and Livney [12], Sanguansri and Augustin [7]
Simple coacervation	Liquid/solid	20–500	40–90	Reservoir	Oil and water emulsions are mixed under turbulent conditions along with actives resulting into three-phase formation followed by cross-linking for increasing stability	Zuidam and Shimoni [4], Đorđević et al. [13], Sanguansri and Augustin [7], Jyothi et al. [3]
Liposome entrapment	Liquid/solid	10–1000	5–50	Various	Phospholipids are dispersed in an aqueous phase	Zuidam and Shimoni [4], Roos and Livney [12], Đorđević et al. [13]

2.2   Ultrasound in Drug Encapsulation

Ultrasound has been used for decades now in various therapeutic applications with focus on targeted drug delivery. However, these targeted deliveries based on cavitation phenomena (acoustic pressure waves bringing about collapse of gas bubbles due to their oscillations) are not the only advantages of ultrasound usage [14]. The energy produced by ultrasonic processes was discovered to be capable of effectively degrading and breaking down biopolymers at a low cost. Ultrasound has grown into a powerful tool for extracting and modifying different biopolymers in order to increase solubility, reduce viscosity, and improve yield in recent years [15]. Ultrasound is also used in the processing stage to prepare microspheres and microparticles through their integration in various conventional processes. Ultrasonic spray drying, ultrasonic spray freeze drying, ultrasound-assisted extrusion, and ultrasonic spray polymerization are the main approaches applied in encapsulation for obtaining microspheres.

Ultrasound (US) is a cyclic sound wave with a frequency above 20 kHz [16], which creates pressure variations in the medium. The main ultrasound parameters that affect the characteristics and levels of benefits obtained in varied applications include frequency, intensity, and duration [17]. Based on the operating frequency, we can identify three distinct sets of applications in the pharmaceutical industry:

(a) High frequency: A low-energy ultrasound with a frequency of 3–10 MHz that is typically used to trigger release at specific points in the body, as well as an analytical method for determining physicochemical properties like composition, structure, particle size, and flow rate [18].
(b) Medium frequency: Therapeutic ultrasound with frequency ranging between 0.7 and 3.0 MHz normally used in physical therapy.
(c) Low frequency: A high-energy power ultrasound with frequency in the range of 20–800 kHz used in various processes like spraying, freezing, extraction, drying, etc. [17, 19].

To carry out an ultrasonic treatment, various approaches based on different configurations can be used. However, certain ways of inserting an ultrasonic probe or submerging in an ultrasonic bath are the most commonly applied ones. Any ultrasound-based system comprises three parts: generator, transducer, and delivery system. To drive the transducer assembly, the generator converts the electricity into the desired alternating current at ultrasonic frequency. The transducer then converts the current into vibrations. Finally, the vibration is relayed to the ultrasonic reactor by the delivery system [18]. Ultrasonic systems may result in a better-quality product, at reduced cost. The costs are lower due to the absence of any moving parts, which leads to less maintenance needs. The technology is also easy to install and can be retrofitted easily.

Ultrasonic Atomization for Spray Drying

Spray drying of biotherapeutics is a well-known technology to enable stabilization and functionality for drug delivery applications. It helps to improve flow properties, increase the solubility of poorly water-soluble drugs, and allows drying heat-sensitive materials [20]. Evaporation from an atomized feed is accomplished by combining the spray with the drying medium. It consists of four steps: atomization, mixing of spray and air, evaporation, and product separation [21]. The atomization phase involves drying leading to the formation of desired particles with required physicochemical and morphological properties [22]. The most critical atomizer characteristics are drop size uniformity, spray homogeneity, and control over droplet size distribution. However, the heterogeneous distribution of particles as a result of conventional encapsulation processes results in irregular drug release characteristics. To avoid this, ultrasonic atomization has been explored in an effort to produce uniform particles [23].

Ultrasonic atomization is a novel spray-drying technique in which fluid is fed into the chamber through an ultrasonic atomizer resulting in the formation of particles of smaller sizes [21]. Ultrasonic atomization is a robust and a novel single-step process that has scale-up potential to generate particles with a reasonably uniform size distribution [24]. It is largely used in the biopharmaceutical and pharmaceutical industries for spray drying with major advantages such as continuous manufacturing and formation of particles with uniform particle size and distribution [1]. Process parameters, liquid physicochemical properties, and equipment parameters are the factors normally used to accurately obtain the desired product characteristics [2]. The tip of a horn has a small orifice that vibrates ultrasonically in a longitudinal mode and is used to feed the fluid at a controlled rate, and thus, small droplets of uniform size can be created [5].

Advantages of Ultrasonic Spray Drying

1. It is a continuous process with good reproducibility and scale-up potential.
2. The obtained particles are uniform and fine resulting in narrow size distribution.
3. Atomization increases the available surface area for the finished product, which improves mass transfer and diffusion.
4. Due to increased particle surface area and increased contact of particles with drying air, operation at lower temperatures is possible.
5. Pressurized fluid is not needed, thus minimizing the energy cost of pressurizing as well as the space for additional equipment.
6. Low velocity atomization decreases the required diameter of drying chamber, thus lowering equipment cost. Low velocity spray has the added benefit of reducing material loss due to particle adhesion to the chamber wall.
7. It has a lower shear and thermal stress compared to the conventional nozzles, thus preserving the chemical and physical integrity of the product.
8. Evaporation rates are higher due to the smaller particle sizes.

9. The particle density is easily controlled.
10. Large apertures can be used in ultrasonic atomizers to solve the problem of nozzle clogging.
11. It is easier to maintain and operate.
12. Better retention of quality of bioactive compounds due to shorter particle residence time [25, 26].

Disadvantages of Ultrasonic Spray drying

Industrial scale operation is limited due to low throughput, heat generation, and lack of suitable large-scale designs. Some of the disadvantages of the ultrasonic spray-drying process include the following:

1. Ultrasonic spray drying is only applicable to the Newtonian fluids with low viscosities.
2. The cavitation efficacy of liquids with a higher viscosity is much lower.
3. The ultrasonic spray units require large quantities of hot air for the evaporation purpose because the decreased pressure is the main driving force for moisture evaporation.
4. Due to their smaller design and low area of vibrating surface, high-frequency atomizers have a limited volume handling ability [25].

Principle

The ultrasonic atomization can be achieved by vibrating a liquid layer using ultrasound transmission into liquid attained using piezoelectric crystal vibrating at a high frequency. Alternatively, an electromechanical device that consists of two piezoelectric disks tightened by a support element and a mechanical amplifying element typically constitutes an ultrasonic atomizer [2]. Normal atomizers use nozzles based on mechanical energy. However, ultrasonic atomizers use just low vibrational energy to produce drops.

Pneumatic nozzles have many disadvantages like inability to generate lower particle size, wide distribution of droplet sizes, partial segregation of the mixture's components, irregular surface morphology, structural defects, unsuitable coating material properties, and clogging problems. Moreover, a correlation can be observed between the particle size and equipment dimensions. An increase in size will see a corresponding increase in associated costs due to requirement of larger equipment. This can be avoided by using ultrasonic energy. Ultrasonic spray drying improves particle formation and leads to a narrow and homogenous particle size distribution [2, 26]. Liquid atomization attempts to break off liquid into tiny droplets from the surface of solids by creating disturbances in the normal direction. These disturbances can be created using various methods. However, if they are induced using vibrations by ultrasonic energy passage, the process is known as ultrasonic atomization [25].

Two kinds of hypothesis have been put forth to explain ultrasonic atomization: capillary and cavitation. The capillary wave hypothesis is based on the Taylor instability. The main consideration of this hypothesis is the capillary wave formation on the vibration surface. These waves are composed of crests and troughs [5]. Typically, during the operation, the first step is the formation of a thin liquid film on the surface. Atomizers are used to circulate this liquid feed at a desired flow rate. Ultrasonic vibrations can be obtained due to piezoelectric crystal vibrations at high frequencies (usually in the 20 kHz to 3 MHz range). During the atomization process, capillary waves will be formed on the liquid surface. Their wavelength is dependent on the ultrasound parameters such as frequency of ultrasound, power supplied, and liquid physicochemical properties. Liquid viscosity, density, concentration, and surface tension are the main properties deciding the capillary wavelength, which ultimately decides the size of droplet formed through ultrasonic atomization. When the vibrations produced are sufficiently higher than the liquid surface tension, waves will begin to pinch off into small droplets and atomization occurs [2, 25].

The cavitation theory, on the other hand, considers that cavitation in the liquid film on the surface is responsible for the formation of droplets. It states that the transmitted wave with its series of compression and rarefaction cycles results into void formation. As they grow, these droplets expand, grow to a maximum, and collapse immediately when they become unstable. When these cavities collapse, particularly near the surface, liquid droplets are ejected immediately. The cavitation hypothesis for atomization is normally applied to high-energy-intensity systems. The governing mechanism is also dependent on many factors like vapor pressure and gas content of the liquid, as well as the presence of luminescence [2, 5].

Equipment

Ultrasonic atomizers are process intensification instruments as they work at low velocities and also generate droplets using lower energy than conventional atomizers [22]. Under certain volumetric flow rate conditions, the use of an ultrasonic atomizer can reduce the energy demand by about 10 MJ/m^3 [5].

A typical ultrasonic atomizer consists of a nozzle for spraying, an extended length for allowing flow, and an ultrasonic generator [23]. A traditional ultrasonic atomizer consists of a vibrating plate with a concentric hole. Liquid feed enters through this hole with the help of a centrifugal or a peristaltic pump and spreads on the surface. There is a need to reduce feed viscosity to prevent clogging in tubes; a pump aids in this process and allows for uniform and reproducible feeding [22, 24]. The vibrating plate is connected to a transducer that is powered by an electric generator which allows the power supplied to the atomizer tip to be varied. Various frequency generators may also be used to regulate the operating frequency to obtain a desired shape [27]. As a conventional ultrasonic atomizer runs risk of blocking immediately after starting the atomization process, a new atomizer with carrier air design can be used (Fig. 1) [26]. Depending on the application, geometric

Fig. 1 Schematic diagram of an ultrasonic atomizer. (1) Connection for oscillator, (2) connection for liquid, (3) connection for carrier air, (4) protecting cap, (5) piezoceramic element, (6) carrier air, (7) actual atomizer, (8) atomizer jet [26]

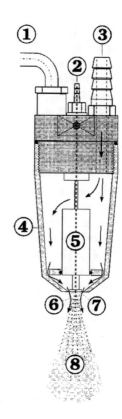

parameters like the diameter of the concentric hole or the disk can also be varied along with operating conditions such as temperature, surface tension, and viscosity of liquid [2].

Applications

Ultrasonic atomization has been used for processes with feed containing low viscous Newtonian fluids. The frequency of operating nozzle ranges from 30 kHz to 2.5 MHz and results in the formation of particles with excellent uniform particle size distribution and a particle size range of 10–100 microns. Due to lower shear stress, it can also be employed widely for pharmaceuticals as their degradation is lowered [25].

Ultrasonic atomization has mainly been utilized in pharmaceutical manufacturing to explore encapsulation techniques for drugs or altering distribution profiles with the aim of creating novel drug delivery systems [2]. Various techniques like coaxial ultrasonic atomization have also been explored for drug encapsulation [23]. Because of the rapid evaporation of the solvent, the temperature of the droplets can be held far below that of the drying air, making spray drying ideal for use in both heat-sensitive and heat-resistant materials [21].

As a specific example, it can be mentioned that darbepoetin alfa, a synthetic type of glycoprotein hormone that regulates red blood cell development, was effectively encapsulated using ultrasonic atomization. Particle production using ultrasonic atomization was found to depend on various parameters like feed flow rate, atomization strength, and form of polymer material. Ultrasonic nozzles were capable of producing droplets of comparable median diameter, around 60 μm or less. The encapsulation efficiencies observed were near 100%. Moreover, it was shown that using ultrasound made the process more robust and reproducible. The synthesized microspheres also reflected excellent physical and chemical characteristics [2]. In another study, it was reported that as compared to atomization using two-fluid nozzles, ultrasound atomization produced higher yields, ranging from a 62% to 77% increase in absolute yield for zirconia to a 47% to 78% increase in absolute yield for ZTA [27]. As another example, Paiva et al. reported collection of about 60% of the atomized feed over the membrane in a dried powder form using the ultrasound spray-drying system. Further, it was found that the product particles were spherical in shape with a diameter size distribution of 0.2–2.6 μm. The mean diameter was found to be about 1.7 μm [21].

Ultrasonic Spray Freeze Drying

Ultrasonic spray freeze drying (USFD), a combination of spray drying and freeze drying, is a newly developed technique used in a diverse range of applications like for the development of drug delivery systems [28]. It is also referred to as lyophilization and is the sublimation process of a frozen solvent (usually water) under reduced pressure. Since it uses a low processing temperature, this method is ideal for heat-sensitive and perishable materials [29]. This method can produce microparticles with a distinctive internal structure and a large specific surface area, which is highly desirable [30].

The steps involved in this process are atomization, rapid freezing, and lyophilization. It works by trapping the solute in a frozen droplet before lyophilization. The rapid freezing step decreases the amount of solute diffusion, which reduces the probability of particles (nano/micro) aggregating [31]. Thus, spray freeze drying has more advantages than spray drying as it results in lesser particle aggregation. It also has other advantages such as uniformity and greater flexibility of controlling particle size and density. It is the most commonly used method for producing stable dry powders of biologics in industry, but it is a time-consuming, complex, and expensive batch process that necessitates a significant financial expenditure due to the requirements of cryogenic facilities. Thus, one should assess the process based on the added advantages obtained for the specific application in question [31].

Advantages

As compared to methods like spray drying or freeze drying, spray freeze drying especially using ultrasonic nozzles has the following advantages:

- Lower temperatures for reduced drying.
- Ability to process extremely heat-sensitive products.
- High process efficiency (yield greater than >90%).
- Particle characteristics can be finely regulated.
- Highly porous particles.
- Processing time is significantly lower.
- It promotes instant rehydration.
- Controlled particle size distribution.
- Particles have high specific surface area.
- Particles retain their spherical shape throughout.
- Excellent compatibility with a variety of excipients and biopharmaceuticals.
- It enhances the apparent solubility of poorly water-soluble drugs.
- Minimization of phase separation between drug and excipients owing to the ultrafast freezing process [28, 32, 33].

Disadvantages

Almost all spray freeze-drying approaches are still experimental and scaled only for laboratory purposes. This is true for ultrasonic spray freeze-drying process too. Industrial and regulatory aspects such as process qualification, scale-up and scale-down potential, and good manufacturing practice have seldom been discussed [33].

Method

The main steps involved in the spray freeze-drying (SFD) process are spraying, freezing, and drying.

(a) Spraying: Dispersion of bulk liquid solutions into droplets.
(b) Rapid freezing: Droplets solidify as they come into close contact with a cold solvent.
(c) Lyophilization: Sublimation drying of the frozen material at a very low temperature and pressure [33].

The main concept behind the spray freeze-drying process is to decrease the drying time. This is done by rapid atomization of a liquid by passing into a low temperature zone that is maintained normally with cryogens (e.g., liquid nitrogen). Following this, the frozen particles are sublimated under atmospheric pressure. This is brought about by a reduction in product dimensions, which leads to an improvement in heat and associated mass transfer, thus reducing freezing and drying times [28]. Precipitation can also be done using an anti-solvent. Precipitated particles are continuously collected in a liquid nitrogen-filled beaker with the help of an ultrasonic atomization probe and then transferred to a freeze dryer to create dry powders [33].

The first step, which is atomization, involves breaking down of a bulk solution, or suspension into smaller droplets takes place. An atomizer is used, which has a significant impact on droplet formation to create a high surface to mass ratio. It determines the particle's form, size, and density as well as provides a wide surface area to aid evaporation. Various nozzles like two-fluid, three-fluid, four-fluid, and ultrasonic nozzles are normally used for the same. Some of the advantages of using ultrasonic nozzles for atomization are the following:

(a) A narrow droplet size distribution that can be controlled.
(b) Since there is no extra air flow, drops are captured easily in a liquid cryogen. [29].

Atomization energy, feed viscosity, surface tension, and feed flow rate are the important factors that affect atomization. Typically, high atomization pressures can be used to attain smaller droplet sizes [28].

After atomization, in the presence of cryogens like liquid nitrogen, freezing can be done at sub-zero temperatures [28]. The following five steps are involved in the freezing of droplets:

(a) Liquid cooling and supercooling: Cooling of the liquid droplet occurs at a temperature below the equilibrium freezing point.
(b) Nucleation: Supercooling to induce spontaneous crystal nucleation.
(c) Recalescence: Rapid kinetic crystal growth from the nuclei is driven by supercooling. Abrupt temperature rise is observed due to liberation of latent heat of fusion with termination of the growth after reaching equilibrium freezing temperature.
(d) Freezing: Further growth is observed till the droplet freezes throughout.
(e) Solid cooling or tempering: The temperature of the frozen droplets falls to a steady-state value similar to that of the ambient air [33].

The size of the particles formed by rapid freezing is determined by the size of the atomized feed droplet, while the solute concentration determines the average particle density. By varying ultrasonic frequencies and power dissipation, particles of varied sizes can be prepared via atomization [32].

Phase separation of solids by lyophilization (sublimation under vacuum) takes place during freezing. This results into void formation in the final dried particles. It is also recognized that the aqueous droplet size dominates the size of particles formed by spray freeze drying at both low and high concentrations. Thus, the size of the frozen droplet determines the final particle size [34]. Furthermore, the amount of solute in each droplet differs depending on the liquid feed's concentration. As a consequence, the particle density is proportional to the starting solution concentration [32]. The process is also reported to result into the formation of highly porous particles with a powder tap density as low as 0.01 g/mL [32].

In normal spray drying, the particle size and shape are determined by the drying step, while in the spray freeze drying, they are determined by the freezing step. The density, compressibility, and friability of the lyophilized microparticles are influenced by the types and concentrations of solids in the starting solution. The obtained particles typically have excellent flow properties, owing to their small size and low density [33].

Equipment

Spray towers with liquid nitrogen cooling jacket can be used for spray freeze drying. This prevents particles from freezing during flight in cold air while preventing contact with liquid nitrogen. Nanoparticle dispersions are also known to be atomized using this method.

The process normally takes place in two main parts:

(a) Freezing chamber: An in-house pressure air supply is used to provide pressurized air, and it is dehumidified. For cooling the air, it can be allowed to flow through a cylindrical pressure chamber filled with dry ice. The outlet air temperature is −85 to −75 °C. After that, the air enters the freezing cabinet from the bottom and exits from the top. To create suitable freezing conditions, an air throughput is used. The spraying nozzle is positioned in the exact center of the chamber's top. This location is strategic to prevent clogging of nozzle owing to its completely exposed-to-the-air position. The droplets freeze during the freezing step, resulting in the formation of crystals within the frozen particle. Liquid nitrogen is normally used to maintain freezing conditions (refer to Fig. 2a).

(b) Drying chamber: The cold air is then warmed to the desired drying temperature. The chamber is double walled, and air enters the drying chamber through the outer walls (blanket). For the purpose of fluidization and drying, the necessary air is directed to the drying chamber. The crystals that have formed are then removed, resulting in porous interconnected particles as opposed to normal spray drying process that forms nonporous particles (Refer Fig. 2b) [35, 36].

The dissolved mixture can be fed into an ultrasonic nozzle that is powered by an ultrasonic generator using a digitally operated syringe pump. The nozzle height has little effect on the size of the drop, but it has to be high enough to keep the solution from freezing in the atomizer. Gravity pulls the atomized droplets into the liquid nitrogen collection vessel. The sprayed mists are instantly frozen and dispersed in the vessel with liquid nitrogen after being trapped by it. The excess liquid nitrogen is later allowed to simmer away after the solution is sprayed. The frozen droplets are lyophilized in a freeze dryer and the resultant USFD microparticles collected and stored [30].

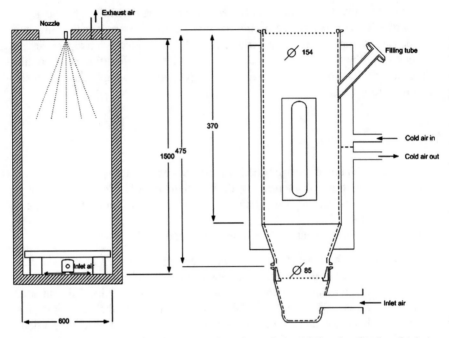

Fig. 2 Schematic representation of ultrasonic spray freeze drying (**a**) Freezing chamber, (**b**) drying chamber [35]

Applications

The highly porous characteristics of powders produced using ultrasonic spray freeze drying are ideal for varied pharmaceutical applications such as improving dissolution of poorly water-soluble drugs and pulmonary delivery [32]. The main advantage of this process is its low temperature spraying operation, which makes it appropriate for formulations such as NCM (nanocomposite microcarriers) that are required for pulmonary inhalation. Another benefit is the porous structure, which enables easy dissolution. Ultrasonic nozzles give an additional benefit of providing greater control over particle size distribution [36]. It results in the formation of porous particles that were shown to facilitate particle deposition in the lungs. Furthermore, in many cases, it was discovered that antigen retention was high, resulting in improved immunogenic responses to the drug [28]. Table 2 gives information about the mean particle diameter observed under different parameters applied in ultrasonic spray freeze drying.

Ultrasound-Assisted Extrusion

Hot melt extrusion has established itself as a very popular and robust process-ing technology for the development of molecular dispersions of varied active

Table 2 Applications of ultrasonic spray freeze drying

Sr. no.	Components	Method	Liquid feed rate	Ultrasonic frequency	Mean particle diameter	References
1	10-Hydroxycampt othecin in tertiary butyl alcohol	Ultrasonic spray into an SS vessel containing liquid N_2	1 mL/min	48 kHz	30–40 μm	Gao et al. [30]
2	Solutions of mannitol, bovine serum albumin, or lysozyme	The atomized droplets are directed into a liquid N_2 collection vessel and lyophilized in a freeze dryer	0.5 mL/min	40 kHz	17.2–30 μm	D'Addio et al. [31]
3	Influenza vaccine preformulation	Formulation sprayed into liquid N_2 taken in an SS pan	1.5 mL/min	60 kHz	30–60 mm	Maa etal. [32]

pharmaceutical ingredients (APIs). Through this technique, modified, extended, time-controlled, and targeted drug delivery through capsules, films, tablets, and implants via transdermal, oral, and transmucosal routes is possible [37].

Extrusion is a transformation process that involves pumping of raw materials into an extruder with counter-rotating or co-rotating screw elements at elevated controlled temperature and pressure. With the help of an extruder, the raw material is melted and mixed to produce desired products [38]. So the extruder serves the role of a pump that pressurizes the raw materials to pass through the nozzle [39]. This technology is normally applied for the preparation of solid dispersions. The material is fed in the solid form and is heated until it reaches the molten state. Later, it leaves the extruder in the desired pre-decided state depending on the applied shape. Some parameters, such as shear, feeding rate, screw rotating speed, and temperature, can be changed to produce final product with a uniform size, shape, and content [37, 40, 41].

The varied applications in the pharmaceutical and other industries of ultrasonic spray freeze drying process are owing to its characteristic features like cost-effective operation, solvent-free nature, green technology, easy scalability, and continuous manufacturing capability as opposed to other conventional technologies. However, certain challenges such as high processing temperatures, high energy input, and non-availability of appropriate grade polymers hamper its usage [38]. The lack of homogeneous dispersion in product particles is also an issue, and to overcome it, an alternative of using ultrasound waves during the extrusion process is widely followed and known as ultrasound-assisted extrusion [39]. The basic advantage of using ultrasonic-assisted extrusion lies in the development of a uniform dispersion of product particles. Rotating screws play a major role behind the agitation and the vigorous mixing. It leads to de-aggregation of drug particles, resulting in the creation of a more uniformly dispersed product that can be either a solid or a liquid solution or a mixture of the both [40].

Advantages

Extrusion offers a number of benefits as opposed to conventional techniques such as the following:

- Fewer processing steps.
- Economical process.
- Solvent-free process.
- Reduced production time.
- Increased solubility and bioavailability of water-insoluble compounds.
- Continuous operation.
- Uniform content in the product.
- Ease of scalability.
- Capabilities of sustained, and targeted drug release.
- Producing a diverse range of performance dosage forms and delivery routes.
- Provision of various screw geometries [37, 40].

Disadvantages

- High process temperatures.
- Unsuitable for heat-sensitive compounds.
- High energy requirement.
- Needs excipients to increase the flow.
- Limited number of suitable grade compounds.
- Requirement of good flow properties for the feed [37, 40].

Concept

Three major zones can be identified in the ultrasound-assisted extrusion process depending on the pressure exerted along the extrusion barrel: the feeding zone, the transition zone, and the dosing zone. The feeding zone is present near the place where the feed enters, and in this zone, gradual compaction occurs at a set speed. Transition zone involves intermediate compression of the present material. Here, fusion takes place and the air that could be trapped escapes through the feed hopper. At the end lies the dosing zone where homogenization of the molten material takes place and it is further pressurized to pass out of the extruder [39].

While melt extrusion itself has many advantages and varied applications, ultrasound-assisted process offers more benefits. The major advantage of ultrasound application in the shaping zone is to reduce the viscosity or decrease the shaping channels' resistance. It also causes an increase in flow rate, a decrease in pressure drop, improved extrudate appearance, reduction in extrusion swell, decreased specific power consumption, and change in molecular weight and its distribution [42]. All this happens because ultrasound vibration makes the configurations of molecular chains random by increasing their motion. The relaxation process of polymer melts is also affected as a reduction in the relaxation time is observed. It leads to an overall weakening of the elastic effect, thus reducing the extrusion swell. A chemical effect is also observed along with the physical effect. An increase in the ultrasound intensity leads to reduction in the molecular weight of compound. Thus, a narrow molecular-weight distribution is observed. As the orientation of the melt molecules changes along the flow direction, the crystallinity decreases. This results into reduction in the non-Newtonian flow characteristics of the melt and a viscosity drop [41, 42].

The mix's thermal and chemical degradation, the extrudate's physicochemical stability, the drug's interaction with the other ingredients in the mixture, and the improvement in drug performance should be considered when designing an extrusion process [41]. The physical state of the active moiety also has a substantial impact on material processing, drug release properties, and drug stability in the final extrudates [40].

Equipment

An extruder requires a feeding system, a melting-plasticizing system, a pumping and pressurizing system, and, ultimately, a device for forming the molten material [39]. Incorporating ultrasound into melt extrusion necessitates a processing system, a sonotrode, and an ultrasonic wave generator in their most basic form (Refer Fig. 3). It's possible to use an extruder with speeds ranging from 50 to 100 rpm [39]. The extruder usually comprises one or two rotating screws operated either in same or opposite directions. These are present inside a stationary cylindrical barrel. Manufacturing of the barrel takes part in sections. This is done to decrease the residence time of molten materials. These sections of barrel are later clamped or

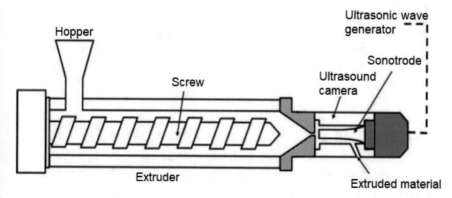

Fig. 3 Schematic representation of an extruder [39]

bolted together. At the barrel's end, a die is connected. Its dimensions and shapes are dependent on the desired shape of the extruded material [37]. A specially designed section generally made of titanium is also attached to the extruder to contain a sonotrode. The chamber also contains a nozzle for the purpose of extraction of nanocomposites, along with a system for temperature control. The ultrasonic generator is connected to the sonotrode, which can run at frequencies ranging from 10 to 100 kHz and with powers up to 1000 W [39].

The screw and the barrel are among the most crucial components in this process because they help to transport, heat, melt, and mix the material. As a result, the screw design has a substantial impact on the process's stability and the quality of the final extrudate product. The screw typically comprises a long cylinder surrounded by a helical fillet [39]. The most important design parameters are length, diameter, angle of the propeller, and thread pitch. If one screw is present, the equipment is referred to as a single-screw extruder, whereas if two screws are present, the equipment is referred to as a double-screw or twin-screw extruder. The number of screws and their configuration have a big impact on the mixing. The screws in twin-screw extruders can be rotated in opposite directions, and they also have varying degrees of interpenetration. A good mixing and degassing capacity with better control of residence time and distribution are important advantages of using twin-screw extruder. The fact that these extruders are more expensive than single-screw extruders and that their performance is difficult to predict are two drawbacks [39].

Application

Ultrasound-assisted extrusion has proven to be a reliable method of producing a variety of drug delivery systems, and as a result, it has been used in the pharmaceutical industry on a large extent. The system allows it to be able to process a wide array of polymers and APIs [37]. It is used in the pharmaceutical industry as a convenient, solvent-free, fast, reproducible, and low-cost manufacturing process for production of a large number of pharmaceutical dosage forms that can be administered via various delivery routes. Some of the specific applications include preparation of nanosystems, improved dissolution of poorly soluble drugs, and sustained release formulations [41].

Several studies of ultrasound-assisted extrusion have reported the preparation of polymer nanocomposites and improved nanoparticle dispersion in polyamide. In addition, there is an improvement in both rheological and mechanical properties after the ultrasonic treatment [39].

3 Sonocrystallization

In the development of solid form active pharmaceutical ingredients (API), crystallization is a key step to decide the characteristics such as purity, type, shape, and size of the particles. The efficacy of getting the desired solid-state property allows solid APIs in the downstream formulation procedure to be processed effectively with the excipient. Cooling or antisolvent crystallization is generally used with application of CSTR (continuous stirred-tank reactors) and mixed-suspension mixed-product removal (MSMPR) as the conventional reactor designs; however, the drawbacks of these traditional routes are the variation in batches and supersaturation design restrictions. In addition, the average particle size of powders produced by traditional crystallization is difficult to monitor and many a time not reproducible. Additional mechanical milling is required in this situation to minimize the size of particles further, but the additional friction often causes issues such as the degradation of surface properties and generation of fines. New crystallization processes including sonocrystallization, oscillatory baffled crystallizers, and non-photochemical laser-induced technologies have been introduced and developed in order to effectively regulate the solid-state property of API and overcome the drawbacks of traditional routes [43]. We will discuss the different aspects of ultrasound-assisted crystallization or the sonocrystallization in this section. The use of ultrasound in crystallization has vastly been reported for a diverse variety of crystalline compounds, but the possible pathways for improvements and scale-up aspects are still unclear [44].

Ultrasound is a frequency-dependent sound wave with a spectrum ranging from 15 kHz to 2 MHz. As ultrasound of adequate amplitude travels through a liquid, the local strength (tensile) of liquid is exceeded by the negative pressure created, resulting in the creation of cavitational bubbles. They form normally near preexisting impurities like dust and gas-filled crevasses, pulsating and expanding at the time of expansion and contraction cycles. The formed bubbles undergo size variations over a normal compression-expansion cycle, reaching a maximum size depending on the resonant size that changes according to the frequency of the applied ultrasound, typically 170 μm is the resonant size for a 20-kHz frequency wave. Bubbles implode finally because they cannot sustain themselves releasing large magnitude of energy [45]. The forming and collapse of bubbles induced by the expansive and compressive acoustic waves applied to the liquid is the phenomenon of acoustic cavitation. The energy released during the process can be used to initiate the nuclei formation, induce crystal size breakdown, and provide faster crystallization based on micro-mixing [46]. Compared to homogeneous systems, the physical impacts of irradiation are more complex in heterogeneous networks due to the favoring of nucleation.

Richards and Loomis were the first to publish on sonocrystallization in 1927. The report looked at the impact of ultrasound on crystallization, as well as other physiochemical factors. Sonocrystallization was widely studied in the Soviet Union from the 1950s to the 1970s. Sonocrystallization of different substances and the alteration of various experimental variables are documented. Because of developments in ultrasonic equipment, industrial applications of sonocrystallization grew in the 1980s, and it is now used to produce crystals in the medicinal and fine chemical industries. Despite extensive research, a thorough knowledge of sonocrystallization, particularly the mechanisms and scale-up strategies, remains elusive.

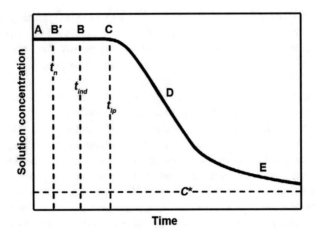

Fig. 4 Variation of solution concentration with time for understanding of induction time

3.1   Crystallization Effects of Ultrasound

Induction Time

The time spent between supersaturation and the formation of crystals is referred to as the induction time (t_{ind}) (Fig. 4). The overall time is divided into three sections: time for relaxation (t_r), time for growth of nucleus (tg), and time for attaining stable nucleus (t_n). Relaxation is the length required to achieve an almost stable distribution of the molecular clusters by the crystallized solution, while the stable time of nucleus development and the time of nucleus growth are the duration it requires for such a stable nucleus to shape and extend to measurable sizes. In certain systems, particularly those with low levels of supersaturation, significant nucleation occurs after a latent period (t_{lp}). During the induction and latent phases, the crystallized solution concentration keeps relatively stable. Following the latent phase, widespread crystal growth occurs, allowing the solution's concentration to change quickly and dramatically. Induction time is affected primarily by turbulence, contaminants, solution viscosity, supersaturation, and other factors [44].

At point A, supersaturation is attained, and after a certain lag duration, crystal nucleation takes place at B'. Nuclei begins developing till crystals of visible dimensions are formed at B. When the concentration of the solution becomes stable at C, growth of crystals lowers solvent concentration rapidly (D region) until balance is achieved (E curve region). C denotes saturation at equilibrium, t_n denotes time for nucleation, t_{ind} denotes time for induction, and t_{lp} denotes duration of latency [44].

Ultrasonic irradiation shortens the induction time due to the intensified mixing and distortion caused by acoustic waves. Cavitation, or the signs associated with it, such as air bubbles and shear due to bubble blowouts and vibrations, was commonly assumed to yield greater formation of crystals during sonication and hence reduction in induction time. The rate of crystal formation accelerates as the induction time

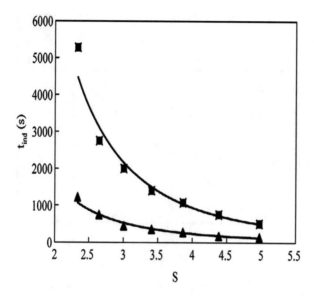

Fig. 5 The induction time of roxithromycin crystallization (t_{ind}) against the supersaturation level (S) when no ultrasound (*squares*) or ultrasound having a frequency of 20 kHz (*triangles*) is used [44]

decreases. As a consequence, the amount of crystals formed grows, and also their size shrinks. Ultrasound effects have been extensively reported for crystallization inductivity. Using saturated roxithromycin solutions, the function of ultrasound in changing the induction time has been analyzed by researchers [44]. In this study, saturated solution of roxithromycin with water through ultrasonication was combined with a laser recording method (He–Ne) to calculate the time of induction. Notably, when sonocrystallization was performed, the induction time was shortened as per the results reproduced in Fig. 5. In addition, the gap in induction period between sonocrystallization and agitation based crystallization increased when the supersaturated ratios of the mixture decreased.

The induction cycle of $BaSO_4$ was also quantified under ultrasonic exposure, and the time of induction for sonocrystallization was observed to be less than the time for agitation based crystallization. Irradiation using high-amplitude ultrasonic waves often shortened the time of induction as compared to the irradiation using low-amplitude waves [45]. Studies also reported the positive effect of ultrasonic power input on induction time before a restricting limit was reached. Surprisingly, supersaturation did not seem to have a noticeable impact on the induction period especially at higher ultrasonic power. While increasing supersaturation is widely reported to reduce induction times during sonication, this effect is often reported to diminish with growing ultrasonic energy. The capability of ultrasound to enable the crystallization process, even at small supersaturation when enough power is applied, is gaining interest as it provides a great deal of flexibility during process expansion [47].

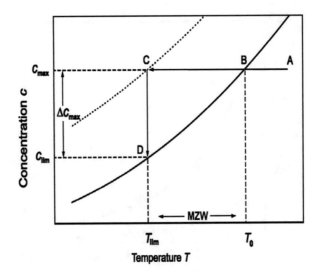

Fig. 6 Temperature-dependent solubility curve showing the metastable zone width (MZW as represented in the figure)

The area between the saturation curve and the experimental supersaturation point at which nucleation exists naturally is defined as the metastable zone width (MSZW) as elucidated in Fig. 6. The MSZW of a solution reduces as it is ultrasonically irradiated. The present heterogeneity due to the cavitating bubbles act as new nucleation places during ultrasound-assisted crystallization, allowing the rate of nucleation to increase. Furthermore, the collapsing of bubbles during sonocrystallization increases microscale mixing and turbulence. It makes solute dissemination easier and enhances nucleation rate. Sonocrystallization reduces the MSZW by increasing nucleation sites and also making nucleation easier by improving the mixing efficiency [45].

The saturation state at equilibrium of the species dissolved in the solution is described by the solid line. As we cool an initially under saturated solution (location A which has concentration C_{max}), at location B, the solution will attain its saturation (T_0); crystals, however, would not form until at a lower temperature the solution is supersaturated. Crystals at a lower temperature are observed (T_{lim}) as the sample is cooled further (location C). The process of crystal growth is repeated until the concentration of solution reaches the solubility curve at equilibrium (location D). For polythermal crystallization, the MSZW is described to be T_0–T_{lim} [44].

Nucleation Rate

When the aim is to create small crystals (a few microns or nanometers in size), nucleation rate is an essential parameter to optimize since high nucleation rates would usually generate a large number of small crystals instead of few particularly large crystals. When aiming for nanocrystals with a small size range, an optimized nucleation rate may be thus critical. Ultrasound can promote nuclei formation by lowering the crucial excessive free energy (G_{crit}). Half of solvent molecules is solvated by the solvent at the bubble–solution interface, as the other half interacts with bubbles which is not solvated. Such interactions decrease the solvation rate. The solute's re-dissolution is then halted, increasing molecule agglomeration in the solution. As a result, G_{crit} for nuclei formation reduces, while the nucleation rate increases. Furthermore, by raising the quantum of secondary sites for nucleation, ultrasound speeds up secondary nuclei formation. Crystals formed by primary nucleation interfere or associate with shockwaves when exposed to ultrasonic irradiation. Existing crystals are destroyed as a result of these events, and they become secondary sites for nucleation [45]. Secondary nuclei formation may also be triggered by violently disrupting already formed crystalline structures or poorly bound agglomerates.

A study with a variety of novel active pharmaceutical ingredients (APIs) revealed that when elevated levels of supersaturation were attained in a typical cooling crystallization, high rates of nuclei formations, along with concurrent poorly controlled crystallization, resulted in the prevalence of a unique needle behavior manifesting itself in poorly shaken slurries and poor material bulk density. An especially promising rhombic or a plate-type pattern was quickly established when a solution was equipped with ultrasonication at very relatively low supersaturation levels. Aside from pattern regulation, cautious insonation regimes enabled for consistent particle shape regulation [48] and the ascribing mechanism to the observation was based on enhanced nucleation rate.

In another study, Nonphotochemical laser-induced nucleation (NPLIN), ultrasonic irradiation, and mechanical damage of specimen vials were used to investigate the formation of nuclei of glycine from supersaturated solution. It was reported that molecules were more susceptible to nuclei formation and produced more of the γ-glycine variant at elevated supersaturation rates. In the presence of ultrasound, there was initiation of relatively high cavitation events, which leads to higher centralized tensions and high saturated concentrations [49].

Polymorphism

Polymorphs are solid forms but have different structural properties, with the same chemical composition. Numerous organic molecules may have several crystalline configurations either through different molecular arrangement in the lattices, which pack the polymorphs, or through a different configuration of the molecules in the lattices. Polymorphs of a substance usually differ according to physical and chemical characteristics such as durability, crystalline structure, compression resistance, density, and rate of dissolution, resulting in changes during the storage and properties of the compound, as well as its shelf life and the degree to which the substance or drug is fully accessible for its biological destination. In the cases where it is impossible to generate the most reliable polymorph, a metastable form with favorable features is used. For any form or type, it is critical for any pharmaceutical industry to maintain efficient and robust procedures as well as compliance with Good Manufacturing Practice. As a consequence, defining the product's potential polymorphic types is crucial and is now also a regulatory necessity [50].

Sonocrystallization can affect polymorphism, and the application of ultrasound generally turns crystals from their preferred kinematic form into a desired thermodynamic form. It is however unclear how exactly ultrasound affects a material's polymorphism [45].

Njegić Džakula, Kontrec, Ukrainczyk, Sviben, and Kralj [51] discussed the formation of precipitate of $CaCO_3$ crystalline forms with various crystal geometries. In contrast to the reference systems, the use of sonication created a variation in distribution of particle sizes and different compositions of the precipitated material. As a result, supersaturation and temperature were discovered to have an impact on the particle size of structures that were under ultrasonic exposure and of those used as reference. At 25 °C, all reference materials produced a combination of calcite, aragonite, and vaterite. The sonication increased the vaterite content at this temperature, but no aragonite was detected. At 80 °C, just aragonite precipitated in reference and ultrasound applied structures. The results further showed that initial supersaturation was the important factor critical for the composition of vaterite with higher concentration resulting in spherical vaterite particles and lower concentration resulting in hexagonal platelets. The observations further revealed different vaterite forms in processes where formation of precipitate began at relatively high saturation concentration: spherulitic vaterite development was observed in ultrasonication systems, whereas primary particle agglomeration was predominant in reference measurements. At lower supersaturation, the effect of concentration ratio of $(Ca^{2+})/(CO_3^{2-})$ mostly on composition of hexagonal shaped platelets of vaterite was also detected. By modifying the concentration ratio of $(Ca^{2+})/(CO_3^{2-})$, significant variations in polymorphic configuration were observed only within ultrasound irradiated structures at 25 °C.

The effects of ultrasonic irradiation on the crystallization behavior of tripalmitoylglycerol (PPP) as well as cocoa butter in terms of rate of nucleation and polymorphic regulation were investigated using a setup having 20 kHz frequency and 100 W power output [52]. To model real fat systems, PPP of high purity having concentration greater than 99% and PPP of low purity having concentration above 80% were used, which typically have higher amounts of secondary components alongside the main ingredient. The use of ultrasound accelerated the nucleation rate in PPPs of both the purities, as measured by the time of induction and the amount of crystals that undergo nucleation. When it came to polymorphism, ultrasound accelerated the nuclei formation of both the β' and β types, but the β'-type nuclei formation was more extreme when PPP of low purity was used. Brief sonication enhanced the crystal growth of Form V in cocoa butter. The results indicate that ultrasonic treatment can be used to tune symmetric crystallization in fats.

The polymorphism in p-amino benzoic acid is classified as occurrence of β-form, which is prismatic in nature, of the occurrence of needle-shaped α-form.

The mechanism is enantiotropic, having a temperature of transition of about 25 °C. Below the temperature of transition, the β-type becomes a thermodynamically stable form, but it is produced through very slow supersaturation development in either water or ethyl acetate. The ultrasonic effect on nuclei formation of p-amino benzoic acid forms was tested using a variety of sonication levels of intensity and schemes [50]. Sonication showed to greatly decrease the induction time for nucleation. Using guided sonication, it was possible to crystallize PPP's β-form more reproducibly and at faster cooling rates. Furthermore, sonication was observed to favor the presence of the β-polymorph very selectively. Above the temperature of transition, it was also possible to produce the pure β-form, which is a metastable state that is difficult to develop without sonication. The α-structure relies upon centro-symmetric dimers created by interaction of groups of carboxylic acid, whereas the β-form is made up of rings (four membered) having hydrogen bonding between alternate amino and carboxylic groups. It is hypothesized that ultrasonic irradiation disrupts dimer formation in solution, allowing the β-form to crystallize.

Sonocrystallization, may sometimes provide a polymorphic form that is less stable in terms of thermodynamic aspects. Paracetamol occurs in stable form I and metastable form II, with form II having greater solubility due to the disparity in stability. In form I, crystals of platelike shape are formed when super-saturated paracetamol mixture was cooled in the absence of sonication. Sonication, on the other hand, culminated in the production of form II crystals that were like needles. Sonocrystallization was thus confirmed to produce less stable forms; however, no specific reasons have been given [45]. It is thus important to decide on the application of ultrasound with an objective to obtain only the desired form of polymorph.

3.2   Variation of Benefits in Crystallization with Ultrasound Parameters

Ultrasonic Frequency

The dynamics of bubble droplets are affected by changes in ultrasound frequencies. Since wavelengths rise as frequencies decrease, cavitation droplets are exposed to ultrasound waves for prolonged time periods at low frequency of waves (100 kHz). As a result, the amplitude of the bubble oscillation is high because the magnitude of the bubble varies significantly during compression and expansion times. Large ultrasonic frequencies (>200 kHz), on the other hand, reduce the wavelength of the ultrasonication applied and decrease the cavity's lifetime. There are usually thick layers of cavitational droplets in all situations; each bubble's power of collapse is proportional to its length: larger for big bubbles at lower frequencies and smaller for small droplets at higher frequencies.

Yamaguchi et al. (2009) used ultrasonic irradiation to create liposomes and studied the influence of irradiation frequency on their scale. At a constant strength of

8 W/cm^2, three separate operating frequencies as 43, 143, and 480 kHz were used. As the sound frequency decreased, liposome size decreased due to changes in bubble dynamics. Another study looked at the impact of frequency of ultrasound wave on the MSZW. Temperature cooled crystallization of paracetamol was measured at various frequencies (from 41 to 1140 kHz) with ultrasonic irradiation, and the difference between temperature of nucleation and saturation was calculated for MSZW. It was reported that MSZW decreased as the ultrasound frequency increased [45].

Among the most essential factors in sonochemical reactors is the choice of an efficient irradiation frequency. A low frequency (10–100) kHz may be used to induce a physical reaction in the environment and also in crystallization under controlled conditions. This frequency range is widely used in biodiesel production, polymer degradation and recovery, fiber production, and other applications including crystallization [53]. Higher frequency can be used in applications such as synthetic chemistry and waste management where an extreme chemical effect is needed. Yamaguchi et al. (2009) investigated the impact of frequency of ultrasound ranging from 19.5 kHz to 1.2 MHz using the seven various sonochemical reactors. It was reported that raising the frequency in the range of 19.5–200 kHz contributes to an improvement in sonochemical effects. However, owing to the low energy dissipation of ultrasound, at a very high frequency, a reverse effect can be explained, leading to an optimum frequency for the beneficial results. It is also important to note that there are several disadvantages to using higher frequency, such as transducer surface deterioration during continuous processing and high power consumption. To avoid these issues, where high cavitation bubble intensities are needed, a singular higher-frequency process may be replaced by dual or multi-low frequency operations. Furthermore, dual or multiple frequency operation may result in more uniform cavitational behavior propagation and better acoustic performance. Combining lower frequencies results in greater effectiveness than a single high frequency. For example, dual frequency sonochemical systems have been reported to produce greater cavitation bubble volume fractions than simple singular frequency sonochemical systems (Servant et al. 2003). Many other studies have also shown that dual or multiple frequency sonochemical systems are more powerful than simple singular frequency sonochemical systems [54].

The systematic method of selection of frequency is affected by the operation scale, controlling mechanism and the required power inputs. Generally, multiple frequency application increases overall cavitational activity. Furthermore, it produces intensities appropriate for the application areas while enhancing energy performance and efficiency. Because of the wavelength combination, the cavitation medium is heavily influenced, resulting in a higher average cavitational intensity as the secondary and primary Bjerkens forces create more cavities and increase droplet-droplet, as well as droplet-acoustic field interaction. Tatake and Pandit (2002) performed computational investigation, modelling a dual frequency structure to explain the dependence of temperature, breakdown stress, period of collapse, and bubble degree on different frequency combinations. According to the reports, multiple frequency activity induced a greater severity of cavitational collapse as compared to single frequency operation at same power dissipation.

Ultrasonic Intensity

Another important operating factor in sonication reactor design is ultrasonic intensity that is determined by the amount of energy dissipated in the liquid per available sonicated surface area. Power dissipation rate influences the volume, duration, and life of bubbles in a liquid medium, as well as temperature increase, and has a clear relationship with solubility of gases and vapor pressure. The calorimetric approach, which is centered on thermodynamics' first law, is widely used to measure the energy dissipation. Calorimetric and electrical energy measurement techniques are used to study energy conversion inside an ultrasonic horn system, and it is found that the extent of energy dissipation was greatly affected by liquid medium characteristics with the power transfer decreasing in volatile and highly viscous medium.

Henglein and Gutierrez studied the effect of output power dissipated on the iodine obtained from potassium iodide oxidative reaction at a constant 20 kHz frequency and discovered an optimum rate of power dissipation of 50 W, as seen in Fig. 7 (reproduced from Asgharzadehahmadi, Abdul Raman, Parthasarathy, & Sajjadi [53]). Many other studies have also confirmed the presence of optimal ultrasonic dissipation, and hence, choosing an optimal rated power not only increases operational efficiency but also reduces operating costs for a given process. Furthermore, the degree of temperature rise in the bulk of a liquid can be described as a function of the rate of output power dissipated, which gradually results in changes in solubility of gases as well as vapor pressure, influencing the ability of producing cavitational activities and the magnitude of the final collapse.

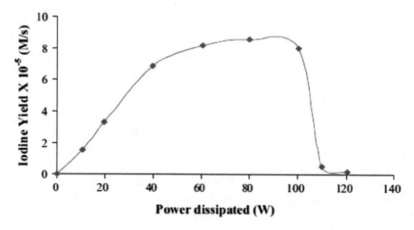

Fig. 7 Iodine yield and power dissipation [53]

Understanding hydrodynamic behavior, such as mixing process, which is based on energy density, is crucial in the design of steady-state sonication reactors. As a result, the amount of real power that has dissipated in the surrounding liquid and needed for generating cavitating effects must be articulated. Due to limitations in the construction equipment, and pulsing piezoelectric material, in large-scale operation and running volume reaching a few hundred liters, it really is difficult to disperse the existing power in the appropriate volume in the reactor using only a singular transducer with excellent efficiency. Furthermore, in sonochemical systems, active areas with the lowest cavitational activity congregate near 2–3 cm away from the surface under sonication. As a consequence, multiple irradiating surfaces will be required to achieve cavitational bubbles with a consistent distribution. Besides that, the placement of transducers in different locations should be optimized. A precise number is determined by the amount of power required for the specified operation, the characteristics of each transmitter, and the volume of operation. For irradiation, the normal range of optimum intensity is 5–20 W/cm^2.

In the case of crystallization, increased sonication intensities result in more intense micro-scale mixing and agitation, allowing solutes to disperse quicker. The increased solute diffusion decreases the time of induction and MSZW, improving the nucleation efficiency. Furthermore, the vigorous blending as well as agitation caused by the micro-scale turbulence assists in the avoidance of crystal agglomeration. The study related to the impact of ultrasound strength on roxithromycin sonocrystallization confirmed that during 10 min. of sonication, when the intensity of sonication was altered from an initial value of 5 to a final value of 15 W/cm^2, crystallographic length could be lowered from about 60 to 15 μm [45].

3.3 Types of Ultrasound Generators

Ultrasonic generating systems are usually made up of irradiating horns, plate transducers, and sonication baths [45]. Having a thorough understanding of the characteristics of sonochemical reactor designs as well as identification of optimum operating conditions plays a crucial role in efficiency improvement depending on the task. We now present some basic overview on the generally applied ultrasonic reactors.

The most widely known type of sonochemical reactor is the ultrasonic horn and is used in several laboratory studies dealing with understanding micro-mixing, or applications such as crystallization, transesterification, membrane filtration, and saccharification, among others. An illustration of a horn reactor used for sonication is illustrated in Fig. 8 [53].

The ultrasonic horn is typically made up of a cylindrical probe that is immersed in fluid and sends the ultrasound directly through the medium. The size of this instrument is typically around 5 mm in diameter and 1.5 cm in length. Ultrasonic horns can generate a high intensity close to the device and are useful for extreme mixing in small-scale operations. When designing horn reactors, the probe's

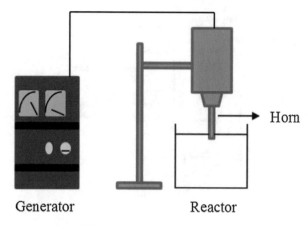

Fig. 8 Ultrasonic horn reactor [53]

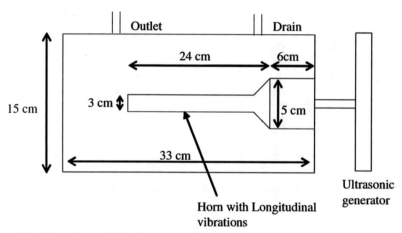

Drain is at 8 cm height from the bottom reactor whereas the outlet is at a
height of 32 cm from the bottom so as to facilitate continuous operation

Fig. 9 Schematic representation of longitudinally vibrating ultrasound horn reactor [54]

penetration depth in the medium and the probe diameter to device diameter ratio
are the crucial factors. Kumar et al. (2006) investigated the effects of such a ratio
on mixing process by adjusting vessel diameter, claiming how an optimum vessel
diameter should be sought regularly to secure consistent stirring. Studies have
also reported that the majority of cavitating bubbles in a sonicating horn reactor
are significantly concentrated nearer the transducer than in other areas indicating
that the prospects of using horn in large-scale operation will be poor (Kanthale,
Gogate, Pandit, Wilhelm, 2003). To increase the cavitationally active volume, a
longitudinally vibrating horn with higher area for sonication can be used in the
media [54]. A schematic of a longitudinal type of horn depicted in Fig. 9 was

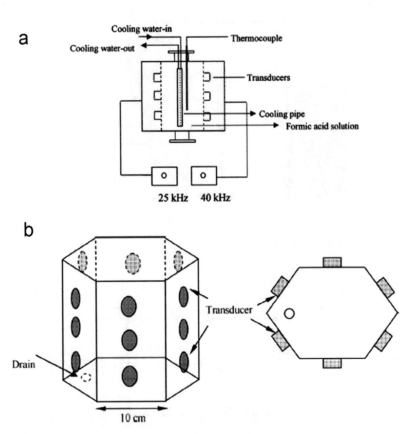

Fig. 10 (**a**) A dual frequency cylindrical flow device. (**b**) Hexagonal flow triple frequency device [53]

indeed reported to be more efficient than the traditional design of horn. The higher irradiation region of the longitudinal horn results in a consistent distribution of acoustic activity in the whole volume of the reactor.

Despite their widespread use in laboratories, ultrasonic horns are not suitable for scale-up because their ability of transmitting acoustic waves into huge tank volumes tends to be lower. Other barriers to industrial implementation of ultrasonic horn generators include cavitational obstruction and probe erosion. As a consequence, in scaled-up applications, another kind of ultrasonic device known as an **ultrasonic bath** or flow cell is typically used. Ultrasound baths are devices, typically operated in batch configurations with the transducers placed at the reactor's bottom. Depending on the required capacity of the vessel, the number of transducers and the total power dissipation can be adjusted. Flow cell is the configuration that can be operated in both batch and continuous modes of irradiation. Flow cell again relies on multiple transducer arrangement on the plates that can be arranged as rectangular or hexagonal configurations (Fig. 10). The reported dual frequency model operates in rectangular cross-section with three transducers on each side, whereas the triple frequency unit has a total of 18 transducers with three on each side. Both the reactors offer multiple frequency operation in different combinations, and this approach provides the necessary flexibility in controlling the cavitational intensity in the reactor. The hexagonal sonication device was reported to produce a much more stable spread of acoustic cavitation activity both along the axis and along the radius. As a consequence, it was reported to outperform traditional sonochemical reactors in terms of cavitation bubble yields and energy performance [53].

Analysis of literature revealed that a wide variety of crystallization devices have been developed in response to the need to tightly control crystallization procedures and the wide variety of crystallized substances. As the market grows increasingly toward continuous operation, continuous crystallization has gained significant attention in recent years [55] and hence it is important to explore the possibility of using ultrasonic reactors in continuous mode of operation. There has been some depiction of operating ultrasound reactor in continuous mode of irradiation. Siddique, Brown, Houson, and Florence [43] presented an approach to transfer a batch operation into continuous processing based on the use of oscillatory baffled crystallizer and sonication. For the first time, continuous sonocrystallization was performed at a throughput of 356 gh^{-1}. The method has shown to be capable of providing close control of particle characteristics at an industrially relevant scale.

3.4 Comparing Different Sonochemical Reactors

It is important to compare the different sonication devices though no such study was seen for the crystallization. Bhirud, Gogate, Wilhelm, and Pandit [54] presented a new design of ultrasound irradiation reactor having a transducer in longitudinal orientation operating at 36 kHz frequency and a peak power input of 150 W. The efficacy of longitudinally vibrating reactor was compared with the conventional designs of horn and bath as well as hexagon-shaped flow cell having triple frequency operation with 18 transducers and dual frequency flow cell with rectangular cross-section. It was demonstrated that the large radiation exposure area of the longitudinally vibrating horn had a significant impact on the uniform distribution of the acoustic cavitation yielding maximum cavitational activity quantified in terms of cavitational yield (Table 3).

Table 3 Comparison of cavitation yield in different types of sonication reactors [54]

Type of ultrasound generator	Cavitational yield (mol/Watt)
Ultrasonic horn	0.0005
Ultrasonic bath	0.01
Dual frequency flow cell	0.011
Triple frequency flow cell	0.018
Longitudinally vibrating reactor	0.077

In the same study, an ultrasound irradiation horn having a frequency of 20 kHz and a power output of 240 W was used. The operating frequency of a sonicating bath having two transducers was 20 kHz with a rated energy output of 220 W. Comparison of the energy efficiency, which denotes the amount of energy efficiently dissipated throughout the device, for ultrasonic horn and bath was also presented. It is important to quantify the energy efficiency as the objective would be to maximize the same which will enable availability of larger energy for cavity production. It was reported that the effective output power is 29.3 W for ultrasonic horn yielding an efficiency of around 12.7%, while the actual output power for bath was 52.4 W giving 24% as energy efficiency. The higher efficiency of ultrasonic bath relative to the ultrasonic horn may be due to larger areas of exposure, resulting in a higher cavitationally activated volume. A general rule that can be established based on this finding is that using higher areas of transducers helps in getting higher energy efficiency, which also means higher energy availability for the specific application.

3.5 Applications

Sonocrystallization can be applied to produce a variety of compounds with a wide variety of sizes and structures. As ultrasound application can tailor crystal dimensions, distribution, and polymorphism, it is commonly used in the manufacture of pharmaceutical agents (PAs). PA size reduction increases solubility and activity, particularly for nanocrystals, and hence, it is desired. Controlling polymorphisms also reduces the likelihood of side effects. Overall controlling polymorphism and size are important for PAs since they have a significant effect on drug propagation and its function. Several pharmaceutical compounds including paracetamol, salicylic acid, carbamazepine, and mefenamic acid have been demonstrated to be positively affected by the use of ultrasound with benefits such as reduction in size, narrow size distribution, and morphology control [45].

Another use for sonocrystallization is the creation of nanostructures and nanocrystals. Qian, Jiang, and Hansen (2003) reported ultrasound application as an innovative technique for creating zinc oxide crystals of size in the range of nanometers. The traditional approach took 2 days; however, sonication (20 kHz) produced nanocrystals in 3 min in the presence of a solvent, heptane. Furthermore, nanocrystals were developed in 25 min. using ultrasound irradiation without any of the presence of heptane as solvent.

4 Concluding Remarks

Microencapsulation in the pharmaceutical industry is an expanding technology that offers several advantages and has countless applications in a large range of industries. Microparticles exhibit a wide range of morphologies that have a great influence on their performance and application. Each microencapsulation technique is a unique method that produces particles with varying type of materials, particle sizes, core loading, and morphologies, while having its own advantages and disadvantages for the indented application. However, the limited array of suitable encapsulants that are permissible for usage is still the most difficult aspect of material selection along with selection of appropriate encapsulation method. High production costs and a scarcity of appropriate grade materials have led to emergence of many limitations in encapsulation processes. To overcome these limitations, more fruitful research is needed. While usage of ultrasound in drug encapsulation does indeed lead to many added benefits like homogeneous dispersion, less maintenance costs, and uniform and narrow particle size distribution, the constraint lies in the opportunities and the profitability of its scaling up for industrial applications. Many a time, a trade-off is established, and conventional processes gain an edge over ultrasound-assisted processes. Thus, the need is to explore better ultrasound processing methods and design efficient equipment.

Recent technological advances, especially the availability of large irradiation cells outfitted with multi-transducers, have extended the potential for using ultrasonic devices in big-scale processes. The ideal configuration, as in most sonication implementations, would irradiate a large system volume from an input energy intensity that is fractionally more than the cavitation bubble minimum level. Recent devices seek to carry out their operation by integrating more than one (multi) transducer; singularly, every transducer generates comparatively less energy response. This process of spreading energy input also assists in minimizing loss of particles and energy. It is seen to have major potential for ultrasonic production and sonocrystallization to be used more extensively in the manufacture of microparticles for cell adhesion and within developing nanomedicine fields.

Centered on a consideration of the intrinsic cavitational behavior of an ultrasonic horn and an ultrasonic bath, it is indeed preferable to pass a comparable quantum of energy over a wider field of irradiation. Furthermore, larger scale designs of sonochemical reactors should be based on the usage of a large number of transducers since cavitational behavior is clustered quite near to the transducing surface and varies greatly at other points in the device. The viability of continuous operation is a crucial element for the implementation of sonochemical circuits for wide-scale operation.

At this phase of sonochemistry's progress, it appears as while there is big scope in sonochemical processes, there are many technical constraints, and therefore, less industrial scale production is in implementation. Without a question, the chemical process industry (CPI) would need the joint efforts of pharmacists, chemical engineers, and machinery manufacturers to exploit ultrasound as a feasible alternative.

References

1. Ziaee, A., Albadarin, A., Padrela, L., Ung, M.-T., Femmer, T., Walker, G., & O'Reilly, E. (2020). A rational approach towards spray drying of biopharmaceuticals: The case of lysozyme. *Powder Technology, 366*(1), 206-215.
2. Gogate. (2021). The use of ultrasonic atomization for encapsulation and other processes in food and pharmaceutical manufacturing. In J. Gallego-Juarez, & K. Graff, *Power Ultrasonics: Applications of High-Intensity Ultrasound (Woodhead Publishing Series in Electronic and Optical Materials)* (1 ed., pp. 911-935). Woodhead Publishing.
3. Jyothi, N., Prasanna, P., Sakarkar, S., Prabha, K., Ramaiah, P., & Srawan, G. (2010). Microencapsulation Techniques, Factors Influencing Encapsulation Efficiency: A Review. *Journal of Microencapsulation, 3*(1), 187–197.
4. Zuidam, N., & Shimoni, E. (2009). Overview of Microencapsulates for Use in Food. In N. Zuidam, & V. Nedovic, *Encapsulation Technologies for Active Food Ingredients and Food Processing* (2010 ed., pp. 3–29). Springer.
5. Dalmoro, A., Barba, A., Lamberti, G., & d'Amore, M. (2012). Intensifying the microencapsulation process: Ultrasonic atomization as an innovative approach. *European Journal of Pharmaceutics and Biopharmaceutics, 80*(3), 471-477.
6. Kirby, C. (1991). Microencapsulation and controlled delivery of food ingredients. *Food Science and Technology Today, 38*(1), 74–80.
7. Sanguansri, L., & Augustin, M. (2010). Microencapsulation in functional food. In J. Smith, & E. Charter, *Functional Food Product Development* (1 ed., pp. 3–23). Wiley-Blackwell.
8. Kita, K., & Dittrich, C. (2011). Drug delivery vehicles with improved encapsulation efficiency: taking advantage of specific drug–carrier interactions. *Expert Opinion on Drug Delivery, 8*(3), 329-342.
9. Tan, M., & Danquah, M. (2012). Drug and protein encapsulation by emulsification: technology enhancement using foam formulations. *Chemical Engineering & Technology, 35*(4), 618-626.
10. Dias, M., Ferreira, I., & Barreiro, M. (2015). Microencapsulation of bioactives for food applications. *Food & Function, 6*(4), 1035-1052.
11. Gurruchaga, H., Saenz del Burgo, L., Ciriza, J., Orive, G., Hernández, R., & Pedraz, J. (2015). Advances in cell encapsulation technology and its application in drug delivery. *Expert Opinion on Drug Delivery, 12*(8), 1251-1267.
12. Roos, Y., & Livney, Y. (2016). *Engineering Foods for Bioactives Stability and Delivery (Food Engineering Series)* (1 ed.). Springer.
13. Đorđević , V., Paraskevopoulou, A., Mantzouridou, F., Lalou, S., Pantić, M., Bugarski, B., & Nedović, V. (2019). Encapsulation Technologies for Food Industry. In V. Nedović, P. Raspor, J. Lević, T. Šaponjac, & G. Barbosa-Cánovas, *Emerging and Traditional Technologies for Safe, Healthy and Quality Food (Food Engineering Series)* (pp. 329-382). Springer.
14. Javadi, M., Pitt, W., Belnap, D., Tsosie, N., & Hartley, J. (2012). Encapsulating Nanoemulsions Inside eLiposomes for Ultrasonic Drug Delivery. *Langmuir, 28*(41), 14720-14729.
15. Wang, W., Feng, Y., Chen, W., Wang, Y., Wilder, G., Liu, D., & Yin, Y. (2020). Ultrasonic modification of pectin for enhanced 2-furfurylthiol encapsulation: process optimization and mechanisms. *Journal of the Science of Food and Agriculture, 100*(5).
16. Fei, J., Cui, Y., He, Q., & Li, J. (2012). Assembly of multilayer capsules for drug encapsulation and controlled release. In G. Decher, & J. Schlenoff, *Multilayer Thin Films: Sequential Assembly of Nanocomposite Materials* (2 ed., pp. 777–799). Wiley-VCH.
17. Yoon, C., & Park, J. (2010). Ultrasound-mediated gene delivery. *Expert Opinion on Drug Delivery, 7*(3), 321-330.
18. Tao, Y., & Sun, D.-W. (2014). Enhancement of food processes by ultrasound: a review. *Critical Reviews in Food Science and Nutrition, 55*(4), 570-594.
19. Pitt, W., & Husseini, G. (2013). Ultrasound-Triggered Release from Micelles. In C. Alvarez-Lorenzo, & A. Concheiro, *Smart Materials for Drug Delivery (Rsc Smart Materials)* (Vol. 1, pp. 148-178). Royal Society of Chemistry.

20. Ré, M.-I. (2006). Formulating drug delivery systems by spray drying. *Drying Technology, 24*(4), 433-446.

21. Priscilla Paiva, L., Pires, A., & Serra, O. (2007). A low-cost ultrasonic spray dryer to produce spherical microparticles from polymeric matrices. *Química Nova, 30*(7), 1744-1746.

22. Cal, K., & Sollohub, K. (2010). Spray Drying Technique. I: Hardware and Process Parameters. *Journal of Pharmaceutical Sciences, 99*(2), 575-586.

23. Graves, R., Poole, D., Moiseyev, R., Bostanian, L., & Mandal, T. (2008). Encapsulation of Indomethacin Using Coaxial Ultrasonic Atomization Followed by Solvent Evaporation. *Drug Development and Industrial Pharmacy, 28*(6), 419-426.

24. Searles, J., & Mohan, G. (2010). Spray Drying of Biopharmaceuticals and Vaccines. In F. Jameel, & S. Hershenson, *Formulation and Process Development Strategies for Manufacturing Biopharmaceuticals* (1 ed., pp. 739–761). Wiley.

25. Khaire, R., & Gogate, P. (2020). Novel approaches based on ultrasound for spray drying of food and bioactive compounds. *Drying Technology*, 1-22.

26. Bittner, B., & Kissel, T. (1999). Ultrasonic atomization for spray drying: a versatile technique for the preparation of protein loaded biodegradable microspheres. *Journal of Microencapsulation, 16*(3), 325-341.

27. Höhne, P., Mieller, B., & Rabe, T. (2020). Advancing spray granulation by ultrasound atomization. *International Journal of Applied Ceramic Technology, 17*(5), 2212-2219.

28. Vishali, D., Monisha, J., Sivakamasundari, S., Moses, J., & Anandharamakrishnan, C. (2019). Spray freeze drying: Emerging applications in drug delivery. *Journal of Controlled Release, 300*, 93-101.

29. Febriyenti Febriyenti, N. Mohtar, Nornisah Mohamed, M. Hamdan, S. N. M. Salleh (2014). Comparison of freeze drying and spray drying methods of haruan extract. *International Journal of Drug Delivery, 6*(3), 286-291.

30. Gao, Y., Zhu, C.-L., Zhang, X.-X., Gan, L., & Gan, Y. (2011). Lipid–polymer composite microspheres for colon-specific drug delivery prepared using an ultrasonic spray freeze-drying technique. *Journal of Microencapsulation, 28*(6), 549=556.

31. D'Addio, S., Kwok, P., Chan, J., Benson, B., Prud'homme, R., & Chan, H.-K. (2013). Aerosol Delivery of Nanoparticles in Uniform Mannitol Carriers Formulated by Ultrasonic Spray Freeze Drying. *Pharmaceutical Research, 30*(11), 2891-2901.

32. Maa, Y.-F., Ameri, M., Shu, C., Payne, L., & Chen, D. (2004). Influenza vaccine powder formulation development: spray-freeze-drying and stability evaluation. *Journal of Pharmaceutical Sciences, 93*(7), 1912-1923.

33. Wanning, S., Süverkrüp, R., & Lamprecht, A. (2015). Pharmaceutical spray freeze drying. *International Journal of Pharmaceutics, 488*(2), 136-153.

34. D'Addio, S., Chan, J., Kwok, P., Prud'homme, R., & Chan, H.-K. (2012). Constant size, variable density aerosol particles by ultrasonic spray freeze drying. *International Journal of Pharmaceutics, 427*(2), 185-191.

35. Leuenberger, H., Plitzko, M., & Puchkov, M. (2006). Spray freeze drying in a fluidized bed at normal and low pressure. *Drying Technology, 24*(6), 711-719.

36. Ali, M., & Lamprecht, A. (2014). Spray freeze drying for dry powder inhalation of nanoparticles. *European Journal of Pharmaceutics and Biopharmaceutics, 87*(3), 510-517.

37. Maniruzzaman, M., Boateng, J., Snowden, M., & Douroumis, D. (2012). A review of hot-melt extrusion: process technology to pharmaceutical products. *ISRN Pharmaceutics, 2012*(436763), 1-9.

38. Sarabu, S., Bandari, S., Kallakunta, V., Tiwari, R., Patil, H., & Repka, M. (2019). An update on the contribution of hot-melt extrusion technology to novel drug delivery in the twenty-first century: part II. *Expert Opinion on Drug Delivery, 16*(6), 567-582.

39. Ávila-Orta, C., González-Morones, P., Valdez, D., González-Sánchez, A., Martinez-Colunga, J., Mata-Padilla, J., & Cruz-Delgado, V. (2019). Ultrasound-Assisted Melt Extrusion of Polymer Nanocomposites. In S. Sivasankaran, *Nanocomposites - Recent Evolutions*. IntechOpen.

40. Repka, M., Shah, S., Lu, J., Maddineni, S., Morott, J., Patwardhan, K., & Mohammed, N. (2012). Melt extrusion: process to product. *Expert opinion on drug delivery, 9*(1), 105–125.

41. Censi, R., Gigliobianco, M., Casadidio, C., & Di Martino, P. (2018). Hot Melt Extrusion: Highlighting Physicochemical Factors to Be Investigated While Designing and Optimizing a Hot Melt Extrusion Process. *Pharmaceutics, 10*(3), 1-27.

42. Chen, J., Chen, Y., Li, H., Lai, S.-Y., & Jow, J. (2010). Physical and chemical effects of ultrasound vibration on polymer melt in extrusion. *Ultrasonics Sonochemistry, 17*(1), 66-71.

43. Siddique, H., Brown, C., Houson, I., & Florence, A. (2015). Establishment of a continuous sonocrystallization process for lactose in an oscillatory baffled crystallizer. *Organic Process Research & Development, 19*(12), 1871-1881.

44. Sander, J., Zeiger, B., & Suslick, K. (2014). Sonocrystallization and sonofragmentation. *Ultrasonics Sonochemistry, 21*(6), 1908-1915.

45. Kim, H., & Suslick, K. (2018). The Effects of Ultrasound on Crystals: Sonocrystallization and Sonofragmentation. *Crystals, 8*(7).

46. Evrard, Q., Houard, F., Daiguebonne, C., Calvez, G., Suffren, Y., Guillou, O., Bernot, K. (2020). Sonocrystallization as an efficient way to control the size, morphology, and purity of coordination compound microcrystallites: application to a single-chain magnet. *Inorganic Chemistry, 59*(13), 9215-9226.

47. Vancleef, A., Seurs, S., Jordens, J., Van Gerven, T., Thomassen, L., & Braeken, L. (2018). Reducing the induction time using ultrasound and high-shear mixing in a continuous crystallization process. *Crystals, 8*(8), 326-336.

48. Ruecroft, G., Hipkiss, D., Ly, T., Maxted, N., & Cains, P. (2005). Sonocrystallization: the use of ultrasound for improved industrial crystallization. *Organic Process Research & Development, 9*(6), 923-932.

49. Liu, Y., van den Berg, M., & Alexander, A. (2017). Supersaturation dependence of glycine polymorphism using laser-induced nucleation, sonocrystallization and nucleation by mechanical shock. *Physical Chemistry Chemical Physics, 19*(29), 19386-19392.

50. Gracin, S., Uusi-Penttilä, M., & Rasmuson, Å. (2005). Influence of Ultrasound on the Nucleation of Polymorphs of p-Aminobenzoic Acid. *Crystal Growth & Design, 5*(5), 1787-1794.

51. Njegić Džakula, B., Kontrec, J., Ukrainczyk, M., Sviben, S., & Kralj, D. (2014). Polymorphic composition and morphology of calcium carbonate as a function of ultrasonic irradiation. *Crystal Research and Technology, 49*(4), 244-256.

52. Higaki, K., Ueno, S., Koyano, T., & Sato, K. (2001). Effects of ultrasonic irradiation on crystallization behavior of tripalmitoylglycerol and cocoa butter. *Journal of the American Oil Chemists' Society, 78*(5), 513-518.

53. Asgharzadehahmadi, S., Abdul Raman, A., Parthasarathy, R., & Sajjadi, B. (2016). Sonochemical reactors: Review on features, advantages and limitations. *Renewable and Sustainable Energy Reviews, 63*, 302-314.

54. Bhirud, U., Gogate, P., Wilhelm, A., & Pandit, A. (2004). Ultrasonic bath with longitudinal vibrations: a novel configuration for efficient wastewater treatment. *Ultrasonics Sonochemistry, 11*(3-4), 143-147.

55. Eder, R., Schrank, S., Besenhard, M., Roblegg, E., Gruber-Woelfler, H., & Khinast, J. (2012). Continuous Sonocrystallization of Acetylsalicylic Acid (ASA): Control of Crystal Size. *Crystal Growth & Design, 12*(10), 4733–4738.

56. Yamaguchi, T., Nomura, M., Matsuoka, T., Koda, S., (2009) Effects of frequency and power of ultrasound on the size reduction of liposome, *Chem Phys Lipids, 160* (1), 58–62.

57. Servant, G. Laborde, J.L., Hita, A., Caltagirone, J.P., Gerad, A. (2003) On the interaction between ultrasound waves and bubble clouds in mono- and dual-frequency sonoreactors. *Ultrasonics Sonochemistry, 10*(3) 47–55

58. Tatake, P.A., Pandit, A.B. (2002). Modeling and experimental investigation into cavity dynamics and cavitational yield: influence of dual frequency ultrasound sources, *Chemical Engineering Science, 57* 49–87

59. Kumar, A., Kumaresan, T., Pandit, A.B., Joshi, J.B., (2006) Characterization of flow phenomena induced by ultrasonic horn. *Chemical Engineering Science, 61*(74) 10–20

60. Kanthale, P.M., Gogate, P.R., Pandit, A.B., Wilhelm, A.M. (2003) Mapping of an ultrasonic horn: link primary and secondary effects of ultrasound, *Ultrasonics Sonochemistry, 10,* 331–335

61. Qian, D., Jiang, J.Z., Hansen, P.L. (2003) Preparation of ZnO nanocrystals via ultrasonic irradiation. *Chemical Communications. 9,* 1078–1079

Nonsmooth Modeling for Simulation and Optimization of Continuous Pharmaceutical Manufacturing Processes

Michael Patrascu and Paul I. Barton

1 Introduction

In this chapter we introduce and demonstrate the use of a new dynamic modeling paradigm, *nonsmooth* modeling, for simulation and optimization of continuous manufacturing processes in the pharmaceutical industry. We specifically address the general problem of dynamic operation, which has large implications on the economical, quality, and safety aspects of any manufacturing plant, especially for continuous manufacturing, as we explain below.

The pharmaceutical industry is undergoing significant adaptation in recent years in pursuit of more reliable, cost-effective, and sustainable manufacturing processes. One of the most promising advancements is moving from the traditional batch-wise to a continuous manufacturing (CM) approach. This requires developments in both the chemistry and the processing technologies. CM offers the opportunity to integrate more efficient and cost-effective intensified processes such as micro-reactors and micro-separators. It creates a more flexible and controllable process, which is less expensive to scale up, has a smaller footprint, reduces wastes, and improves overall yields.

In contrast to most traditional continuous processes, CM of pharmaceuticals is likely to be characterized by short operation times (campaigns), on the order of a few hours to weeks. Thus, the relatively long unproductive start-up and shutdown phases become more significant compared to other industries. This is one of the most

M. Patrascu (✉)
Department of Chemical Engineering, Technion-Israel Institute of Technology, Haifa, Israel
e-mail: michael@technion.ac.il

P. I. Barton
Process Systems Engineering Laboratory, Massachusetts Institute of Technology, Cambridge, MA, USA
e-mail: pib@mit.edu

challenging problems CM of pharmaceuticals is facing in making CM technologies economically attractive. Thus optimal dynamic campaigns are sought, where the production is optimized over the entire time horizon, including the start-up and shutdown phases [23, 25].

In the transition from batch to CM it is most valuable to implement process systems engineering tools for modeling, simulation, and optimization. This is essential in order to design and validate the improved performance in terms of yield, productivity, energy consumption and other important process attributes. In recent years, various studies have focused on the dynamics of individual process units, e.g. crystallization, granulation, and blending [15, 18, 37, 42], where the time to steady-state, the interaction of unit operations, the effect of process upsets and process optimization were studied. Plant-wide models and simulations of integrated continuous pharmaceutical plants have also been reported [7, 22].

Many relevant phenomena to pharmaceuticals manufacturing processes exhibit a mixture of continuous and discrete behavior which can cause failure of standard modeling and simulation methods [5, 6]. These include, for example, thermo-dynamic phase changes, switching between kinetic modes, flow reversals, safety instrumentation operation, and more. Most dynamic processes have been tradi-tionally described as hybrid (discrete/continuous) systems, exhibiting both discrete and continuous behavior [4, 5]. Typically, the more abstract the hybrid system formalism, the more universal its applicability, but more limited its solvability and therefore practical usefulness, as depicted in Fig. 1. Such modeling paradigms can exhibit pathological behavior that is unphysical and difficult to exclude a priori, contributing to an absence of appropriate theoretical results guaranteeing regularity of solutions. Difficulties in always obtaining meaningful sensitivity information from hybrid dynamic models prevents the use of gradient-based optimization schemes [2, 10]. Smoothing approximations are often used, but these typically

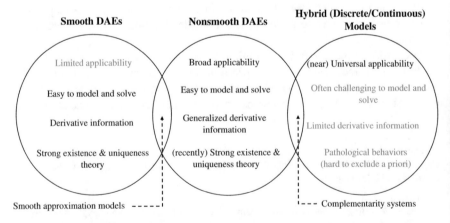

Fig. 1 Dynamic modeling frameworks in PSE depicting the trade-off between applicability vs. ease of modeling and solving

depend on user-defined (unphysical) parameters with the purpose of avoiding nondifferentiability.

This is no longer necessary thanks to recent advancements, which enable a direct and tractable treatment of nonsmooth systems, in steady-state and transient [3]. Many of the relevant transient phenomena can be formulated in a nonsmooth differential-algebraic-equations (DAEs) framework [31–33], rather than (the more general) hybrid framework. The nonsmooth DAE modeling framework is broadly applicable in both equation-oriented and modular approaches [35].

Here, we give a brief overview of the fundamentals of the new nonsmooth modeling paradigm, and demonstrate its applicability to simulation and optimization of continuous pharmaceuticals manufacturing processes, including dynamic optimization of an end-to-end continuous plant.

2 Fundamentals of Nonsmooth Dynamic Modeling

Most of the transient operations and phenomena in the pharmaceutical industry may be modeled by a set of nonsmooth DAEs. The mathematical structure of an autonomous nonsmooth, semi-explicit, DAE system is given by the following equations:

$$\dot{\mathbf{x}}(t, \mathbf{p}) = \mathbf{f}(\mathbf{p}, \mathbf{x}(t, \mathbf{p}), \mathbf{y}(t, \mathbf{p})), \tag{1a}$$

$$\mathbf{0}_{n_y} = \mathbf{g}(\mathbf{p}, \mathbf{x}(t, \mathbf{p}), \mathbf{y}(t, \mathbf{p})), \tag{1b}$$

$$\mathbf{x}(t_0, \mathbf{p}) = \mathbf{f}_0(\mathbf{p}), \tag{1c}$$

where t is the independent variable, $\mathbf{p}$ is a vector of the problem parameters, and $\mathbf{x}$ and $\mathbf{y}$ are the differential and algebraic state variables, respectively. In the nonsmooth setting $\mathbf{f}$, $\mathbf{g}$, and $\mathbf{f}_0$ are not necessarily differentiable in their entire respective domains. It is possible to extend the results described hereafter to the case when $\mathbf{f}$ and $\mathbf{g}$ are non-autonomous, including with $\mathbf{f}$ being discontinuous with respect to t [36]. $\mathbf{f}$, $\mathbf{g}$, and $\mathbf{f}_0$ are locally Lipschitz continuous functions defined on open sets, with respect to state variables and parameters. Therefore, the functions $\mathbf{f}$, $\mathbf{g}$, and $\mathbf{f}_0$ may be piecewise differentiable (PC^1) [28] functions of parameter and state variables. PC^1 functions are an important class of functions, as they include all C^1 functions as well as min, max, the absolute value function, mid, and all compositions of PC^1 functions.

2.1 Well-Posedness of a Nonsmooth DAE Model

The notion of a regular solution of (1) is presented here, which requires generalized derivatives concepts from nonsmooth analysis since $\mathbf{g}$ does not need to be differentiable everywhere. With a generalized notion of differentiation index 1, Eq. (1) now possesses regularized mathematical properties similar to the classical theory for smooth DAEs, i.e. well-posedness [36] and a sensitivity analysis theory [34], in the form of generalized derivative information.

A regular solution of the nonsmooth DAE system (1) (which implies generalized differentiation index 1), $(\mathbf{x}, \mathbf{y})$, corresponding to a reference parameter value $\mathbf{p} = \mathbf{p}_0$ must satisfy that every $n_y \times n_y$ matrix in the set

$$\pi_{\mathbf{y}} \partial \mathbf{g}(\mathbf{p}_0, \mathbf{x}(t, \mathbf{p}_0), \mathbf{y}(t, \mathbf{p}_0)) \tag{2}$$

is nonsingular for all $t \in [t_0, t_f]$. This condition corresponds to the classical differentiation index 1 when $\mathbf{g}$ is continuously differentiable. Equation (2) is the *projection of the* Clarke *Jacobian* with respect to $\mathbf{y}$ at $(\mathbf{p}_0, \mathbf{x}_0, \mathbf{y}_0)$ which is defined as follows:

$$\begin{aligned} \pi_{\mathbf{y}} \partial \mathbf{g}(\mathbf{p}_0, \mathbf{x}_0, \mathbf{y}_0) \\ \equiv \{\mathbf{Y} \in \mathbb{R}^{n_y \times n_y} : \exists [\mathbf{P} \quad \mathbf{X} \quad \mathbf{Y}] \in \partial \mathbf{g}(\mathbf{p}_0, \mathbf{x}_0, \mathbf{y}_0)\}, \end{aligned} \tag{3}$$

and is a nonsmooth analogue of a partial Jacobian matrix allowing to define a generalized differentiation index for Eq. (1). Note that $\pi_{\mathbf{y}} \partial \mathbf{g}(\mathbf{p}_0, \mathbf{x}_0, \mathbf{y}_0)$ is the set of $n_y \times n_y$ matrices $\mathbf{Y}$ such that there exists a corresponding matrix $[\mathbf{P} \quad \mathbf{X} \quad \mathbf{Y}] \in \partial \mathbf{g}(\mathbf{p}_0, \mathbf{x}_0, \mathbf{y}_0)$. In the smooth case, $\pi_{\mathbf{y}} \partial \mathbf{g}(\mathbf{p}_0, \mathbf{x}_0, \mathbf{y}_0) = \{\frac{\partial \mathbf{g}}{\partial \mathbf{y}}(\mathbf{p}_0, \mathbf{x}_0, \mathbf{y}_0)\}$.

Clarke's generalized *Jacobian* [9] of $\mathbf{g}$ at $(\mathbf{p}_0, \mathbf{x}_0, \mathbf{y}_0)$ is defined as the convex hull of the limiting Jacobian; i.e.,

$$\partial \mathbf{g}(\mathbf{p}_0, \mathbf{x}_0, \mathbf{y}_0) \equiv \text{conv } \partial_B \mathbf{g}(\mathbf{p}_0, \mathbf{x}_0, \mathbf{y}_0),$$

and satisfies a number of useful calculus properties (including a nonsmooth implicit function theorem for use in analyzing a nonsmooth DAE system). The limiting Jacobian is the set of limits of nearby Jacobian matrices, which is a nonempty set of $n_y \times (n_p + n_x + n_y)$ real-valued matrices. The limiting Jacobian (often called the *B-subdifferential*) of $\mathbf{g}$ at $(\mathbf{p}_0, \mathbf{x}_0, \mathbf{y}_0)$ is well-defined for any locally Lipschitz continuous function and is equal to

$$\begin{aligned} \partial_B \mathbf{g}(\mathbf{p}_0, \mathbf{x}_0, \mathbf{y}_0) \\ = \left\{ \mathbf{Jg}_{(i)}(\mathbf{p}_0, \mathbf{x}_0, \mathbf{y}_0) : i = 1, \ldots, n_{ac} \right\}, \end{aligned} \tag{4}$$

where $\mathbf{Jg}_{(i)}(\mathbf{p}_0, \mathbf{x}_0, \mathbf{y}_0)$ is the Jacobian matrix of $\mathbf{g}_{(i)}$ evaluated at $(\mathbf{p}_0, \mathbf{x}_0, \mathbf{y}_0)$ and n_{ac} is a positive integer corresponding to the number of (essentially active) C^1 selection functions. If $\mathbf{g}$ is continuously differentiable at $(\mathbf{p}_0, \mathbf{x}_0, \mathbf{y}_0)$ the limiting Jacobian contains only one element, $\{\mathbf{Jg}(\mathbf{p}_0, \mathbf{x}_0, \mathbf{y}_0)\}$.

Generalized differentiation index 1 is therefore a local characteristic along a solution trajectory, and it can often be verified a priori in a global manner based on the functional form of $\mathbf{g}$. For example, given an algebraic equation $0 = g(p, x, y) \equiv |x| + |y| - p$ with reference parameter value $p_0 = 1$,

$$\pi_y g(p_0, x, y) = \begin{cases} \{1\}, & \text{if } y > 0, \\ [-1, 1] & \text{if } y = 0, \\ \{-1\}, & \text{if } y < 0, \end{cases}$$

for any $x \in \mathbb{R}$. Hence, if a solution $(x(t, p_0), y(t, p_0))$ of (1) satisfies $y(t, p_0) \neq 0$ for all $t \in [t_0, t_f]$, then it is regular. In general it may be challenging to analyze the generalized differentiation index or regularity of a solution associated with the nonsmooth DAE system (1), but this is also true for a nonlinear smooth DAE system.

2.2   Sensitivity Information of a Nonsmooth DAE Model

In the traditional case of a smooth DAE set the sensitivity system of Eq. (1) is given by

$$\dot{\mathbf{S}}_{\mathbf{x}}(t) = \frac{\partial \mathbf{f}}{\partial \mathbf{p}} + \frac{\partial \mathbf{f}}{\partial \mathbf{x}} \mathbf{S}_{\mathbf{x}}(t) + \frac{\partial \mathbf{f}}{\partial \mathbf{y}} \mathbf{S}_{\mathbf{y}}(t),$$

$$\mathbf{0}_{n_y \times n_p} = \frac{\partial \mathbf{g}}{\partial \mathbf{p}} + \frac{\partial \mathbf{g}}{\partial \mathbf{x}} \mathbf{S}_{\mathbf{x}}(t) + \frac{\partial \mathbf{g}}{\partial \mathbf{y}} \mathbf{S}_{\mathbf{y}}(t), \tag{5}$$

$$\mathbf{S}_{\mathbf{x}}(t_0) = \mathbf{Jf}_0(\mathbf{p}_0),$$

where the partial derivatives of $\mathbf{f}$ and $\mathbf{g}$ are evaluated at $(\mathbf{p}_0, \mathbf{x}(t, \mathbf{p}_0), \mathbf{y}(t, \mathbf{p}_0))$. The sought functions $\mathbf{S}_{\mathbf{x}}(t) = \frac{\partial \mathbf{x}}{\partial \mathbf{p}}(t, \mathbf{p}_0)$ and $\mathbf{S}_{\mathbf{y}}(t) = \frac{\partial \mathbf{y}}{\partial \mathbf{p}}(t, \mathbf{p}_0)$ are the forward parametric sensitivity functions. The smooth DAE sensitivity system (5) is linear and admits a unique continuous solution and initialization. However, system (5) is not valid for a nonsmooth DAE system. In the nonsmooth case a regular solution $(\mathbf{x}, \mathbf{y})$ may vary nonsmoothly with respect to parameter so that $\mathbf{S}_{\mathbf{x}}(t)$ and $\mathbf{S}_{\mathbf{y}}(t)$ may not be well-defined for all t. In this case we will search for elements of the Clarke Jacobians $\partial \mathbf{x}_t(\mathbf{p}_0)$ and $\partial \mathbf{y}_t(\mathbf{p}_0)$ (i.e. for fixed t and varying $\mathbf{p}$). These elements provide sensitivity information with respect to $\mathbf{p}$ at $\mathbf{p} = \mathbf{p}_0$ for differential and algebraic variables, respectively, and guarantee attractive convergence properties in nonsmooth optimization and equation-solving methods (see [3] and the references therein). A new theory enables the calculation of such elements, as described hereafter.

The *lexicographic directional (LD-)derivative* [12] is a nonsmooth analogue of the classical directional derivative. It satisfies sharp calculus rules, which makes it a useful tool for automatic evaluation, and is applicable to a wide class of nonsmooth functions including PC^1 functions, convex functions, the Euclidean norm, and all compositions of such functions. The LD-derivative is defined with respect to a point and a directions matrix whose columns represent different directions to systematically probe local sensitivity information. Given that $\mathbf{P}$ is square and nonsingular, the LD-derivatives of $\mathbf{x}_t$ and $\mathbf{y}_t$ of Eq. (1) at $\mathbf{p}_0$ (for some fixed time $t \in [t_0, t_f]$) in the directions $\mathbf{P} \in \mathbb{R}^{n_p \times n_p}$ (denoted $[\mathbf{x}_t]'(\mathbf{p}_0; \mathbf{P})$ and $[\mathbf{y}_t]'(\mathbf{p}_0; \mathbf{P})$) can be used to build the computationally relevant generalized derivative elements, $\mathbf{S}_\mathbf{x}(t)$ and $\mathbf{S}_\mathbf{y}(t)$, in the following way:

$$[\mathbf{x}_t]'(\mathbf{p}_0; \mathbf{P}) = \mathbf{S}_\mathbf{x}(t)\mathbf{P},$$
$$[\mathbf{y}_t]'(\mathbf{p}_0; \mathbf{P}) = \mathbf{S}_\mathbf{y}(t)\mathbf{P}, \tag{6}$$

where $\mathbf{S}_\mathbf{x}(t)$ and $\mathbf{S}_\mathbf{y}(t)$ are the Jacobian-like sensitivities[1] of the differentiable and algebraic variables at time t, respectively. These are a nonsmooth analogue of the forward parametric sensitivity functions of the smooth case. The Jacobian-like objects $\mathbf{S}_\mathbf{x}(t)$ and $\mathbf{S}_\mathbf{y}(t)$ can be calculated once the LD-derivatives $[\mathbf{x}_t]'(\mathbf{p}_0; \mathbf{P})$ and $[\mathbf{y}_t]'(\mathbf{p}_0; \mathbf{P})$ are available. Explicit LD-derivative calculus rules for basic nonsmooth functions have already been established [3, 12].

Given a regular solution $(\mathbf{x}, \mathbf{y})$ of (1) on $[t_0, t_f]$ associated with the reference parameter value $\mathbf{p}_0$ that passes through the point $(t_0, \mathbf{p}_0, \mathbf{x}_0, \mathbf{y}_0)$, the nonsmooth DAE sensitivity system associated with Eq. (1) is given by the following nonsmooth DAE system [34]:

$$\dot{\mathbf{X}}(t) = \mathbf{f}'(\mathbf{p}_0, \mathbf{x}(t, \mathbf{p}_0), \mathbf{y}(t, \mathbf{p}_0); (\mathbf{P}, \mathbf{X}(t), \mathbf{Y}(t))),$$
$$\mathbf{0}_{n_y \times n_p} = \mathbf{g}'(\mathbf{p}_0, \mathbf{x}(t, \mathbf{p}_0), \mathbf{y}(t, \mathbf{p}_0); (\mathbf{P}, \mathbf{X}(t), \mathbf{Y}(t))), \tag{7}$$
$$\mathbf{X}(t_0) = [\mathbf{f}_0]'(\mathbf{p}_0; \mathbf{P}),$$

for some directions matrix $\mathbf{P} \in \mathbb{R}^{n_p \times n_p}$ chosen a priori (which is a sequence of directions exploring the parameter space). Here

$$\mathbf{f}'(\mathbf{p}_0, \mathbf{x}(t, \mathbf{p}_0), \mathbf{y}(t, \mathbf{p}_0); (\mathbf{P}, \mathbf{X}(t), \mathbf{Y}(t)))$$

is the LD-derivative of $\mathbf{f}$ at $(\mathbf{p}_0, \mathbf{x}(t, \mathbf{p}_0), \mathbf{y}(t, \mathbf{p}_0))$ in the directions of the matrix

$$(\mathbf{P}, \mathbf{X}(t), \mathbf{Y}(t)) = \begin{bmatrix} \mathbf{P} \\ \mathbf{X}(t) \\ \mathbf{Y}(t) \end{bmatrix}.$$

Equation (7) admits a unique solution on the time horizon $[t_0, t_f]$ given by

$$\mathbf{X}(t) = [\mathbf{x}_t]'(\mathbf{p}_0; \mathbf{P}), \quad \mathbf{Y}(t) = [\mathbf{y}_t]'(\mathbf{p}_0; \mathbf{P}),$$

---

[1] Formally, $\mathbf{S}_\mathbf{x}(t) = \mathbf{J}_L[\mathbf{x}_t](\mathbf{p}_0; \mathbf{P})$ and $\mathbf{S}_\mathbf{y}(t) = \mathbf{J}_L[\mathbf{y}_t](\mathbf{p}_0; \mathbf{P})$ are the *lexicographic (L-)derivatives* [21] of $\mathbf{x}_t$ and $\mathbf{y}_t$ at $\mathbf{p}_0$ in the directions $\mathbf{P}$.

which satisfies $\mathbf{X}(t_0) = [\mathbf{f}_0]'(\mathbf{p}_0; \mathbf{P})$ such that $\mathbf{Y}(t_0) = \mathbf{Y}_0 \in \mathbb{R}^{n_y \times n_p}$ is the unique solution of the nonsmooth equation system

$$0 = \mathbf{g}'(\mathbf{p}_0, \mathbf{x}_0, \mathbf{y}_0; (\mathbf{P}, \mathbf{X}(t_0), \mathbf{Y}_0)).$$

For a detailed procedure to obtain generalized derivative information, including numerical examples, the reader is referred to [33].

3 Applications in Pharmaceuticals Manufacturing

Nonsmooth formulations are useful in modeling many processes in chemical engineering and other disciplines. Plant-wide dynamic simulation and optimization tools are essential to improve yields, productivity, energy consumption and other important process attributes. In recent years, various studies have focused on the dynamics of individual process units, e.g. crystallization, granulation, and blending [15, 18, 37, 42], where the time to steady-state, the interaction of unit operations, the effect of process upsets and process optimization were studied. We recently studied the optimal performance of a fully integrated end-to-end continuous pharmaceutical plant over the entire time horizon of the campaign, rather than only the steady-state operation [22–24].

In this section we describe a few important examples with wide applications in the pharmaceutical industry. We demonstrate the usefulness of the nonsmooth modeling framework using an equation-oriented approach in the form of Eq. (1). Such examples include multi-phase systems such as single and multi-component thermodynamic vapor-liquid equilibrium (VLE) and liquid-liquid equilibrium (LLE). Another multi-phase example models changes in kinetic modes, such as between growth and dissolution in crystallization processes.

3.1 Liquid-Liquid Extraction

Here, we look at a separation process conducted in a membrane based continuous microfluidic liquid-liquid extraction device [14], which separates a multi-component stream (denoted by LLE) to an organic phase (denoted by org) and an aqueous phase (denoted by aq). We assume there exist five components: $\mathbf{C}_1$ and $\mathbf{C}_2$ are raw material, $\mathbf{C}_3$ is the product, $\mathbf{I}_1$ is a byproduct and cat is the acidic catalyst, all of which flow from an upstream reactor to the continuous separation device. Pure organic and aqueous solvents (S_1 and S_2) are added prior to feeding to the separation device. The total number of components is thus $n_c^{\text{LLE}} = 7$. A process flow diagram of this system is depicted in Fig. 2.

The mass and component balances are expressed by the nonsmooth formulation (8) that was originally developed for VLE systems [41] and whose thermodynamical

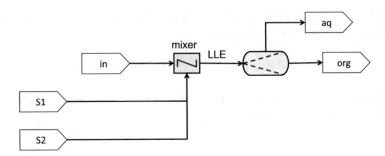

Fig. 2 Process flow diagram of a continuous liquid-liquid separation device

correctness was proven in [26]. This formulation uses the nonsmooth mid function, which picks the median out of three arguments. Due to the short residence time we can assume a pseudo steady-state, equilibrium-limited separation, where K_i^{LLE} are constant partition coefficients, and perfect separation of the organic and aqueous phases is simulated.

$$F^{\mathrm{org}}(t)w_i^{\mathrm{org}}(t) + F^{\mathrm{aq}}(t)w_i^{\mathrm{aq}}(t) = F^{\mathrm{in}}(t)w_i^{\mathrm{in}}(t)+ \tag{8a}$$

$$F^{S_1}(t)w_i^{S_1}(t) + F^{S_2}(t)w_i^{S_2}(t), \quad i = 1, \dots, n_c^{\mathrm{LLE}},$$

$$F^{\mathrm{org}}(t) + F^{\mathrm{aq1}}(t) = F^{\mathrm{in}}(t) + F^{S_1}(t) + F^{S_2}(t), \tag{8b}$$

$$0 = \mathrm{mid}\left(\frac{F^{\mathrm{org}}(t)}{F^{\mathrm{org}}(t) + F^{\mathrm{aq}}(t)} - 1, \sum_{i=1}^{nc^{\mathrm{LLE}}} w_i^{\mathrm{aq}}(t) - \sum_{i=1}^{nc^{\mathrm{LLE}}} w_i^{\mathrm{org}}(t), \tag{8c}\right.$$

$$\left.\frac{F^{\mathrm{org}}(t)}{F^{\mathrm{org}}(t) + F^{\mathrm{aq}}(t)}\right),$$

$$w_i^{\mathrm{org}}(t) = K_i^{\mathrm{LLE}}w_i^{\mathrm{aq}}(t), \quad i = 1, \dots, n_c^{\mathrm{LLE}}. \tag{8d}$$

The feed flow rates of the solvents are assumed to be perfectly controlled to obtain 0.12 %w of the desired component $\mathbf{C}_3$ in the organic phase and 20 %w of $\mathbf{C}_2$ in the aqueous phase. A naive approach will be to simply write $F^{\mathrm{in}}w_{\mathbf{C}_3}^{\mathrm{in}} = 0.12 F^{\mathrm{org}}$; however, this formulation may result in a high index system or an unphysical solution, since F^{org} is determined from the nonsmooth equation (8c), and may equal to zero if only the aqueous phase exists. Furthermore, the concentration $w_{\mathbf{C}_3}^{\mathrm{in}}$ might be too small to enable the desired 0.12 %w. Therefore, we use a direct nonsmooth formulation using the max function to determine F^{S_1} and F^{S_2}, depending on the inlet composition w_i^{in}, as follows:

$$F^{S_1}(t) = F^{\mathrm{in}}(t) \max\left(0, \frac{w_{\mathbf{C}_3}^{\mathrm{in}}(t)}{0.12} - \left(w_{\mathbf{C}_3}^{\mathrm{in}}(t) + w_{\mathbf{I}_1}^{\mathrm{in}}(t) + w_{\mathbf{C}_1}^{\mathrm{in}}(t)\right)\right), \tag{9}$$

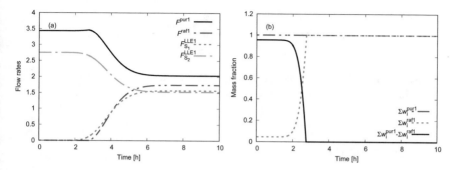

Fig. 3 Nonsmooth dynamics associated with continuous liquid-liquid extraction. Inlet solvent flow rates and outlet flow rates (**a**) and composition of the organic (raf1) and aqueous (pur1) phases (**b**) during the start-up process

$$F^{S_2}(t) = F^{in}(t) \max\left(0, \frac{w^{in}_{C_2}(t)}{0.2} - \left(w^{in}_{C_2}(t) + w^{in}_{cat_1}(t)\right)\right). \tag{10}$$

We can now simulate (solve) the nonsmooth model, Eqs. (8)–(10). Note that this is a pure algebraic system of equations, however, it is a dynamic one since it is connected to an upstream dynamic unit, i.e. the inlet stream to this unit changes with time (rate and composition).

Figure 3 depicts a start-up process of an example system (more details can be found in [22]). Initially, pure C_2 (in practice the solvent from the upstream reactor) flows into the membrane separator and is mixed with a water stream, at a flow rate, F^{S_2}, determined by Eq. (10). Temporarily, only one flowing phase exists, F^{aq}, and the flow rate of the raffinate, F^{org}, is zero. Equation (8c) picks the correct argument (or selection function) of the mid function and becomes:

$$0 = \frac{F^{org}(t)}{F^{org}(t) + F^{aq}(t),}$$

because the expression

$$\sum_{i=1}^{n_c^{LLE}} w^{aq}_i(t) - \sum_{i=1}^{n_c^{LLE}} w^{org}_i(t)$$

is between 0 and 1, as illustrated in Fig. 3b. The other argument equals -1 in this case. Two phases will exist only when the above expression equals zero. At this time the mass fractions associated with F^{org} are *pseudo* mass fractions, because the organic phase does not exist. As flow of organic components from the reactor increases, the liquid solution approaches the two-phase thermodynamic regime, the expression above rapidly approaches zero, reaching it at $t \sim 2.75$ h. At this point the mid function switches between the selection functions, and Eq. (8c) reads:

$$0 = \sum_{i=1}^{n_c^{\text{LLE}}} w_i^{\text{aq}}(t) - \sum_{i=1}^{n_c^{\text{LLE}}} w_i^{\text{org}}(t),$$

which simulates the existence of two phases, reaching the steady-state of this example system.

3.2 Crystallization

Next we look at crystallization processes [17, 19, 43]. In these processes the solid phase of component C is formed from a liquid phase (a solution of C, a solvent, and often other components). This is a relatively slow process and is usually represented by a concentration dependent kinetic expression. The reverse process, dissolution, is usually much faster compared to crystallization. These two modes, formation-growth and dissolution-disappearance, are important to take into account when modeling the dynamics of crystallizers, especially when changes in the operating conditions (such as temperature or feed composition) may lead to switching between the modes. This is accomplished by the following nonsmooth equations (min, max and $|\cdot|$ all being examples of nonsmooth functions) [22]:

$$G(t) = \max\left(k_G(t)s(t)\,|s(t)|^{n_G-1}, 0\right), \tag{11a}$$

$$D(t) = \min\left(0, k_D(t)s(t)\,|s(t)|^{n_D-1}\right), \tag{11b}$$

$$B(t) = G(t)\frac{k_B(t)}{k_G(t)}\,|s(t)|^{n_B-n_G} + \frac{D(t)}{2\Delta L}n_1(t). \tag{11c}$$

Here, the absolute function is necessary to avoid the undefined operation of raising a negative number to a positive but non-integer power. D, G, and B are the dissolution, growth, and nucleation (birth) rates of crystals, which are functions of the supersaturation, s, defined as:

$$s(t) = \frac{w_C^l(t) - w_C^{\text{sat}}(T(t))}{w_C^{\text{sat}}(T(t))}, \tag{12}$$

where the saturation mass fraction, w_C^{sat}, is assumed to be temperature dependent. k_G and k_D are temperature-dependent empirical rate constants calculated from:

$$k_G = k_{G,0}\exp\left(-k_{G,1}/(T+273)\right), \tag{13a}$$

$$k_D = 10k_G, \tag{13b}$$

and k_B is a constant. n_D, n_G, and n_B are empirical rate orders.

These kinetic rate equations are coupled to dynamic continuous flow models of mass and component balances, known as *mixed suspension mixed product removal* (MSMPR) models. Here, the occupied volume, V, is allowed to change freely.

$$\frac{dM_i}{dt}(t) = F_{\text{in}}(t)w_{i,\text{in}}(t)$$

$$- F_{\text{out}}(t)\left(\varepsilon_w(t)w_i^l(t) + (1 - \varepsilon_w(t))w_i^s(t)\right), \quad i = 1, \ldots, n_c, \tag{14}$$

$$M_i(t) = M\left(\varepsilon_w(t)w_i^l(t) + (1 - \varepsilon_w(t))w_i^s(t)\right), \quad i = 1, \ldots, n_c, \tag{15}$$

$$\rho_m(t) = \varepsilon(t)\rho_l + (1 - \varepsilon(t))\rho_s, \tag{16}$$

$$\varepsilon_w(t) = \varepsilon(t)\rho_l/\rho_m(t), \tag{17}$$

$$\varepsilon(t) = 1 - k_v\mu_3(t), \tag{18}$$

$$M(t) = \rho_m(t)V(t), \tag{19}$$

$$\sum_{i=1}^{n_c} w_i^l(t) = 1, \tag{20}$$

where F_{in} and F_{out} are the mass flow rates in and out, respectively, ε and ε_w are the liquid volume and mass fractions, respectively (which are calculated based on the crystal size distribution, as described below). ρ_l and ρ_s are the (constant) density of the mother liquor and the crystals, respectively, k_v is the shape factor of the crystals and μ_3 is the third moment of the crystal size distribution (CSD), determined from a solid particle population balance, as follows:

The mass of solid at a given time is calculated from a dynamic population balance for the MSMPR configuration. Assuming the McCabe law is valid (growth rate is independent of size) a general population balance takes the PDE form:

$$\frac{\partial(Vn)}{\partial t}(t, z) + (G(t) + D(t))\frac{\partial(Vn)}{\partial z}(t, z) = Q_{\text{in}}(t)n_{\text{in}}(t, z) - Q_{\text{out}}(t)n(t, z), \tag{21a}$$

$$(Vn)(t, 0) = B(t)V(t), \tag{21b}$$

$$(Vn)(t, +\infty) = 0, \tag{21c}$$

$$(Vn)(0, z) = n_0(z), \tag{21d}$$

where $Q_{\text{in}}(t) = F_{\text{in}}(t)/\rho_l$ and $Q_{\text{out}}(t) = F_{\text{out}}(t)/\rho_m(t)$ are the volumetric flow rates in and out, respectively, n is the *population density* of crystals. Equation (21), which is a PDE, is often discretized by an upwind finite volume method to obtain a set of DAEs to be solved numerically by a DAEs solver.

F_{out} should be a degree of freedom to determine the optimal residence time and enable to drain and fill the vessel during shutdown and start-up steps. This can also be modeled by a nonsmooth equation:

$$F_{out}(t) = u(t)C_v \frac{V(t) - V_{min}}{\sqrt{|V(t) - V_{min}| + \epsilon}}, \tag{22}$$

where u is a valve position, C_v is the flow coefficient of the valve, V_{min} is a small liquid volume below which flow is not permitted (similar to a weir), and ϵ is a small positive number used to make the function Lipschitz continuous.

Let us demonstrate the nonsmooth behavior associated with the transition between crystal growth and dissolution in continuous crystallizers with an example which was first discussed in [22]. Figure 4 illustrates nonsmooth dynamics. First, the vessel is almost empty and contains no crystals ($\varepsilon_w = 1$), and the concentration of C is zero, so the supersaturation s is negative. Hence, the nonsmooth equations (11) set the growth rate to zero and the dissolution rate, D, is negative (but ε_w stays constant, since there is no solid phase). At time $t \approx 1.2$ h concentrated solution of C flows into the vessel (followed by volume increase) and the supersaturation rapidly becomes positive, switching from dissolution to growth mode ($D = 0$, $G > 0$), leading to crystal formation, such that ε_w falls below one.

In this example, at time $t = 4$ h two control actions are initiated which lead to dilution of C in the liquid phase. These actions cause the mass fraction w^l to decrease, lowering the supersaturation to a small negative value, switching back to a dissolution mode and increasing ε_w slightly. As long as a solid phase exists the supersaturation will be very close to zero, especially when dissolution occurs, which is very fast. After a few minutes the supersaturation crosses zero again, switching back to crystal growth mode. This example illustrates that a crystallizer can switch

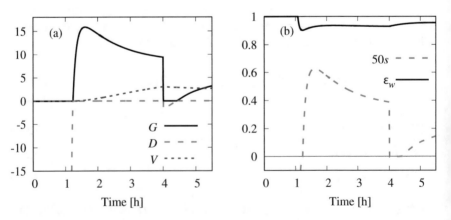

Fig. 4 Nonsmooth dynamics in a crystallizer during a start-up step. (a) Growth rate, dissolution rate, and the holdup volume. (b) the supersaturation (s), which is scaled by a factor of 50 for clarity, and the liquid mass fraction (ε_w)

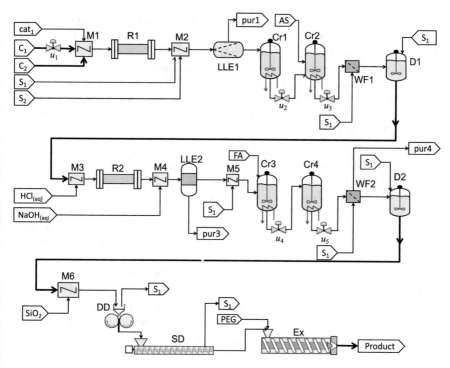

Fig. 5 Process flow diagram of the continuous manufacturing pilot plant. The control valves chosen for the dynamic optimization of the production process, $u_1 - u_5$, are highlighted. Some of the unit and stream names, as labeled here, are referred to in the text

between dissolution and growth several times during start-up, and this sequence of switches is hard to predict a priori.

4   Dynamic Optimization Using Nonsmooth Formulation

The parametric sensitivity information of nonsmooth DAE models introduced in Sect. 2.2 enables the rigorous optimization of continuous pharmaceuticals manufacturing processes, using gradient-based algorithms. Plant-wide dynamic models of a full production line have been reported in the literature [7, 22], and have been used to find optimal production procedures, including start-up and shutdown phases [23, 24]. These models have been developed for a pilot plant which was operated at the Novartis-MIT Center for Continuous Manufacturing [19]. Next, we demonstrate how nonsmooth DAE models can be used to optimize the dynamics of entire production campaigns.

A schematic process flow diagram of the pilot unit, which includes reaction, separation, and formulation steps is depicted in Fig. 5. The raw material, C_1, is fed to a mixer (M1), together with excess of the second reactant, C_2, and the catalyst, cat1. The mixed stream enters a PFR type reactor (R1) to produce the intermediate C_3 and impurity I_1. Solvents S_1 and S_2 are added in Mixer M2. C_2 and cat1 are dissolved in S_2 while unreacted C_1, C_3, and I_1 are dissolved in S_1. LLE1 separates the two liquid phases. The organic phase continues downstream for separation. The intermediate compound C_3 is crystallized in two sequential mixed suspension mixed product removal (MSMPR) crystallizers (Cr1, Cr2). The filter cake is collected and transported into a well-mixed vessel (D1) to which S_1 is added to dissolve and reduce the concentration of C_3 to the desired level.

A T-mixer (M3) is used to mix the slurry with aqueous HCl to synthesize C_4 by removing the protecting Boc group in Reactor R2 at room temperature where the impurity I_2 is formed. Next the acid is neutralized by adding NaOH. The organic phase with C_4 is subsequently separated from the aqueous phase inside a mixer-settler (LLE2) and diluted with S_1 in a T-mixer downstream of LLE2. The mixture with C_4 is diluted with S_1 and mixed with fumaric acid (FA) in a two-stage reactive crystallization (Cr3, Cr4) to crystallize the API. The crystals of API are separated from the mother liquor in a continuous washing and filtration stage (WF2) and then diluted in a well-mixed buffer tank (D2). The slurry with API is mixed with a slurry of silicon dioxide before being fed to a two-stage continuous dryer, which consists of a drum dryer (DD) followed by a tubular dryer with a rotating screw to convey the powder (SD). Finally, the API powder is mixed with polyethylene glycol (PEG) in the extruder (Ex). On-spec product must satisfy the following critical quality attributes: At least 34 %w of the API. Maximum of 0.3 %w of I_2 and maximum 0.5 %w of the total of I_1 and I_2.

4.1 Problem Formulation

In the pharmaceutical industry achieving a high yield is most often extremely important as the raw materials are very expensive. Thus, we would usually like to find the optimal yield of a manufacturing campaign given some desired productivity (i.e. total volume/mass of final product produced).

The following problem formulation is motivated by the detailed discussion in [25]. It also makes use of nonsmooth models, as demonstrated below. The entire time horizon of the manufacturing campaign is divided into 3 epochs; off-spec, on-spec and off-spec again, on time intervals $[0, t_{on})$, $[t_{on}, t_{off}]$ and $(t_{off}, t_f]$, respectively. On-spec production is only accounted for during the second epoch, and is guaranteed by enforcing appropriate quality constraints, $\mathbf{q}$. This ensures computable sensitivities of the resulting hybrid (discrete/continuous) system by fixing the mode sequence [10, 25]. t_{on} and t_{off} are included in the decision variables, enabling the optimizer to find the longest on-spec production phase (epoch) possible. The concept is similar to the classical approach of a start-up, steady-state (on-spec) operation and shutdown sequence but with a major difference; the on-spec epoch does not have to be steady. Consequently, this formulation is a relaxation of the steady-state constraint, making it superior to the traditional direct steady-state optimization approach [16]. The formulation is:

$$\max_{\mathbf{p} \in \mathcal{P}} \quad Y(\mathbf{p}, t_f) \tag{23a}$$

$$\text{s.t.} \quad \text{model (1),} \quad \forall t \in [0, t_f],$$

$$\mathbf{q}(\mathbf{p}, t) \leq 0, \quad \forall t \in [t_{\text{on}}, t_{\text{off}}], \tag{23b}$$

$$P - M_{\text{on} - \text{spec}}^{\text{Pr}}(\mathbf{p}, t_f) \leq 0, \tag{23c}$$

$$\mathbf{p}^l \leq \mathbf{p} \leq \mathbf{p}^u, \tag{23d}$$

where $\mathbf{p} \in \mathbb{R}^{n_p}$ is the vector of decision (optimization) variables, including t_{on} and t_{off}, with lower and upper bounds, $\mathbf{p}^l$ and $\mathbf{p}^u$, respectively, and $\mathbf{q}$ are the quality constraints defining an on-spec product. Overall, the campaign duration will be discretized into n_t time intervals. In general the decision variables are the valve positions at the discretized time intervals. In this example there are 5 valves, thus the total number of decision variables will be $(5 + 1) \times n_t$. For more details on the normalized and discretized formulation see [23].

The overall yield is optimized in this formulation. It is defined by:

$$Y = \frac{\text{mass of on-spec product}}{\text{mass of raw material fed}}, \quad \forall t \in (0, t_f]. \tag{24}$$

If M^{rm} is the total mass of the raw material fed to the process. It can be calculated from the following ODE:

$$\frac{dM^{rm}}{dt}(\mathbf{p}, t) = F^{rm}(\mathbf{p}, t), \quad \forall t \in [0, t_f], \tag{25}$$

$$M^{rm}(0) = 0.$$

If $M^{\text{on-spec}}$ is the total on-spec product produced in the campaign, it can be calculated from:

$$\frac{dM^{\text{on-spec}}}{dt}(\mathbf{p}, t) = \begin{cases} 0, & t \in [0, t_{\text{on}}), \\ F^{pr}(\mathbf{p}, t), & t \in [t_{\text{on}}, t_{\text{off}}], \\ 0, & t \in (t_{\text{off}}, t_f], \end{cases} \tag{26}$$

$$M^{\text{on-spec}}(0) = 0,$$

where F^{pr} is the mass flow rate of the product. Notice that product accumulation is only considered during the on-spec production epoch, but the consumption of the main reactant is considered over the entire campaign. In general, other end-point constraints can be added, for example, to enforce shutdown specifications, according to the specific requirements of the campaign. Nonetheless, as we show later, optimizing over the yield (instead of the total production) results in optimal shutdown procedures without the need to add explicit constraints.

The quality constraints, $\mathbf{q}$, of the on-spec product are path constraints, which are handled by introducing auxiliary variables, x_α, transforming them to endpoint equality constraints in terms of the auxiliary variables, using the hybrid and nonsmooth formulation equation:

$$\frac{dx_\alpha}{dt}(\mathbf{p}, t) = \begin{cases} 0, & t \in [0, t_{on}), \\ \max\left(0, q_\alpha(\mathbf{p}, t)\right), & t \in [t_{on}, t_{off}], \\ 0, & t \in (t_{off}, t_f], \end{cases} \quad \alpha \in \{a, b, c, d\}, \quad (27)$$

$$x_\alpha(0) = 0,$$

where q_α is the original path constraint. The new end-point constraints are:

$$x_\alpha(\mathbf{p}, t_f) = 0, \qquad \alpha \in \{a, b, c, d\}. \quad (28)$$

4.2 Optimal Dynamic Operation

Here, we look at an example problem which was optimized by the above approach. An end-to-end continuous manufacturing plant, as depicted in Fig. 5, was modeled by a nonsmooth DAE system (composed of 2132 equations), and the yield of the production campaign was optimized, given a limited campaign duration [23, 24].

Consider the solution of Formulation (23) with $P = 120$ kg for a campaign time of 200 h ($t_f = 200$). The time horizon is discretized into 4 sub-epochs; one for the first off-spec epoch, two for the on-spec epoch and another one for the last off-spec epoch, such that $n_t = 4$. We assume piecewise constant decision variables over the time horizon based on this discretization. Integration and sensitivity analysis was performed by DAEPACK [38]. The local optimization was performed by IPOPT with C++ interface [40].

We examine the results in terms of the objective function (the yield) and the constraints (overall on-spec productivity and impurity levels). Figure 6a presents the yield and the productivity, and Fig. 6b depicts the final product impurity profiles. A few interesting details are revealed by inspecting the optimal solution:

1. The overall productivity for the campaign is exactly 120 kg (i.e. Constraint (23c) is active).
2. The impurity levels were pushed to the maximum specified by the quality path constraints (23b), and were not violated during the entire campaign. Thus, essentially all the product produced is on-spec, and no product is wasted.
3. It takes about 17 h for an on-spec product to flow and to obtain a positive yield, which then increase monotonically throughout the campaign time. However,

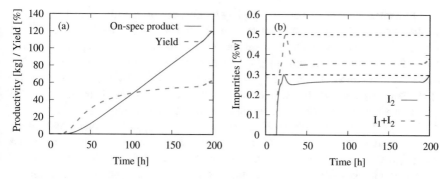

Fig. 6 (**a**) On-spec productivity and yield. (**b**) The impurity mass fractions in the final product. The specification levels are indicated by thin dashed lines

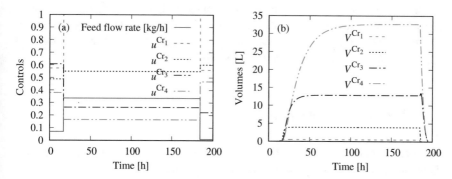

Fig. 7 Solution of the optimization problem (23) with $P = 120\,kg$ and campaign time of 200 h. (**a**) Optimal control profiles. (**b**) Holdup volumes in the crystallizers

some process attributes reach a steady-state much later (e.g. the holdup volume of Cr4 reaches steady-state after more than 75 h, see Fig. 7b).

4. A jump in the slope of the yield is apparent at $t = 186.1$ h, together with some change of the impurity levels of the product. The final (optimal) yield obtained is 63 %.

The optimal control trajectories and the resulting holdup volumes in the crystallizers are depicted in Fig. 7. The most important decision variables are the sub-epoch durations, τ_k, with optimal values: $\tau_1 = 16.8$ h, $\tau_2 = 167.5$ h, $\tau_3 = 15.7$ h and $\tau_4 = 0.0$ h. The final off-spec epoch, therefore, has been reduced to its lower bound, practically zero. The on-spec epoch is $t \in [16.8, 200]$ ($[\tau_1, \sum_{i=1}^{3} \tau_i]$). The relatively short initial off-spec epoch, $t \in [0, 16.8)$, is necessary because of the time required for the appearance of the API at the required concentration in the product stream. The optimal start-up procedure is characterized by a relatively short time to produce the API at the required concentration in the final product, while keeping the impurity mass fraction peaks below the specification levels.

More interesting details are revealed by looking at Fig. 7, which shows the values of the dynamic decision variables for the optimal solution. The feed flow rate of the reactant C_1 is reduced to its lower bound and the vessels are depleted towards the end of the time horizon. In practice this is a shutdown procedure. Shutting down while maintaining on-spec production was enabled by discretizing the on-spec epoch by more than just one sub-epoch, and optimizing their duration. The resulting shutdown procedure is a consequence of maximizing the yield; there is no justification to continue feeding reactants to the system if there will be no time to process them. The crystallizers are completely depleted by the end of the campaign (by appropriately adjusting their valve positions), while satisfying the product quality constraints. The optimizer finds the optimal time towards the end of the campaign to make this switch. It is important to emphasize that vessel depletion was not enforced by any end-point constraint. It is a property of the optimal solution when optimization of the yield is considered. The fact that a "shutdown" procedure was achieved while satisfying the on-spec quality path constraints shows the importance of setting all of the sub-epoch durations as decision variables, as opposed to only the main epochs (on/off-spec) [25].

4.3 Multi-Objective Optimization

The performance characteristics of the process depend on the design and the dynamic operating procedures. Often, more than one objective is of interest to the decision maker, such as yield and productivity. In many processes there is a trade-off between the optimal productivity and the optimal yield. In such cases, results may be presented as Pareto curves (or surfaces)[1, 8, 27], representing a set of non-inferior solutions.

Pareto curves may be generated by varying P in Formulation (23) and solving the optimization problem for each value. This is called the ϵ-constraint method [8]. After obtaining a solution to one problem we solve a similar problem, changing the value of P slightly, using the solution from the previous iteration as initial guess for the decision variables and the multipliers (see the IPOPT documentation). The results for campaigns of 150–250 h are presented in Fig. 8. The maximum yield that can be achieved for various campaign durations is comparable, around 67%, although this decreases slightly as the time horizon decreases. The optimal steady-state yield is shown for comparison as well. The campaign yield gets closer to this optimal value as the productivity constraint is decreased, and as the campaign duration is increased. The on-spec productivity, however, changes significantly with the time horizon. Better results are obtained in terms of yield and productivity for longer campaigns, as expected.

Although here we focused on the yield and the productivity as the performance objectives, other performance characteristics can be evaluated and optimized by introducing appropriate quality constraints or objective functions, such as the environmental factor (E-factor) [30] or the total energy consumption. Furthermore,

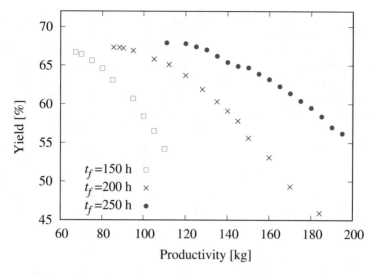

Fig. 8 Pareto curves of optimal solutions of Formulation (23) for various campaign durations of the end-to-end continuous pilot plant

the minimization of the campaign time could be performed readily by defining t_f as the objective function. This information should be available to the decision makers when deciding on the desired performance and appropriate procedures.

5   Conclusions and Outlook

The nonsmooth formulation approach demonstrated here is capable of simulating a wide range of dynamic phenomena such as switching between different physical regimes (e.g., between thermodynamic phases or kinetic regimes), control valve limitations, and nonsmooth changes in stream compositions. The nonsmooth DAEs framework guarantees the existence of meaningful sensitivity information, which can be computed by appropriate sensitivity analysis, and used by optimization algorithms to find optimal dynamic procedures, as exemplified here even for end-to-end continuous manufacturing plants.

Optimization problems for nonsmooth systems are traditionally handled by introducing cumbersome, unphysical reformulations in the frameworks of mixed-integer and complementarity system approaches. These methods lead to additional (probably unnecessary) parameters, artificial variables, binary variables, constraints, and considerations. Consequently, mixed-integer reformulations of nonsmooth problems may be inaccurate. Furthermore, the introduction of artificial numerical parameters/binary variables may significantly increase the solver's running time. Now, thanks to the developments presented in this chapter, these can be formulated and solved in a more straightforward approach that is mathematically sound. Moreover, local-optimization solvers for nonsmooth problems exist and provide an approach to find local solutions of larger problems that are outside the scope of global nonconvex mixed-integer solvers. Extension of deterministic global optimization methods to nonsmooth DAEs should be immediate since relaxations of nonsmooth functions can be computed using McCormick's framework [13, 29, 39]. For dynamic simulation of nonsmooth DAEs, process simulators need to be extended to include a library of nonsmooth elemental functions (e.g. the Euclidean norm, min, max, mid, mid with n arguments). The Jacobian software [11], used for the simulations presented in Sect. 3, already supports most of these nonsmooth elemental functions. Now, there exists a potential of implementing such nonsmooth dynamic formulations in online economic optimization and control systems, known as nonlinear model predictive control [20]. In such systems, an updated optimal control profile will be calculated based on real-time measurements. These systems should also be robust and take parametric uncertainty into account.

The dynamic optimization formulation presented in Sect. 4.1 outperforms the traditional steady-state optimization approach. This is accomplished by enforcing the quality constraints on an internal epoch and optimizing its duration, allowing an overall transient behavior (relaxing the steady-state constraint). Importantly, by allowing the switching times of the controls to vary by the optimizer it is possible to find optimal start-up and shutdown procedures. Here, we showed that the optimal solution completely eliminated off-spec production, achieving high levels of yield for campaigns of 150–250 h. Performance maps of the manufacturing process may be expressed by Pareto curves, where optimal yield and optimal productivity are considered as opposing objectives.

Traditionally, the pharmaceutical industry has adopted batch processes as the main manufacturing approach. These unit operations involve unsteady flow, time-dependent conditions and are disconnected from the rest of the plant. Continuous flow processes allow for higher level of process integration, control, and efficiency. Sometimes these processes are (wrongly) defined as steady-state processes. However, this is not necessarily the case, and an optimal continuous operation may exhibit significant transients, as demonstrated here. In this sense, the pharmaceutical industry may evolve to operate manufacturing processes which hold both batch and continuous type properties (continuous flow with significant transients).

References

1. David Acevedo, Yanssen Tandy, and Zoltan K. Nagy. Multiobjective Optimization of an Unseeded Batch Cooling Crystallizer for Shape and Size Manipulation. *Ind. Eng. Chem. Res.*, 54(7):2156–2166, 2015.
2. Paul I Barton, Russell J Allgor, William F Feehery, and Santos Galán. Dynamic Optimization in a Discontinuous World. *Ind. Eng. Chem. Res.*, 37(3):966–981, 1998.
3. Paul I. Barton, Kamil A. Khan, Peter Stechlinski, and Harry A.J. Watson. Computationally relevant generalized derivatives: theory, evaluation and applications. *Optim. Methods Softw.*, 33(4-6):1030–1072, nov 2018.

4. Paul I Barton and Cha Kun Lee. Modeling, simulation, sensitivity analysis, and optimization of hybrid systems. *ACM Trans. Model. Comput. Simul.*, 12(4):256–289, 2002.
5. Paul I Barton and Cha Kun Lee. Design of process operations using hybrid dynamic optimization. *Comput. Chem. Eng.*, 28(6-7):955–969, jun 2004.
6. Paul I. Barton, Cha Kun Lee, and Mehmet Yunt. Optimization of hybrid systems. *Comput. Chem. Eng.*, 30(10-12):1576–1589, sep 2006.
7. Brahim Benyahia, Richard Lakerveld, and Paul I Barton. A Plant-Wide Dynamic Model of a Continuous Pharmaceutical Process. *Ind. Eng. Chem. Res.*, 51(47):15393–15412, nov 2012.
8. Vira Chankong and Yacov Y Haimes. *Multiobjective decision making: theory and methodology*. Courier Dover Publications, Mineola, New York, 2008.
9. Frank H Clarke. *Optimization and nonsmooth analysis*. SIAM, Philadelphia, 1990.
10. Santos Galán, William F Feehery, and Paul I Barton. Parametric sensitivity functions for hybrid discrete/continuous systems. *Appl. Numer. Math.*, 31(1):17–47, 1999.
11. RES Group Inc. http://www.resgroupinc.com/, 2019.
12. Kamil A Khan and Paul I Barton. A vector forward mode of automatic differentiation for generalized derivative evaluation. *Optim. Methods Softw.*, 30(6):1185–1212, nov 2015.
13. Kamil A Khan and Paul I Barton. Generalized Derivatives for Hybrid Systems. *IEEE Trans. Automat. Contr.*, pages 1–16, 2017.
14. Jason G Kralj, Hemantkumar R Sahoo, and Klavs F Jensen. Integrated continuous microfluidic liquid-liquid extraction. *Lab Chip*, 7(2):256–263, 2007.
15. Ashish Kumar, Jurgen Vercruysse, Valérie Vanhoorne, Maunu Toiviainen, Pierre Emmanuel Panouillot, Mikko Juuti, Chris Vervaet, Jean Paul Remon, Krist V Gernaey, Thomas De Beer, and Ingmar Nopens. Conceptual framework for model-based analysis of residence time distribution in twin-screw granulation. *Eur. J. Pharm. Sci.*, 71:25–34, apr 2015.
16. Richard Lakerveld, Brahim Benyahia, Richard D. Braatz, and Paul I. Barton. Model-Based Design of a Plant-Wide Control Strategy for a Continuous Pharmaceutical Plant. *AIChE J.*, 59(10):3671–3685, 2013.
17. Richard Lakerveld, Brahim Benyahia, Patrick L Heider, Haitao Zhang, Aaron Wolfe, Christopher J Testa, Sean Ogden, Devin R Hersey, Salvatore Mascia, James M B Evans, Richard D Braatz, and Paul I Barton. The Application of an Automated Control Strategy for an Integrated Continuous Pharmaceutical Pilot Plant. *Org. Process Res. Dev.*, 19(9):1088–1100, 2015.
18. Zhen Li, Matthias Kind, and Gerald Gruenewald. Modeling the Growth Kinetics of Fluidized-Bed Spray Granulation. *Chem. Eng. Technol.*, 34(7, SI):1067–1075, jul 2011.
19. Salvatore Mascia, Patrick L. Heider, Haitao Zhang, Richard Lakerveld, Brahim Benyahia, Paul I. Barton, Richard D. Braatz, Charles L. Cooney, James M B Evans, Timothy F. Jamison, Klavs F. Jensen, Allan S. Myerson, and Bernhardt L. Trout. End-to-end continuous manufacturing of pharmaceuticals: Integrated synthesis, purification, and final dosage formation. *Angew. Chemie - Int. Ed.*, 52(47):12359–12363, 2013.
20. Ali Mesbah, Joel A Paulson, Richard Lakerveld, and Richard D Braatz. Model Predictive Control of an Integrated Continuous Pharmaceutical Manufacturing Pilot Plant. *Org. Process Res. Dev.*, 21(6):844–854, 2017.
21. Yu Nesterov. Lexicographic differentiation of nonsmooth functions. *Math. Program.*, 104(2-3):669–700, 2005.
22. Michael Patrascu and Paul I. Barton. Optimal campaigns in end-to-end continuous pharmaceuticals manufacturing. Part 1: Nonsmooth dynamic modeling. *Chem. Eng. Process. - Process Intensif.*, 125:298–310, 2018.
23. Michael Patrascu and Paul I. Barton. Optimal campaigns in end-to-end continuous pharmaceuticals manufacturing. Part 2: Dynamic optimization. *Chem. Eng. Process. - Process Intensif.*, 125:124–132, 2018.
24. Michael Patrascu and Paul I. Barton. Optimal Dynamic Continuous Manufacturing of Pharmaceuticals with Recycle. *Ind. Eng. Chem. Res.*, 58(30):13423–13436, 2019.
25. Ali M Sahlodin and Paul I Barton. Optimal campaign continuous manufacturing. *Ind. Eng. Chem. Res.*, 54(45):11344–11359, 2015.

26. Ali M. Sahlodin, Harry A. J. Watson, and Paul I. Barton. Nonsmooth model for dynamic simulation of phase changes. *AIChE J.*, 62(9):3334–3351, sep 2016.
27. Debasis Sarkar and Jayant M Modak. Pareto-optimal solutions for multi-objective optimization of fed-batch bioreactors using nondominated sorting genetic algorithm. *Chem. Eng. Sci.*, 60(2):481–492, 2005.
28. Stefan Scholtes. *Introduction to Piecewise Differentiable Equations*. SpringerBriefs in Optimization. Springer New York, New York, NY, 2013.
29. Joseph K. Scott and Paul I. Barton. Convex and Concave Relaxations for the Parametric Solutions of Semi-explicit Index-One Differential-Algebraic Equations. *J. Optim. Theory Appl.*, 156(3):617–649, mar 2013.
30. Roger A Sheldon. The E Factor: fifteen years on. *Green Chem.*, 9(12):1273–1283, 2007.
31. Peter Stechlinski and Paul I. Barton. Nonsmooth Hessenberg differential-algebraic equations. *J. Math. Anal. Appl.*, 495(1):124721, 2021.
32. Peter Stechlinski, Michael Patrascu, and Paul I. Barton. Nonsmooth DAEs with Applications in Modeling Phase Changes. pages 243–275. sep 2018.
33. Peter Stechlinski, Michael Patrascu, and Paul I. Barton. Nonsmooth differential-algebraic equations in chemical engineering. *Comput. Chem. Eng.*, 114:52–68, jun 2018.
34. Peter G Stechlinski and Paul I Barton. Generalized derivatives of differential–algebraic equations. *J. Optim. Theory Appl.*, 171(1):1–26, 2016.
35. Peter G. Stechlinski and Paul I. Barton. Generalized derivatives of optimal control problems with nonsmooth differential-algebraic equations embedded. In *2016 IEEE 55th Conf. Decis. Control. CDC 2016*, pages 592–597. Institute of Electrical and Electronics Engineers Inc., 2016.
36. Peter G Stechlinski and Paul I Barton. Dependence of solutions of nonsmooth differential-algebraic equations on parameters. *J. Differ. Equ.*, 262(3):2254–2285, 2017.
37. Qinglin Su, Zoltan K Nagy, and Chris D Rielly. Pharmaceutical crystallisation processes from batch to continuous operation using MSMPR stages: Modelling, design, and control. *Chem. Eng. Process. Process Intensif.*, 89:41–53, mar 2015.
38. John Tolsma and Paul I Barton. DAEPACK: An open modeling environment for legacy models. *Ind. Eng. Chem. Res.*, 39(6):1826–1839, 2000.
39. A. Tsoukalas and A. Mitsos. Multivariate McCormick relaxations. *J. Glob. Optim.*, 59(2-3):633–662, apr 2014.
40. Andreas Wächter and Lorenz T. Biegler. On the implementation of an interior-point filter line-search algorithm for large-scale nonlinear programming. *Math. Program.*, 106(1):25–57, 2006.
41. Harry A.J. Watson and Paul I. Barton. Modeling phase changes in multistream heat exchangers. *Int. J. Heat Mass Transf.*, 105:207–219, 2017.
42. M. Wulkow, A. Gerstlauer, and U. Nieken. Modeling and simulation of crystallization processes using parsival. 56(7):2575–2588, apr 2001.
43. Haitao Zhang, Justin Quon, Alejandro J Alvarez, James Evans, Allan S Myerson, and Bernhardt Trout. Development of continuous anti-solvent/cooling crystallization process using cascaded mixed suspension, mixed product removal crystallizers. *Org. Process Res. Dev.*, 16(5):915–924, 2012.

Integrated Synthesis, Crystallization, Filtration, and Drying of Active Pharmaceutical Ingredients: A Model-Based Digital Design Framework for Process Optimization and Control

Daniel J. Laky, Daniel Casas-Orozco, Francesco Destro, Massimiliano Barolo, Gintaras V. Reklaitis, and Zoltan K. Nagy

1 Introduction

Over the past two decades, initiatives such as quality-by-design (QbD) [1] and quality-by-control (QbC) [2] have accelerated a modernization in pharmaceutical manufacturing. These paradigms require quantitative interpretation of an operating region of the process, often branded as the *design space*. The *design space* has been previously characterized as "the multidimensional combination and inter-action of input variables and process parameters that have been demonstrated to provide assurance of quality" [3]. Naturally, incorporation of Industry 4.0 standards [4] accompanies modernization via digitalization and computerization of manufacturing, especially during identification/quantification, and maintenance of a robust operating region through process design and online process management, respectively.

Standard computational methods for design space identification typically fall into three categories: (1) data-driven sampling [5, 6], (2) fully mechanistic, direct optimization [7], and (3) data-driven modeling with optimization [8, 9], or a combination of such methods [10, 11]. Each technique requires high-quality mechanistic models, quantified uncertainty of model parameters, and high-quality data for meaningful justification of process digitalization.

Design space identification through mechanistic modeling may be applied to a single unit operation or larger pieces of a manufacturing process. Certain key operations in pharmaceutical manufacturing, for instance, the crystallization-

D. J. Laky · D. Casas-Orozco · G. V. Reklaitis · Z. K. Nagy (✉)
Davidson School of Chemical Engineering, Purdue University, West Lafayette, IN, USA
e-mail: znagy@purdue.edu

F. Destro · M. Barolo
CAPE-Lab—Computer-Aided Process Engineering Laboratory, University of Padova, Padova (PD), Italy

filtration-drying steps, are highly coupled subprocesses and should be considered simultaneously while identifying optimal process design. Achieving such an optimal operation while considering the interaction of these process steps will be at least as good as considering the units separately, of which the latter often requires some heuristic blending of qualitative and quantitative conclusions.

Even with implementations achieving computational tractability with quality design space identification, there is still much work to be done with regard to the accessibility and standardization of traditional pharmaceutical unit operations. Currently, one may use a commercial software, such as gPROMS FormulatedProducts [12], to analyze integrated design and control of pharmaceutical processes. However, limitations exist on user flexibility for automated simulation and analysis techniques, the availability of models in the provided model library, the ease of implementing custom models, and robustness with respect to hybrid modelling (i.e., batch, semibatch, and continuous manufacturing steps in the same process).

Given this drawback, when developing intensified or novel processing steps, collaboration with commercial developers or usage of a more accessible coding framework (i.e., Python or MATLAB) is often required. For this reason, an open-source pharmaceutical manufacturing package, PharmaPy [13], has been developed to supplement other (commercial) software packages, as a tool for simulation and optimization of pharmaceutical processes, focusing on allowing process design and analysis through automated simulation, custom modeling, and hybrid modeling capabilities.

Creating and maintaining a process digital twin is a key step while analyzing and optimizing a given process through digital design. In fact, once a digital twin is realized, one may perform digital tests of active control loops for model-based control applications. This paradigm begins pushing the QbD approach to an online QbC approach, employing the same or similar models and modeling techniques. In Yu et al. [14], this move has been defined by the FDA as the final step in the modernization of pharmaceutical manufacturing. Even yet, both approaches provide the ability for online analysis, requiring user scrutiny when deciding under which paradigm process-specific design space identification and maintenance fall.

In this work, we present mathematical models relevant to the synthesis, crystallization, filtration, and drying steps of an active pharmaceutical ingredient (API). Each step encourages QbD by utilizing an integrated simulation framework for process analysis and optimization. The rest of the chapter is organized as follows. In Sect. 2, we present the relevant model implementations utilized in the case studies. In Sect. 3, we present a case study for synthesis-crystallization of paracetamol using experimental data available from existing literature. Then, a case study showcasing an intensification of filtration-drying steps within an integrated carousel is presented as well. Also, to encourage the movement toward QbC, we test an active control strategy on the digital twin of the integrated filtration-drying carousel.

2 Mathematical Modeling of API Synthesis, Crystallization, Filtration, and Drying

In this section, we present four subsections describing the mathematical modeling employed for each step: synthesis, crystallization, filtration, and drying. Further information on the modeling environments used for each model is discussed with the case studies in Sect. 3.

2.1 Synthesis Modeling

For the first case study, a plug flow reactor (PFR) for the synthesis of paracetamol is modeled under the following assumptions: (1) no radial gradients, (2) negligible axial dispersion, and (3) constant heat transfer fluid temperature T_{ht}. The model is represented below as Eq. (1):

$$\frac{\partial C_j}{\partial t} = -\dot{F}_{in}\frac{\partial C_j}{\partial V} + v_j \cdot r \quad j = A, B, C, D,$$

$$\sum_{j=1}^{n_{comp}} C_j C_{p,j}\frac{\partial T}{\partial t} = -\dot{F}_{in}\sum_{j=1}^{n_{comp}} C_j C_{p,j}\frac{\partial T}{\partial V} + \Delta H_{rxn}(T)\cdot r - Ua(T - T_{ht}),$$

$$(1)$$

where U is the heat transfer coefficient (W m^{-2} K^{-1}), a is the heat transfer area (m^2 m^{-3}), and $C_{p,j}$ is the heat capacity of component j (J mol^{-1} K^{-1}), given by

$$C_{p,j}(T) = A_j + B_j T + C_j T^2 + \dots \quad (2)$$

Heat of reaction ΔH_{rxn} (J mol^{-1}) was computed from data taken from literature [15, 16]. For simulation purposes, the model is translated to a set of ordinary differential equations (ODEs) via an upwind discretization in the V dimension (Eq. (3)):

$$\frac{dC_j^n}{dt} = -\dot{F}_{in}\frac{C_j^n - C_j^{n-1}}{\Delta V} + v_j \cdot r\left(C_A^n, C_B^n, T^n\right) \quad j = A, B, C, D, \quad n = 1, \dots, n_{discr},$$

$$C_{p,vol}\frac{dT^n}{dt} = -\dot{F}_{in}C_{p,vol}\frac{T^n - T^{n-1}}{\Delta V} + \Delta H_{rxn}\left(T^n\right)\cdot r - Ua\left(T^n - T_{ht}\right),$$

$$(3)$$

with boundary and initial conditions for concentrations:

$$C_j^0 = C_{j,in} \quad j = A, B, C, D$$
$$C_j (V, 0) = 0 \quad j = A, B, C, \tag{4}$$
$$C_D (V, 0) = 55 \text{ mol L}^{-1},$$

and

$$T^0 = T_{in}, \tag{5}$$
$$T (V, 0) = 298.15 \text{ K}$$

for temperature. Volumetric heat capacity $C_{p, vol}$ (J m^{-3} K^{-1}) is given by

$$C_{p,vol} = \sum_{j=1}^{n_{comp}} \left[C_j^n \cdot C_{p,j} \left(T^n \right) \right]. \tag{6}$$

2.2 Crystallization Modeling

For continuous crystallization, a one-dimensional population balance with size-independent growth is used to represent the crystal phase, as shown in Eq. (7).

$$\frac{\partial f (t, x)}{\partial t} + G \frac{\partial f (t, x)}{\partial x} = B \cdot \delta (x - x_0) - \dot{F}_{in} (f_{in} - f), \tag{7}$$

where f represents the crystal size distribution (CSD) of the solids present in suspension (# μm^{-1} m^{-3}). The crystallization model shown in Eq. (7) is converted to a system of ODEs by discretizing the spatial coordinate x using a high-resolution method ([17, 18]). The change in crystal size distribution (CSD) can then be written as the following semi-discretized equation system ($n = 1, \cdots, n_{discr}$):

$$\frac{d f_n}{dt} = \frac{F_{n+1/2} - F_{n-1/2}}{\Delta x}, \tag{8}$$

where fluxes F are given by

$$F_{1-1/2} = B,$$
$$F_{n-1/2} = G \left[f_{n-1} + \tfrac{1}{2} (f_n - f_{n-1}) \varphi_{n-1} \right] + D \left[f_n + \tfrac{1}{2} (f_{n-1} - f_n) \varphi_n \right]$$
$$+ \dot{F}_{in} \left(f_{n,in} - f_n \right), \quad n = 2, \ldots, n_{discr}, \tag{9}$$
$$F_{n_{discr}+1/2} = 0.$$

Van Leer flux limiters φ_n were used to incorporate the high-resolution component of the discretization method:

$$\varphi_n = \frac{|\theta_n| + \theta_n}{1 + |\theta_n|},$$

$$\theta_n = \frac{f_n - f_{n-1}}{f_{n+1} - f_n}. \tag{10}$$

Material balance on the continuous phase is represented by

$$\frac{dC_j}{dt} = \frac{1}{\varepsilon}\left(\frac{\dot{F}_{in}}{V}\left(\varepsilon_{in}C_{j,in} - \varepsilon C_j\right) - tr\left(\delta_{j,tg} - \frac{C_j}{\rho_s}\right)\right),$$

$$tr = 3\,k_v\,\rho_s\,\mu_2\,G,$$

$$\varepsilon = 1 - k_v\mu_3, \tag{11}$$

where ρ_s is the crystal density (kg m^{-3}) and $\delta_{j,tg}$ is the Kronecker delta that relates species j and the target crystallizing component, indexed as tg ($j = 1 \ldots, n_{comp}$):

$$\delta_{j,tg} = \begin{cases} 1 & j = tg \\ 0 & j \neq tg \end{cases} \tag{12}$$

The nth moment of the CSD, f, is given by

$$\mu_n = \int_0^\infty x^n f(x,t)\,dx, \tag{13}$$

which can be computed numerically from the model solution given a specified size grid in the x dimension.

Regarding batch and semibatch operation, solid-phase population balances are computed for the CSD expressed as total particle number $\tilde{f}$ (# μm^{-1}). On the other hand, liquid-phase material balances for batch and semibatch operation can be obtained from Eqs. (7) and (11) by appropriate manipulation, which requires including an expression for the change in liquid volume (dV_L/dt), as described elsewhere [19, 20].

Furthermore, energy balances for the different operation modes analyzed for crystallizers are given by

$$\left(mC_p\right)_{sl}\frac{dT}{dt} = \dot{F}_{in}\left[\left(\varepsilon\rho_l h_l + (1-\varepsilon)\rho_s h_s\right)_{in} - \left(\varepsilon\rho_l h_l + (1-\varepsilon)\rho_s h_s\right)\right]$$

$$- \Delta H_{cry} tr - UA(T - T_{ht}) - \frac{dm}{dt}h(T),$$

$$\left(mC_p\right)_{sl} = \begin{cases} V\left[\varepsilon\rho_l C_{p,l} + (1-\varepsilon)\rho_s C_{p,s}\right], & \text{(MSMPR)} \\ V_L\left[\rho_l C_{p,l} + \frac{(1-\varepsilon)}{\varepsilon}\rho_s C_{p,s}\right]. & \text{(Batch and semibatch)} \end{cases} \tag{14}$$

where $C_{p,l}$ and $C_{p,s}$ are the heat capacity of the liquid and solid phase, respectively (J kg^{-1} K^{-1}), and ΔH_{cry} is the latent heat of fusion of the target compound (J kg^{-1}).

Table 1 Kinetic constants for CR01

Constant	Value	Unit
k_b	16.034	$\# \, s^{-1}(kg \ m^3)^{-b}$
b	6.23	–
k_g	6.56E-03	$\mu m \ s^{-1}(kg \ m^3)^{-g}$
g	1.54	–
k_d	6.56E-03	$\mu m \ s^{-1}(kg \ m^3)^{-d}$
d	1.54	–

Operation of batch and mixed suspension-mixed product removal (MSMPR) crystallizers is assumed at constant mass $dm/dt = 0$, whereas for semibatch crystallizers,

$$\frac{dm}{dt} = \dot{F}_{in} \left(\varepsilon \rho_{l,in} + (1 - \varepsilon) \rho_{s,in} \right). \tag{15}$$

Crystallization kinetics are represented as power law expressions for nucleation, growth, and dissolution depending on absolute supersaturation (Eq. 16):

$$S = C - C_{sat} \tag{16}$$

Nucleation rate is expressed as the sum of primary and secondary nucleation rates [21]:

$$
\begin{aligned}
B &= B_p + B_s, \\
B_p &= k_p \exp\left(-E_p/RT\right) S^p, \\
B_s &= k_s \exp\left(-E_s/RT\right) \, S^{s_1} (k_v \mu_3)^{s_2}, \\
B &= \max(B, 0).
\end{aligned}
\tag{17}
$$

Growth and dissolution rates are expressed similarly:

$$G = \max \left(k_g \exp\left(-E_g/RT\right) S^g, 0 \right) \tag{18}$$

$$D = \min \left(k_d \exp\left(-E_d/RT\right) S|S|^{d-1}, 0 \right). \tag{19}$$

The operators *max* and *min* in Eqs. (17)–(19) dictate which crystallization kinetics are active during the growth regime (growth and nucleation) and dissolution regime (only dissolution). Kinetic constants used in Sect. 3 were adapted from Nagy et al. [22] (Table 1).

Paracetamol solubility in a mixture of water and acetic anhydride + acetic acid was modeled according to a polynomial expansion [23]:

$$C_{sat} = 4.442 \times 10^3 - 30.86 \, T + 5.368 \times 10^{-2} \, T^2. \tag{20}$$

Finally, the influence of chemical species other than paracetamol on growth kinetics was modeled using a simplified multi-impurity adsorption model (MIAM), which can be written as [24]

$$p_{imp} = 1 - \alpha \frac{K_j C_j}{1 + \sum_i K_i C_i}, \tag{21}$$

where K_j (m^3 kg^{-1}) is the adsorption constant of species j and α is the effectiveness factor [25].

The Holding tank operation model depends on the presence/absence of crystals in the incoming material. For material coming from a crystallizer, the holding tank acts as an adiabatic, semibatch crystallizer, for which material and energy balances can be adapted, as explained above. On the other hand, for streams composed only by liquid, the balances shown in Eq. (22) are used:

$$\frac{dw_j}{dt} = \frac{\dot{m}_{in}}{m_{tot}} \left(w_{j,in} - w_j \right),$$

$$\frac{dm_{tot}}{dt} = \dot{m}_{in}(t), \tag{22}$$

$$\frac{dT}{dt} = \frac{\dot{m}_{in}}{m_{tot} \sum_j C_{p,j} w_j} \left(h_{in}(T_{in}) - h(T) \right),$$

where w_j represents the mass fraction of component j, $\dot{m}_{in}$ is the entering mass flow (kg s^{-1}), and m_{tot} is the instantaneous accumulated liquid mass (kg). Specific enthalpy (J kg^{-1}) is calculated as

$$h(T) = \sum_{j=1}^{n_{comp}} w_j \left[\int_T^{T_{ref}} C_{p,j} \, dT \right]. \tag{23}$$

2.3 Filtration Modeling

We predict ε and α from the crystal size and shape distribution of the slurry being filtered according to the following models. The porosity model is based on the work of Yu, Zou, and Standish [26], who proposed and validated a modified linear packing model for predicting the porosity of nonspherical particle mixtures. Given the CSD expressed as percentage volume distribution $f(d_i)$, with respect to particle size d_i, the modified linear packing model assumes that one bin of size d_i is the controlling component, determining the porosity of the whole mixture. Under this assumption, the cake specific volume V (with $\varepsilon = 1 - 1/V$) is given by

$$V = \max \left(V_i^C \right) \tag{24}$$

where V_i^C is the specific volume calculated assuming that the ith component of the CSD is the controlling one. Arranging the bins in decreasing size order, V_i^C is obtained with the following set of equations, for every ith component:

$$V_i^C = V_i + \sum_{j=1}^{i-1} \left[V_j - \left(V_j - 1\right) g(r) - V_i \right] x_{v,j} + \sum_{j=i+1}^{n} \left[V_j - V_j \ f(r) - V_i \right] x_{v,j},$$

(25)

$$r = \begin{cases} \frac{d_{p,i}}{d_{p,j}} & \text{if } j < i, \\ \frac{d_{p,j}}{d_{p,i}} & \text{if } j > i, \end{cases}$$

(26)

$$f(r) = (1-r)^{3.3} + 2.8 \ r \ (1-r)^{2.7},$$

(27)

$$g(r) = (1-r)^2 + 0.4 \ r \ (1-r)^{3.7},$$

(28)

where V_i is the specific volume of a cake composed only by particles of size d_i, $g(r)$ and $f(r)$ are interaction functions between two components of size ratio r, $x_{v,i}$ is the volumetric fraction of the ith component in the mixture (calculated from $f(d_i)$), and $d_{p,i}$ is the equivalent packing diameter of the ith component (calculated following Yu et al. [26]). The effect of the shape distribution on ε is accounted for by calculating V_i with the relations proposed by Zou and Yu [27].

We calculate α following a resistance additivity hypothesis [28], considering the contribution of every component of the particle mixture:

$$\alpha = \sum f(d_i) \ 180 \frac{1-\varepsilon}{\varepsilon^3} \frac{1}{\phi_i^2 d_i^2} \frac{1}{\rho_s},$$

(29)

where ρ_s is the solid mass density and Φ_i is the sphericity of the ith component of the particle mixture, calculated as

$$\Phi_i = \frac{\pi^{\frac{1}{3}} (6 \ k_V \ (d_i))^{\frac{2}{3}}}{k_S \ (d_i)},$$

(30)

in which $k_V(d_i)$ and $k_S(d_i)$ are the surface and the volume shape factors of the crystals of size d_i, respectively. We neglect the cake compressibility, as the cakes processed in the carousel are not particularly subject to this phenomenon due to small cake size and relatively low applied ΔP. Suitable power law relations [29] can be introduced for compressible systems. The cake permeability k is then defined from α as

$$k = \frac{1}{\alpha_m \ \rho_s \ (1 - \varepsilon)}, \tag{31}$$

with cake properties established; batch filtration is modeled under the following rules. At the end of filtration, the cake saturation S (ratio between volume of liquid in the cake porosity and pore volume) is equal to one in every point of the cake, and the liquid composition is the same as in the fed slurry. The remaining outputs of the filtration model to be calculated are the filtration duration $\Delta t_{filtration}$, the final cake height H_{cake}, and the dynamic profile of filtrate V_{filt}, which are obtained according to the following discussion. The driving force for filtration ΔP is equal to the sum of the pressure drops through the cake ΔP_{cake} and the pressure drops through the filter mesh ΔP_{filter}:

$$\Delta P = \Delta P_{cake}(t) + \Delta P_{filter}(t) \tag{32}$$

Factoring the Darcy law [30] into Eq. (32) and rearranging, the instantaneous filtrate flow rate is

$$\frac{dV_{filt}}{dt} = \frac{\Delta P}{\frac{\alpha \ \mu_l}{A^2} \frac{V_{slurry} \ c_{slurry}}{V_{filt, \ final}} V + \frac{R_m \mu_l}{A}}, \tag{33}$$

where μ_l is the liquid viscosity, A is the filter cross-section, V_{slurry} is the slurry volume loaded in the carousel at every cycle, c_{slurry} is the crystal concentration in the slurry, R_m is the filter mesh resistance, and $V_{filt, \ final}$ is the volume of filtrate at the end of filtration, which is calculated with a mass balance:

$$V_{filt, \ final} = V_{slurry} \left(1 - \frac{c_{slurry}}{\rho_s} \left(1 + \frac{\varepsilon}{1 + \varepsilon} \right) \right). \tag{34}$$

The integration of Eq. (33) assuming constant ΔP yields the quadratic law for $V_{filt}(t)$:

$$\frac{\alpha \ \mu_l}{2 \ A^2} \frac{V_{slurry} \ c_{slurry}}{V_{filt, \ final}} V_{filt}^2(t) + \frac{R_m \mu_l}{A} V_{filt}(t) - \Delta P \ t = 0 \tag{35}$$

Imposing V_{filt} equal to $V_{filt, \ final}$ in Eq. (35), $\Delta t_{filtration}$ is obtained as

$$\Delta t_{filtration} = \frac{\mu_l \ \alpha \ V_{slurry} \ c_{slurry} \ V_{filt, \ final}}{2 \ A^2 \Delta P} + \frac{\mu_l R_m V_{filtrate, final}}{A \ \Delta P}. \tag{36}$$

At the end of filtration and during all the subsequent carousel processing, H_{cake} and ΔP_{cake} correspond to Eqs. (37) and (38), respectively,

$$H_{cake} = \frac{V_{slurry} C_{slurry}}{\rho_s (1 - \varepsilon) A},$$ (37)

$$\Delta P_{cake} \left(t \geq \Delta t_{filtration} \right) = \Delta P \left(1 - \frac{R_m}{\alpha \ H_{cake} \ \rho_s (1 - \varepsilon) + R_m} \right).$$ (38)

At the end of filtration, cake deliquoring immediately starts, consisting of the mechanical removal of the liquid retained in the pores under the action of ΔP. Due to capillary forces, there is a minimum pressure threshold P_b to be applied to the cake to initiate liquid removal. Because of capillarity, there is also an equilibrium saturation of the cake S_∞, at which deliquoring stops, and further cake desaturation can be carried out only through thermal drying. For this study, we calculate P_b and S_∞ with literature equations [31] for cakes of mono-sized particles, to which we introduce an additive hypothesis to account for the CSD in the cake as follows:

$$P_b = \sum f(d_i) \ \frac{4.6 \ (1 - \varepsilon) \ \sigma}{\varepsilon \ d_i},$$ (39)

$$S_\infty = \sum f(d_i) \ 0.155 \ \left(1 + 0.031 \ N_{cap}^{-0.49} \right),$$ (40)

where σ is the liquid surface tension and N_{cap} is the capillary number, calculated as

$$N_{cap} = \frac{\varepsilon^3 d_i^2 \ (\rho_l \ g \ H_{cake} + \Delta P_{cake})}{(1 - \varepsilon)^2 \ H_{cake} \ \sigma}.$$ (41)

The local velocity of the liquid u_l is given by the Darcy law for multiphase flow [30]:

$$u_l = - \frac{k \ k_{rl}}{\mu_l} \frac{dP_l}{dz},$$ (42)

in which P_l is the local pressure of the liquid and k_{rl} is the liquid relative cake permeability. We calculate k_{rl} with the following relations [32]:

$$k_{rl} = k \ S_R^{2+3\lambda},$$ (43)

$$S_R = \frac{S - S_\infty}{1 - S_\infty} = \left(\frac{P_b}{P_g - P_l} \right)^\lambda,$$ (44)

where λ is the pore size distribution parameter (usually assumed equal to 5), S_R is the local reduced saturation, and P_g is the local gas pressure. In Eq. (42), we calculate P_l through Eq. (44), assuming linear and constant gas pressure gradient during the process, with total gas pressure drop through the cake equal to ΔP_{cake} (Eq. 32). With this assumption, we neglect the initial deliquoring transient for a fully saturated cake, during which there is no gas at the outlet of the bed, to avoid solving the gas mass balance and the Darcy law for the gas phase. This initial transient is relatively fast compared to process dynamics and has little impact on the process.

We develop a one-dimensional dynamic model for deliquoring, along the cake axial coordinate z. The liquid phase mass balance reads

$$\frac{\partial S}{\partial t} = -\frac{1}{\varepsilon}\frac{du_l}{dz}. \tag{45}$$

We account for initial gradients in the liquid composition by including in the model the liquid phase species mass balances, assuming absence of species diffusion in the liquid:

$$\frac{\partial c_{i,l}}{\partial t} = -\frac{u_l}{\varepsilon S}\frac{\partial c_{i,l}}{\partial z}, \text{ for } i = 1, \ldots, N_L. \tag{46}$$

The boundary conditions are

$$\begin{cases} S(t, z = 0) = 0, & \forall t > 0, \\ \frac{\partial c_{i,l}(t,z=0)}{\partial z} = 0, & \forall t > 0. \end{cases} \tag{47}$$

The model of Eqs. (39)–(46) presents $1 + N_L$ partial differential equations (PDEs), which we semi-discretize with a high-resolution finite volume approach [33] along the z dimension.

2.4 Thermal Drying Modeling

A one-dimensional dynamic model is developed for dead-end convective cake drying, based on the following equations. The local drying rate $\dot{m}_i^{L \to G}$ [kg/(m^3 s)] for the $N_{L, vol}$ volatile species still present in the liquid phase is [34]

$$\dot{m}_i^{L \to G} = h_{M,i} a \left(P_{i,sat} - P_{i,g}\right) \eta_i, \text{ for } i = 1, \ldots, N_{L,vol}, \tag{48}$$

where $h_{M,i}$ is the mass transfer coefficient, calculated with correlations or from experimental data; a is the cake specific surface, either computed as $a = 6/d_p$ (where d_p is the Sauter diameter from the CSD) or measured; and for species i, $P_{i,sat}$ is the saturation pressure (from the Antoine equation), $P_{i,g}$ is the partial pressure, and η_i is a factor accounting for mass transfer limitations occurring, mostly due to capillarity, when the mass fraction of i in the cake ($w_{i,cake}$) becomes lower than a critical value $w_{i,cake}^{crit}$ (falling rate period). η_i is instead equal to one when $w_{i,cake}$ is greater than $w_{i,cake}^{crit}$ (constant rate period). In the falling rate period, η_i is typically linearly or quadratically dependent on $w_{i,cake}$, and it should be estimated with experiments. More than one falling rate period (and the corresponding critical solvent content) can be identified for certain systems. The species mass balance with respect to the concentration of i in the cake $c_{i,cake}$ is

$$\frac{\partial c_{i,cake}}{\partial t} = -\dot{m}_i^{L \to G}, \text{ for } i = 1, \dots, N_{L,vol}. \tag{49}$$

Equation (49) is not solved for non-volatile species, as their concentration in the cake does not vary during drying. In addition, in the equation, both $c_{i,cake}$ and $\dot{m}_i^{L \to G}$ are functions of time and z. The local cake saturation is related to the species concentrations in the cake with

$$S = \frac{\sum_{i=1}^{N_L} c_{i,cake}/\rho_{i,l}}{\varepsilon}, \text{ for } i = 1, \dots, N_L, \tag{50}$$

where $\rho_{i,l}$ is the liquid density of pure i. The species mass balances in the gas phase for the volatile solvents and impurities read, in terms of mass fraction $w_{i,g}$,

$$\rho_g \varepsilon (1-S) \frac{\partial w_{i,g}}{\partial t} = -\rho_g u_g \frac{\partial w_{i,g}}{\partial z} + \dot{m}_i^{L \to G} - w_{i,g} \sum_{i=1}^{N_L} \dot{m}_i^{L \to G}, \text{ for } i = 1, \dots, N_{L,vol}, \tag{51}$$

where ρ_g is the density of the gas and u_g is the gas velocity, calculated with the Darcy law for mono-phase gas flow in a porous medium [30].

Inter-phase energy transfer is very fast for the process, as found from experiments on the carousel and literature correlations [35]. Hence, we assume local thermal equilibrium among phases for the development of the differential energy balance:

$$\left(\rho_s c_{p,s} (1-\varepsilon) + \rho_l c_{p,l} \varepsilon S + \rho_g c_{p,g} \varepsilon (1-S)\right) \frac{\partial T}{\partial t} = -\sum_i \left(\dot{m}_i^{L \to G} \lambda_i\right) - u_g c_{p,g} \rho_g \frac{\partial T}{\partial z} + \dot{Q}, \tag{52}$$

where ρ_l is the liquid phase density, $c_{p,g}$ is the gas phase specific heat, $c_{p,l}$ is the liquid phase specific heat, $c_{p,s}$ is the solid phase specific heat, T is the local temperature, λ_i is the latent heat of vaporization of species i, and $\dot{Q}$ is the heat exchange with the environment, namely, the heat loss through the dryer walls (assumed equal to zero for the purposes of this study). The boundary conditions are given by the drying gas inlet composition and the drying gas inlet temperature T_{drying}, both inputs of the model. The drying model of Eqs. (48)–(52) presents $1 + N_{L, vol}$ PDEs, which we semi-discretize along z dimension with a first-order upwind scheme for a resulting system of ODEs.

3 Case Studies

3.1 Case Study 1: Synthesis-Crystallization

In the first case study, paracetamol will be synthesized and purified using a two-unit manufacturing process. The final reaction step of paracetamol synthesis [36] is modeled in a PFR using Eq. (3) described in Sect. 2.1. Crystallization is then utilized as a recovery mechanism for the synthesized paracetamol. To emphasize integrated analysis, this case study analyzes optimal operation of both units in tandem. Also, we analyze an end-to-end continuous operation, PFR followed by a MSMPR crystallizer, and how it compares to a hybrid manufacturing alternative, PFR followed by a batch crystallizer. The MSMPR is modeled using Eqs. (8)–(19), and batch crystallizer is modeled under the considerations described in Sect. 2.2. In the case of the batch crystallizer, a linear cooling profile is used. All simulations in case study 1 were modeled and simulated in Python utilizing PharmaPy, an open-source framework for pharmaceutical process development [13]. Automated analysis on the proposed process alternatives was performed by coupling PharmaPy with other open-source Python tools.

Synthesis Step Parameter Estimation

Parameter estimation is performed for a reaction where p-aminophenol (A) reacts with acetic anhydride (B) to produce paracetamol (C) and acetic acid (D), in water as a solvent. The reaction is described with elementary kinetics taking place in a batch reactor (Eq. 53):

$$\frac{dC_j}{dt} = v_j \cdot r, \ j = A, B, C, D,$$
$$r = kC_A^{\alpha_A} C_B^{\alpha_B}, \tag{53}$$
$$k = A \cdot \exp\left(-\frac{E_a}{RT}\right).$$

In order to improve conditioning of the Jacobian passed to the optimization algorithm, parameters of the temperature-dependent term k in Eq. (53) were reformulated as [37, 38]

Table 2 Parameter constraints

	Original parameters		Reparametrization		
Parameter	Lower bound	Upper bound	Lower bound	Upper bound	Seed
A (L mol^{-1} s^{-1})	0	10	-25.724	0.318	0.5
E_a (J mol^{-1})	5000	30,000	6.399	8.191	10,000
α_1	0.5	2	–	–	1
α_2	0.5	2	–	–	1

$$k = \exp\left(\varphi_1 + \varphi_2\left(\frac{1}{T_{ref}} - \frac{1}{T}\right)\right),$$
$$\varphi_1 = \ln(A) - \frac{E_a}{T_{ref}}, \tag{54}$$
$$\varphi_2 = \ln\left(\frac{E_a}{R}\right).$$

Experimental data for parameter estimation were taken from Lee, Lin, and Lee [23]. The reported time variation in temperature was modeled through a logistic function (Eq. 55):

$$T(t) = \frac{T_\infty}{1 + e^{-k(t-t_0)}}, \tag{55}$$

with $k = 0.007$ s^{-1}, $T_\infty = 353.15$ K, and $t_0 = -241$ s. The specified temperature trajectory was entered to PharmaPy via a control function.

Precise gradient information for parameter estimation was provided via dynamic parametric sensitivity [39, 40]. State-dependent sensitivities are represented as

$$\frac{\partial r}{\partial C_j} = k\alpha_j \frac{C_A^{\alpha_A} C_B^{\alpha_B}}{C_j}, \quad j = A, B, \tag{56}$$

and parametric sensitivities are given by

$$\frac{\partial r}{\partial \varphi_1} = r,$$
$$\frac{\partial r}{\partial \varphi_2} = r\left(\frac{1}{T_{ref}} - \frac{1}{T}\right)\exp(\varphi_2), \tag{57}$$
$$\frac{\partial r}{\partial \alpha_j} = \ln\left(C_j\right) r, \quad j = A, B.$$

Given the limited amount of reaction data, constrained optimization through IPOPT [41] was used, allowing bounded kinetic parameter values. Numerical values of the parameter limits and initial estimates are shown in Table 2.

Results from the fitting are shown in Fig. 1, where the dynamic concentration data is correctly described by the reactor model using the converged parameter estimates. Numerical parameter estimates and asymptotic confidence intervals obtained by constrained optimization were $\varphi_1 = -5.121 \pm 5.785$, $\varphi_2 = 6.828 \pm 26.102$, $\alpha_1 = 1.713 \pm 3.452$, and $\alpha_2 = 2.0 \pm 14.478$, which translate into nominal

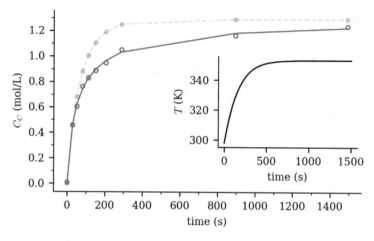

Fig. 1 Parameter estimation results on experimental paracetamol concentration. *Dashed lines*: model prediction with seed parameters, *continuous line*: model prediction with converged parameters, *circles*: experimental results. *Inset*: modeled temperature trajectory

parameter values of $k = 0.126$ L mol^{-1} s^{-1}, $E_a = 7676.1$ J mol^{-1}, $\alpha_1 = 1.71$, and $\alpha_2 = 2.0$. Given the small amount of data available and the relatively small confidence in the nominal parameters, more experiments should be performed on varying reaction conditions (temperature, reactant/product concentration) to better understand the underlying reaction mechanism and to estimate parameters with greater confidence. Nevertheless, the capabilities of the software PharmaPy to perform constrained parameter estimation and to support control variables are clearly exemplified through the proposed case study, which are valuable tools for the analysis of reaction or crystallization data.

Synthesis-Crystallization, Simulation

Once reaction kinetics parameters were estimated, a flowsheet model representation of each of the two processes was constructed in PharmaPy. Design and operating conditions for the PFR and batch crystallizer are described in Fig. 2. The MSMPR crystallizer was constantly cooled with an external source of cooling water at a specified temperature. The MSMPR crystallizer is initially loaded with pure solvent, and its volume is considered constant. For the hybrid process, the material resulting from operating R01 continuously is collected in HOLD01 and then transferred to CR01 to perform cooling crystallization. HOLD01 is initialized as an empty tank for both operation modes.

Results for the continuous reactor R01 are shown in Fig. 3. It can be seen how different time scales must be resolved for this distributed system, as the transient period of concentration spans about half an hour, whereas temperature dynamics progresses within the first minute. It is also noteworthy how temperature evolves

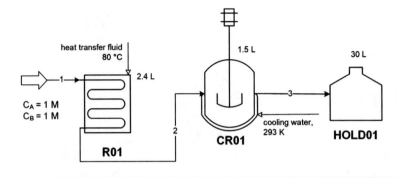

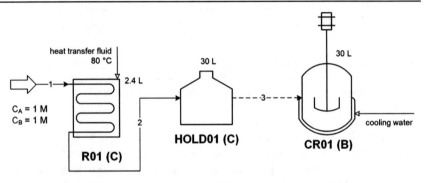

Fig. 2 Top: continuous process. Bottom: hybrid process. *Continuous lines*: material flow, *dashed line*: material transfer after the operation is completed. (*C*): continuous unit, (*B*): batch unit

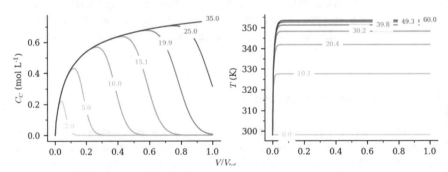

Fig. 3 Transient behavior of R01 for API concentration (left) and liquid temperature (right). Time tags for concentration are in minutes, whereas those of temperature are in seconds

as a flat profile with respect to volume. This is caused by the relatively high heat transfer component in the energy balance compared to the flow and reaction terms in Eq. (3). Moreover, steady-state paracetamol concentration at the outlet of R01 is 0.75 mol L^{-1}, which represents a 75% conversion of A.

The behavior of CR01 and HOLD01 is shown in Fig. 4. Relatively fast nucleation and growth kinetics made it necessary to use a nonuniform, geometric crystal size

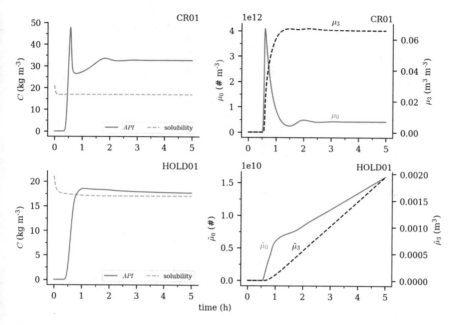

Fig. 4 Dynamic behavior of the CR01-HOLD01 pair

grid to better capture the change in CSD, especially at low particle sizes. This avoids numerical error to propagate in the calculation of the CSD moments, which compounds with increasing moment order. Regarding dynamic behavior for CR01, a strong growth inhibition by the presence of acetic acid and acetic anhydride is reflected in the considerably high remaining supersaturation at steady state, top right of Fig. 4. Low growth kinetics are also responsible for the high concentration peak after the system reaches the solubility curve for CR01, which causes a large amount of fines to be produced at high supersaturation (large number of particles at the onset of crystallization, top right plot in Fig. 4) for the start-up of the unit operation.

In general, slower dynamics are observed for HOLD01, bottom plots in Fig. 4. Firstly, concentration reaches the solubility curve a little later than the observed concentration in CR01, given that this tank starts receiving liquid without any API at the start-up of the process. This first material accumulated in HOLD01, composed only by solvent, acts as a buffer that dilutes the incoming stream, causing the concentration dynamics to slow down. It also results in slower API crystal volume production, observed when comparing the third moment profiles, right plots in Fig. 4. The interaction of units involving solids in the continuous flowsheet is comparatively shown in Fig. 5 for their corresponding kinetics. Both nucleation and liquid-solid mass transfer get delayed in HOLD01 compared to CR01. An interesting first period of negative mass transfer is observed in the right plot of Fig. 5 (*dotted line*), which results from the incoming slurry and present liquid in HOLD01 having total API concentration below the solubility curve, triggering dissolution

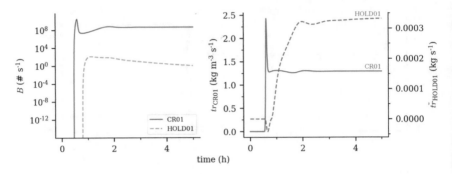

Fig. 5 Kinetics of the CR01-HOLD01 pair

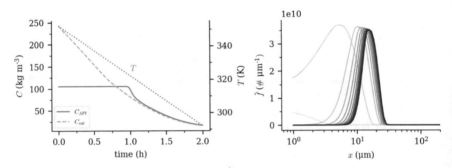

Fig. 6 Left: Concentration-temperature evolution in CR01 for batch operation. Right: CSD within the period 0.7–2 h, for 0.1 h increments

kinetics (Eq. 19). At the end of 5 hours of continuous operation, a total of 2.46 kg of paracetamol crystals are present in HOLD01 with mean crystal size $\mu_1/\mu_0 = 30$ μm.

Crystallization results for the hybrid process are shown in Fig. 6. The linear cooling profile employed for this operation mode reaches 293.15 K (-30 K h^{-1} cooling rate), or the same temperature used for the cooling water in CR01 of the continuous process. A relatively rapid depletion in supersaturation is observed in Fig. 6 (left plot), caused by fast paracetamol concentration drop due to the linear cooling profile. CSD smoothly changes to reach a final mean particle size of 17 μm, as observed at the right-hand side of Fig. 6. After hybrid operation, a total of 2.73 kg of crystals are recovered from the slurry in CR01.

Synthesis-Crystallization, Integrated Design and Analysis

In order to optimize performance and compare the two process candidates, the following procedure was employed. First, each flowsheet was optimized using a gradient-free, evolutionary-type approach implemented in the open-source Never-

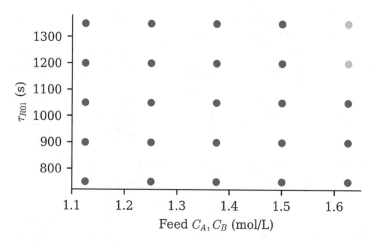

Fig. 7 Process constraint visualization for supersaturation limit within the PFR as a design space. *Green points*: >20% below supersaturation limit, *orange points*: <20% below supersaturation limit

grad package for Python [42]. Next, a uniform grid in the critical process parameters was generated around the optimal point to perform a search to qualitatively analyze the solution quality. Each uniform grid point represents a unique operating or design condition and was simulated in PharmaPy. Particularly, the trade-off between mass production rate and mean particle size of the purified paracetamol was weighed to attain a reasonable operating point for comparison of both process alternatives. To achieve this goal, the following objective was supplied to the gradient-free algorithm:

$$\max_{\tau_{PFR}, \tau_{CR}, C_{feed}, T_{CR}} m_{PCM} + \alpha d_{avg} \tag{58}$$

where m_{PCM} is the mass production rate of paracetamol in kg/h, d_{avg} is the mean particle size of the crystallized paracetamol, and α is a multi-objective weight of 0.01 for this study. The manipulated process parameters are the PFR residence time, τ_{PFR}; crystallizer residence time (MSMPR) or cycle time (batch crystallization), τ_{CR}; initial feed concentration to the PFR of species A in which B is fed in 10% excess, C_{feed}; and the temperature of the cooling medium (MSMPR) or the final temperature (batch crystallization), T_{CR}. A penalty for exceeding the supersaturation limit for paracetamol in the PFR was considered; however, it was not active for this set of explored operating conditions, as shown in Fig. 7.

The base process models from Sect. 3.1.2 were generalized as to be called by a gradient-free optimization method within Python. Nevergrad was then called on the PharmaPy model to perform a gradient-free simulation-optimization of both the continuous and hybrid flowsheets. A small budget of 50 nodes was given during the optimization, since the parameter sweep with the uniform grid of critical process parameters will capture local behavior surrounding the gradient-

Table 3 Bounds for critical process parameters during gradient-free optimization and optimal point with a budget of 50 nodes for both processes

	PFR-MSMPR		PFR-batch	
Parameter	Bounds	Optimum	Bounds	Optimum
τ_{PFR} (min)	(15, 45)	15	(15, 45)	15
τ_{CR} (min)	(12.5, 45)	41.3	(60, 300)	300
C_{feed} (mol/L)	(0.5, 1.5)	1.5	(0.5, 1.5)	1.5
T_{CR} (K)	(283, 313)	283	(283, 313)	283

Table 4 Bounds and optimal point for parameter sweep approach using a uniform grid

	PFR-MSMPR		PFR-batch	
Parameter	Bounds	Optimum	Bounds	Optimum
τ_{PFR} (min)	(12.5, 22.5)	12.5	(12.5, 22.5)	12.5
τ_{CR} (min)	(33.3, 50)	50	(60, 300)	300
C_{feed} (mol/L)	(1.125, 1.625)	1.625	(1.125, 1.625)	1.625
T_{CR} (K)	(273, 313)	283	(273, 313)	293

free optimal operating condition. The results summarized and shown in Table 3 for the PFR-MSMPR system were {15 min, 41.3 min, 1.5 mol/L, 283 K}, and for the PFR-batch system, the results were {15 min, 5 h, 1.5 mol/L, 283 K} for {τ_{PFR}, τ_{CR}, C_{feed}, T_{CR}}.

Following optimization, a uniform grid on the critical parameter space was generated with values within the ranges included in Table 4. The utilized grid has five equally spaced points including the endpoints of each critical process parameter, or a total of 625 points simulated for each of the two analyzed processes. Following simulation, results on mass production and mean particle size were compiled for both flowsheets, as seen in Fig. 8. A qualitative discussion may result from this figure, as it is seen that operating below 283 K represents diminishing returns, possibly due to limitations in the modeled solubility polynomial. Overall, running at higher residence times produces larger particles for the MSMPR in the top left subfigure of Fig. 8. The batch crystallization yields a smaller average crystal size at higher run times, with only 35 μm compared to 55 μm with the MSMPR. Overall solid paracetamol production rate has similar maxima for both process alternatives; however, the startup procedure to generate a consistent particle size distribution in the end-to-end continuous process alternative requires nearly 12 h of operation to achieve steady state in the MSMPR, whereas less than 1 h is required to achieve steady state in the PFR. Due to this factor, if particle sizes of less than 30 μm are acceptable, the hybrid operating procedure will immediately produce more paracetamol. However, with the given objective function, the end-to-end continuous operation provides a slightly higher maximum value.

The optimum operating point, with respect to the objective value, Eq. (58), for both process alternatives using the parameter sweep approach is shown in Table 4 for completeness.

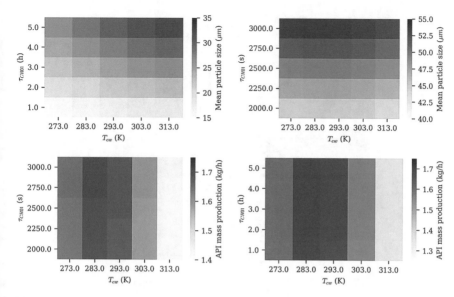

Fig. 8 Heatmaps of objective contributions for MSMPR, left, and batch crystallization, right, describing mean particle size, top, and mass production rate of the API, paracetamol, bottom

3.2 Case Study 2: Carousel Case Study

In this section, we present a workflow for the digital design of integrated filtration-drying. The unit operation that we consider is a novel intensified carousel (Fig. 9), representing a breakthrough technology in continuous filtration-drying [43, 44]. The main cylindrical body of the carousel contains multiple ports, each aligned to a certain processing station, where a processing step is carried out batchwise. For every fixed cycle duration, the main body of the carousel rotates, moving each port to the following station and enabling continuous operation. All the stations present a filter mesh at the bottom, except for the last one, open for cake discharge. The pressure drop acting as driving force for the process is either supplied by a vacuum pump or by connecting the top part of the ports to an overpressure source. In the first station, the slurry from the crystallizer is loaded and filtered, leading to cake formation. In the second station, cake washing is carried out, followed by a cake deliquoring step that continues into the third station. From the fourth station onward and prior to cake discharge, the cake is dried through a hot air flow. This drying stage further decreases the cake saturation level below the deliquoring equilibrium. The actual number of drying ports before the cake discharge varies from carousel to carousel, and it can be designed based on the needs of the process of interest.

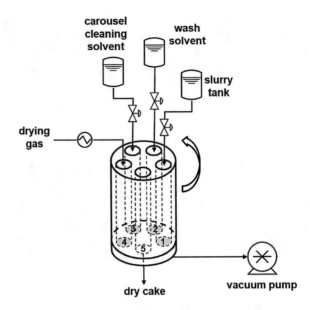

Fig. 9 Schematic diagram of the five-stations prototype carousel installed at Purdue University. Filter meshes are installed at the bottom of stations 1–4 and are connected to the vacuum pump. Station 1: slurry loading and filtration. Station 2: cake washing and deliquoring. Station 3: deliquoring. Station 4: thermal drying. Station 5: cake discharge. Production scale carousels present additional drying stations to reduce the cycle duration and increase the throughput. A cleaning-in-place procedure is automatically triggered when significant mesh fouling is detected, allowing the cleaning solvent stored above station 3 into the carousel

Carousel Design Space Optimization

In this case study, we develop a mathematical model of the carousel, and we exploit it for different purposes. The considered sample process consists of the separation of paracetamol crystals from a slurry whose liquid phase is composed at 95% by isopropyl alcohol (mother liquor) and at 5% by a non-volatile impurity, with cake washing carried out through pure ethanol. First, we calculate the probabilistic DS of the process, referring to a prototype carousel installed in the Crystallization Systems Engineering laboratory at Purdue University. The carousel has five stations (only one for drying), each of 10 mL capacity. After DS identification, we use the model for optimizing the operating conditions, to maximize the carousel throughput. Then, we consider the general design problem for which a carousel is not already available, and the number of stations has to be selected. Finally, we present a strategy for active control of the critical quality attributes (CQAs), and we demonstrate how the mathematical model can be used for testing the closed-loop response to disturbances. The control system is based on a hierarchical three-level approach recently proposed within the quality-by-control framework [2].

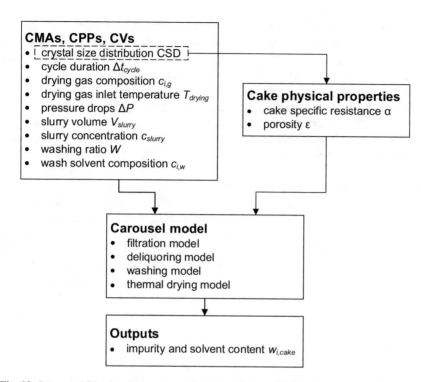

Fig. 10 Integrated filtration-drying carousel mathematical model: input/output structure

The developed mathematical model of the carousel presents the input/output structure reported in Fig. 10. Given a set of inputs (critical material attributes (CMAs), critical process parameters (CPPs) and control variables (CVs)), the model provides as outputs the solvent and impurities contents in the discharged cake (CQAs). A cake physical properties module is also implemented within the carousel model to (approximately) predict the cake porosity and specific resistance from the slurry CSD, if their experimental measurements are not available. The core of the carousel simulator is obtained by combining together the stand-alone models of the four processes occurring in the carousel: (a) slurry filtration, (b) cake deliquoring, (c) cake washing, and (d) thermal drying. The models are implemented in the MATLAB/Simulink environment as functions, called by an external wrapper to mimic the operation sequence of a physical carousel. The deliquoring and drying models are coded in C and interfaced with MATLAB through C-MEX functions to reduce the computational burden. The simulator is flexible and robust: it can simulate carousels with different number of drying stations, and it accounts for limiting cases in which filtration and/or washing last for more than one cycle duration due to poor cake filterability or unfavorable operating conditions. The model was calibrated to the sample process involving paracetamol isolation through experimental activities reported elsewhere [43].

The DS is determined with a probabilistic approach [5], accounting for modeling uncertainty by assigning a probability distribution to selected model parameters. First, we build a grid of CPPs (cycle duration Δt_{cycle} and amount of loaded slurry per cycle V_{slurry}) and CMAs (crystal concentration in the slurry c_{slurry}), uniformly sampling the points among reference operation boundaries. For every point of the grid, we calculate the probability of meeting the target CQAs through Monte Carlo simulations (400 realizations). For each realization, the uncertain parameters are sampled from their probability distributions, and the CQAs of the discharged cake are calculated with the carousel model. The percentage of realizations satisfying the CQA requirements (residual solvents and impurity content in the discharged cake below 0.5%) in a grid point corresponds to the probability of meeting the quality target for the corresponding combination of CPPs and CMAs. The uncertain parameters are the mass transfer coefficient, the filter mesh resistance, the specific cake resistance, and the cake porosity. They are all considered normally distributed, with mean value coming from model calibration and standard deviation set to 5% of the mean. The only exception is the filter mesh resistance, for which we adopt a uniform distribution to reproduce the increase of fouling occurring during carousel operation (filter meshes undergo a cleaning-in-place procedure only after a certain fouling threshold is reached). We introduce two additional normally distributed parameters: additive process noise coefficients for c_{slurry} and V_{slurry}, to simulate the small fluctuations around their set points occurring from cycle to cycle. Overall, the selected uncertain parameters aim at accounting on the calculated probability for the effect of the model error and of the unmodelled disturbances (e.g., small changes in the CSD of the fed slurry) that can occur during carousel processing.

The calculated probabilities in the CPPs and CMAs grid are reported in Fig. 11. After having set the minimum acceptable probability to 90%, we obtain the following expression for the DS through multiple linear regression on the calculated probabilities:

$$DS = \left\{ \left(V_{slurry}, \ \Delta t_{cycle}, c_{slurry} \right) | \Delta t_{cycle} \ \geq \ a_1 \ V_{slurry} + a_2 \ c_{slurry} + \ a_3 c_{slurry} \ V_{slurry} + a_4 \right\}$$
(59)

where 1 mL $< V_{slurry} <$ 10 mL and 50 kg/m^3 $< c_{slurry} <$ 200 kg/m^3 (boundaries of the calibration domain) and with $a_1 = -2.78E6$ s/m^3, $a_2 = -1.05E-1$ s m^3/kg, $a_3 = 3.06E5$ s/kg, and $a_4 = 5.14E1$ s. The surface at the boundary of the region described by Eq. (59) effectively delimits the DS (Fig. 11) in all the domain. As a note, the linearity of the DS boundary for fixed c_{slurry} in Eq. (59) is due to the low specific resistance of the cakes obtained from the paracetamol crystal mixture used for model calibration. For the general case, linear and bilinear terms, as seen with V_{slurry} and c_{slurry} in Eq. (59), may be insufficient to produce a reasonable fit of the DS. Thus, the use of higher-order terms may be desired to accurately fit the DS boundary.

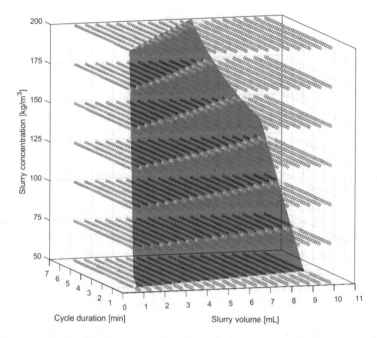

Fig. 11 Integrated filtration-drying carousel case study: probabilistic DS, representing the probability of meeting the target CQAs for a given combination of CPPs and CMAs. Green triangles: probability ≥90%, *yellow circles*: 80% ≤ probability <90%, *orange squares*: 60% ≤ probability <80% and red diamonds: probability <60%. The dark surface represents the DS boundary calculated with Eq. (59)

The maximum throughput T_{max} within the DS, namely, the maximum amount of paracetamol crystals with acceptable quality that can be isolated with the carousel per unit of time, is given by the following optimization problem:

$$T_{max} = \max_{V_{slurry}, \Delta t_{cycle}, c_{slurry}} T, \qquad (60)$$

subject to

$$T = \frac{c_{slurry} \ V_{slurry}}{\Delta t_{cycle}},$$

$$\Delta t_{cycle} \geq a_1 \ V_{slurry} + a_2 \ c_{slurry} + a_3 c_{slurry} \ V_{slurry} + a_4, \qquad (61)$$

$$50 \ \text{kg/m}^3 < c_{slurry} < 200 \ \text{kg/m}^3,$$

$$1 \ \text{mL} < V_{slurry} < 10 \ \text{mL},$$

where T is the throughput processed in the carousel. Since the optimum of Eqs. (60)–(61) lies on the DS boundary, the problem can be re-expressed by eliminsinating the explicit dependence of T_{max} on Δt_{cycle}:

$$T_{max} = \max_{V_{slurry}, \Delta t_{cycle}, c_{slurry}} T, \tag{62}$$

subject to

$$T = \frac{c_{slurry}\ V_{slurry}}{a_1\ V_{slurry} + a_2\ c_{slurry} + a_3 c_{slurry}\ V_{slurry} + a_4},$$

$$50\ kg/m^3 < c_{slurry} < 200\ kg/m^3, \tag{63}$$

$$1\ mL < V_{slurry} < 10\ mL.$$

The gradients of the objective function T with respect to c_{slurry} and V_{slurry} are always positive under the constraint domain. Hence, T_{max} is achieved at the boundary point defined by $c_{slurry} = 200$ kg/m^3 and $V_{slurry} = 10$ mL, where $T = T_{max} = 195$ mg of crystals per minute. The obtained analytical solution of Eqs. (62)–(63) is confirmed by the plots of the throughput at the DS boundary (Fig. 12). In other case studies of integrated filtration-drying with the carousel, T_{max} was achieved in between the grid bounds, rather than at the bounds themselves [45], possibly due to higher nonlinearity of the DS boundary. Looking at Fig. 12, a stationary point of maximum would eventually be reached if the maximum port capacity were larger than 10 mL. As a final remark, it is recommended to conduct the process inside the DS and close to the conditions of T_{max}, rather than on the optimal point itself (located on the DS boundary). This choice reflects the greater importance that product quality compliance has with respect to economic optimality in pharmaceutical manufacturing.

In the general case in which a new carousel has to be designed for a process, the simulator can be used for sensitivity analyses on the variations of the CQAs and of T_{max} with the design variables, such as the station diameter, the maximum port capacity, and the number of stations. In the simulation activity, model uncertainty can be computed with the aforementioned Monte Carlo approach or neglected, in first approximation. Considering again the paracetamol isolation process, we repeat the probabilistic DS calculation varying the number of drying ports (Fig. 13). For the sake of simplicity, the other design variables are considered to be the same as in the carousel prototype, and c_{slurry} is fixed to 125 kg/m^3. The DS surface considerably widens passing from one to two drying stations, and an additional (smaller) gain is obtained, adding a third drying station. The fourth and the fifth drying stations do not allow increasing the DS area much more, as filtration becomes the limiting step (filtration duration against V_{slurry} is reported as *solid line* in Fig. 13). Also on the maximum throughput side, the fourth and fifth drying stations allow a smaller improvement: T_{max} is 189 mg/min with one drying station, 349 mg/min with two, 517 mg/min with three, 652 mg/min with four, and 790 mg/min with five. However, the actual selection of the number of drying stations depends on the throughput requirements of the overall manufacturing line.

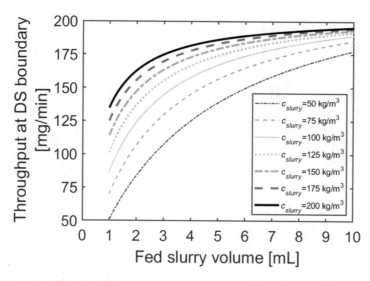

Fig. 12 Integrated filtration-drying carousel case study: throughput T at the design space boundary (Eq. 59) for varying V_{slurry} and c_{slurry}

Carousel Active Control Strategy

Controlling carousel operation is an intrinsically challenging task, given the intensified nature of the unit. An approach to control system design recently proposed within the QbC initiative [2] includes three hierarchical levels, following the ISA-95 Enterprise-Control System Integration Standard. Level 0 consists of simple PID control and of the built-in control system of the units (sensors, controllers, and PLCs). Level 1 is made up of advanced PID control loops, while Level 2 relies on model-based control. The developed carousel model is a useful tool for the development of all the levels of the control system, as it can be used (a) for model-based control at Level 2 and (b) as digital twin of the physical unit for quickly and safely testing different control strategies, either model-free (Levels 0–1) or model based (Level 2). In the rest of this section, after having described the carousel Level 0 control system, we demonstrate the effectiveness of a Level 1 control strategy for disturbance rejection through simulations with the carousel model. Thorough discussion of Level 2 implementation will be covered in the future work.

The built-in control system of the carousel and of the accessory equipment is sketched in Fig. 14, inside the Level 0 box. All Level 0 controllers (except for pressure controllers) are contained in the carousel PLC. Each carousel station is represented as an independent tank (V104–108), instead of being included in the main carousel body, for the sake of clarity. The transfer of material upon carousel rotation is given by the streams among tanks V104–108 (controller FC102 opens the stream valves at each cycle switch). V109 is, instead, the wash solvent tank. The carousel cleaning solvent vessel is not reported for conciseness. V101 is the

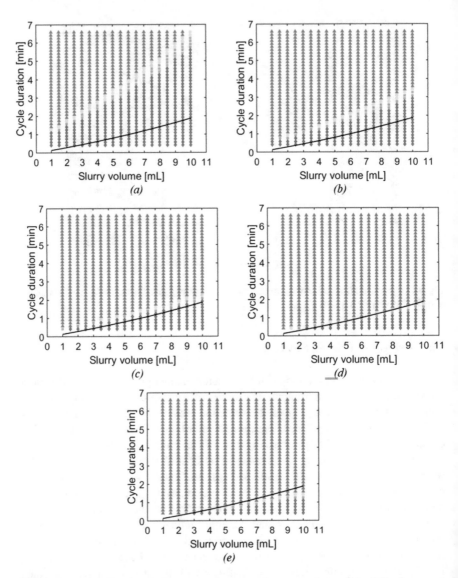

Fig. 13 Integrated filtration-drying carousel case study: comparison of the DS of carousel configurations with different number of drying stations: (**a**) one station, (**b**) two stations, (**c**) three stations, (**d**) four stations, and (**e**) five stations. The *solid line* represents the filtration duration. The marker's legend is as in Fig. 11, and c_{slurry} is 125 kg/m^3

upstream crystallizer, from which the slurry is moved into an intermediate storage tank (V102) with a peristaltic pump (P101). At the beginning of every cycle, the set V_{slurry} (controlled by FC101) is drawn into the charge cell V103 through the action of vacuum pump P102. P102 is connected to V103 only during this charging

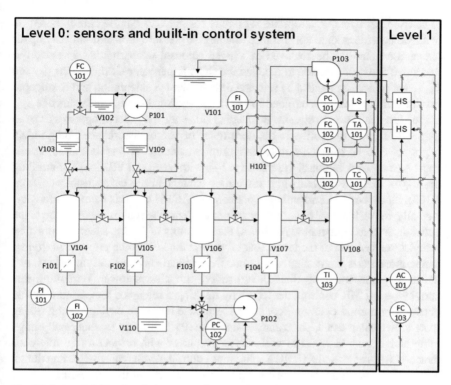

Fig. 14 Integrated filtration-drying carousel case study: P&ID with Level 0 (built-in control) and Level 1 (advanced PID) control systems

phase, through a three-way valve. During the rest of the cycle, P102 is connected to the filtrate receiver V110 and, hence, to the bottom of V104–107, providing the driving force for liquid and gas displacement. The fan P103 can be used for increasing the pressure drops in each station, or the top portion of V104–107 can be directly connected to the atmosphere (i.e., eliminating F103 from the P&ID). PC101 and PC102 are, respectively, the built-in pressure controllers of P103 and P102. TC101 manipulates the heater (H101) jacket temperature to control the temperature of the drying air entering V107. TA101 and the connected low selector take care of preventing the jacket temperature to go beyond 150 °C for safety reasons. Additional sensors are available for monitoring and control applications. PI101 measures the pressure at the bottom of the carousel stations, FI101 measures the air flow rate entering the carousel, FI102 (a scale installed below V110) measures the flow rate of filtrate entering V110, and TI101–103 are, respectively, the thermocouples for jacket temperature, gas temperature at the dryer inlet, and gas temperature at the dryer outlet.

Operating the carousel requires fixing the set points of the Level 0 controllers, namely, of the CPPs Δt_{cycle} and V_{slurry} and of multiple CVs: the pressure drop in the ports, the inlet temperature of the drying air, and the amount of wash solvent to be used per cycle. Appropriate set points for the CVs can be chosen based on heuristic considerations. For instance, the largest pressure drop and inlet drying air temperature that can be achieved in a given carousel setup should be selected to maximize their contribution to meeting the CQA target values. Suitable Δt_{cycle} and V_{slurry} set points can instead be selected through the DS calculation and throughput maximization procedures outlined earlier in this section, based on the value of c_{slurry} in the slurry fed from upstream. Proceeding this way, the process operates as open loop with respect to quality. In the occurrence of severe disturbances, the product might have to be rejected due to compromised quality. To tackle this issue, we conceived a Level 1 control system (Fig. 14), with advanced PID loops controlling the CQAs (i.e., the solvents and impurities content in the cake discharged from V108). Since the CQAs are not measured online, AC101 controls them by inference. Actually, the residual solvents and impurities content in the cake are correlated to the outlet drying gas temperature profile. At the beginning of drying, a temperature drop is registered because of the latent heat of vaporization. With the progress of drying, temperature starts increasing back, since the residual solvents and impurities, and the energy consumed by their volatilization, are always lower. Exploiting this correlation, AC101 controls the CQAs by tracking a reference temperature profile obtained in normal operating conditions. Suppose that cake drying is progressing more slowly than usual, for example, due to F104 fouling or to abnormally large initial solvent content. TI103 will measure an error with respect to the reference temperature profile, and AC101, a split range controller, will react, increasing the set points of one or more of the following: the pressure drop in the processing stations (PC101), the drying gas inlet temperature (TC101), and/or Δt_{cycle} (FC102). At first, only the pressure drop set point will be increased. If this is not enough to compensate for the disturbance, AC101 will then increase the drying gas inlet temperature set point. The set point of Δt_{cycle} will be increased only as last resource, as a higher cycle duration causes a reduction of the process throughput. On the other hand, if drying is progressing faster than in the reference conditions, AC101 will react in the opposite direction, eventually reducing Δt_{cycle} and increasing the throughput. Control of the CQAs is also achieved at Level 1 through the action of flow rate controller FC103. FC103, another split-range controller, controls the filtrate flow rate by increasing/decreasing the set points of the pressure drop and/or of Δt_{cycle}, with the same heuristics adopted for AC101 to maximize the throughput. FC103 compensates for disturbances increasing the filtration duration, such as fouling of F101–104, or cake resistance increase. Since both AC101 and FC103 act on the pressure drop and Δt_{cycle} set points, two high selectors are included in the Level 1 control system (Fig. 14).

Figure 15 shows the response of Level 1 control system to a fouling disturbance (complete process conditions are not reported for conciseness). Shortly after the process onset, the filter mesh resistance starts increasing with a linear ramp, until the cleaning-in-place procedure is triggered, restoring the initial fouling conditions (150 min after the beginning of the process). As detailed above, filter mesh resistance was considered an uncertain parameter with uniform distribution for the purposes of DS calculation, accounting for the increase of mesh fouling during

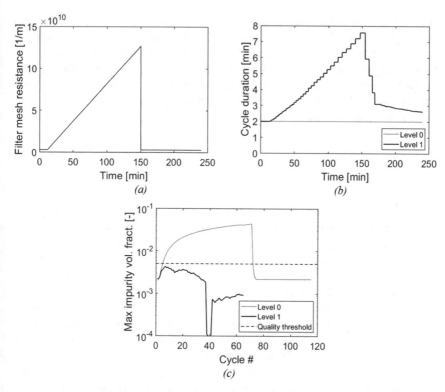

Fig. 15 Integrated filtration-drying carousel case study: control system response to (**a**) a fouling disturbance, including (**b**) Δt_{cycle} (manipulated variable) and (**c**) the CQA (controlled-by-inference variable). Both Level 0 (built-in control, open loop) and Level 1 (advanced PID control, closed-loop) responses are reported

operation. As a result, the values of Δt_{cycle} in the DS for given V_{slurry} and c_{slurry} conditions are conservative by considering many fouling conditions, among those the highest fouling conditions before cleaning is triggered. When the filter meshes are clean, smaller Δt_{cycle} values could be used, increasing the throughput. In Fig. 15, a Δt_{cycle} of 2 min meets the desired quality target with the clean meshes. However, with a Level 0 control system (open loop), the cakes produced in Cycles 7–71 have to be rejected, as they do not meet the desired quality (Fig. 15c). The quality target is eventually reached again, from Cycle 72 onward, only after the meshes are cleaned. Instead, Level 1 controllers react very fast to the abnormal CQAs, at first by increasing the pressure drop and the inlet drying air temperature. A few minutes after the disturbance onset, the set points of the pressure drop and of the drying air inlet temperature saturate, and Level 1 controllers start increasing Δt_{cycle} (Fig. 15b). Due to the increased Δt_{cycle}, with Level 1 control, only 65 cycles are completed in the same amount of time in which Level 0 control completes 115 cycles (Fig. 15b). However, with Level 1 control, the CQAs always adhere to the quality threshold. Upon filter mesh cleaning, Level 1 controllers automatically start decreasing Δt_{cycle}

(Fig. 15b), effectively increasing the throughput again. This example shows that the proposed Level 1 control system is capable of rejecting disturbances known to occur during carousel operation, such as fouling, trying to (suboptimally) maximize the throughput at the same time. Improved throughput maximization in the presence of disturbances can also be obtained, manipulating V_{slurry}. However, achieving this goal through PID control loops is a cumbersome procedure. A Level 2 control system is required for proper real-time optimization.

4 Conclusions

In pharmaceutical manufacturing, QbD and QbC provide key benchmarks for digital analysis of pharmaceutical manufacturing systems. Although QbD may be implemented on single unit operations in pharmaceutical manufacturing systems, as manufacturing practices proceed to end-to-end continuous or hybrid batch-continuous operation, integrated analysis is required to implement meaningful process control schemes and maintain the design space dynamically.

To highlight the advantages of integrated design and optimal operation of pharmaceutical manufacturing systems, we presented two case studies on multiple-unit subprocesses for the synthesis-crystallization and filtration-drying of paracetamol, using an integrated process simulation and optimization framework utilizing digital twins. In the first case study, we showed process optimization of the synthesis-crystallization of paracetamol utilizing gradient-free optimization followed with a narrowed uniform grid search for optimal operating points. We utilized the new, open-source simulation tool, PharmaPy, to understand whether end-to-end continuous or hybrid batch-continuous operation was optimal. We found that in this case, the end-to-end continuous process provided a nearly equivalent mass output rate, but for the optimal operating conditions, it provided larger crystal sizes, favoring a PFR-MSMPR setup to a hybrid, PFR-batch crystallization setup. As process integration and modernization continue, more detailed frameworks and metrics for direct comparison of such operating mode choices will become an important analysis tool for the automated comparison potential manufacturing routes.

In the second case study, we analyzed the behavior of the filtration-drying process of a paracetamol slurry in an integrated carousel unit. The probabilistic design space was quantified and successfully identified feasible operating regions for critical process parameters of the carousel. For this particular case, a function describing the relevant probabilistic front can be fit and justified, resulting in a closed-form equation that is vital for quantitative validation that CQAs are satisfied within the operating region. Then, an online control system was implemented and shown to successfully control the carousel operation.

This model-based framework for process optimization and control showcases process digital twins and the capability of generating optimal operating conditions, quantifying feasible design spaces, and controlling integrated processing systems.

As process modernization and computerization continue, adoption of such digital frameworks for new and improved manufacturing schemes is a key part to quantitatively optimal and qualitatively feasible operation.

References

1. FDA (2004) 'Pharmaceutical cgmps for the 21 st century-a risk-based approach final report'.
2. Su, Q., Ganesh, S., Moreno, M., Bommireddy, Y., Gonzalez, M., Reklaitis, G. V., *et al.* (2019) 'A perspective on Quality-by-Control (QbC) in pharmaceutical continuous manufacturing', *Computers and Chemical Engineering*. Elsevier Ltd, 125, pp. 216–231. doi: https://doi.org/10.1016/j.compchemeng.2019.03.001.
3. FDA (2009) 'Guidance for Industry Q8(R2) Pharmaceutical Development'. Available at: http://www.fda.gov/Drugs/GuidanceComplianceRegulatoryInformation/Guidances/default.htm.
4. Rojko, A. (2017) 'Industry 4.0 concept: Background and overview', *International Journal of Interactive Mobile Technologies*. International Association of Online Engineering, 11(5), pp. 77–90. doi: https://doi.org/10.3991/ijim.v11i5.7072.
5. García-Muñoz, S. *et al.* (2015) 'Definition of Design Spaces Using Mechanistic Models and Geometric Projections of Probability Maps', *Organic Process Research and Development*, 19(8), pp. 1012–1023. doi: https://doi.org/10.1021/acs.oprd.5b00158.
6. García-Muñoz, S., Dolph, S. and Ward, H. W. (2010) 'Handling uncertainty in the establishment of a design space for the manufacture of a pharmaceutical product', *Computers and Chemical Engineering*, 34(7), pp. 1098–1107. doi: https://doi.org/10.1016/j.compchemeng.2010.02.027.
7. Ochoa, M. P. *et al.* (2019) 'Flexibility Analysis For Design Space Definition', in *Computer Aided Chemical Engineering*. Elsevier Masson SAS, pp. 323–328. doi: https://doi.org/10.1016/B978-0-12-818597-1.50051-5.
8. Boukouvala, F., Muzzio, F. J. and Ierapetritou, M. G. (2010) 'Design space of pharmaceutical processes using data-driven-based methods', *Journal of Pharmaceutical Innovation*, 5(3), pp. 119–137. doi: https://doi.org/10.1007/s12247-010-9086-y.
9. Wang, Z., Escotet-Espinoza, M. S. and Ierapetritou, M. (2017) 'Process analysis and optimization of continuous pharmaceutical manufacturing using flowsheet models', *Computers and Chemical Engineering*. Elsevier Ltd, 107, pp. 77–91. doi: https://doi.org/10.1016/j.compchemeng.2017.02.030.
10. Bano, G. *et al.* (2019) 'Design space maintenance by online model adaptation in pharmaceutical manufacturing', *Computers and Chemical Engineering*, 127, pp. 254–271. doi: https://doi.org/10.1016/j.compchemeng.2019.05.019.
11. Laky, D. *et al.* (2019) 'An optimization-based framework to define the probabilistic design space of pharmaceutical processes with model uncertainty', *Processes*, 7(2). doi: https://doi.org/10.3390/pr7020096.
12. Process Systems Enterprise (2020) *Process Systems Enterprise, gPROMS*. Available at: www.psenterprise.com/products/gproms (Accessed: 24 December 2020).
13. Casas-Orozco, D. *et al.* (2021) 'PharmaPy: an object-oriented tool for the development of hybrid pharmaceutical processes', *In Review*.
14. Yu, L. X. *et al.* (2014) 'Understanding pharmaceutical quality by design', *AAPS Journal*, 16(4), pp. 771–783. doi: https://doi.org/10.1208/s12248-014-9598-3.
15. National Institute of Standards and Technology (2015) *Libro del Web de Química del NIST*. Available at: http://webbook.nist.gov/chemistry/ (Accessed: 20 May 2015).
16. Picciochi, R., Diogo, H. P. and Minas Da Piedade, M. E. (2010) 'Thermochemistry of paracetamol', *Journal of Thermal Analysis and Calorimetry*, 100(2), pp. 391–401. doi: https://doi.org/10.1007/s10973-009-0634-y.

17. Gunawan, R., Fusman, I. and Braatz, R. D. (2004) 'High resolution algorithms for multidimensional population balance equations', *AIChE Journal*, 50(11), pp. 2738–2749. doi: https://doi.org/10.1002/aic.10228.
18. LeVeque, R. J. (2002) *Finite Volume Methods for Hyperbolic Problems*. New York: Cambridge University Press.
19. Rachah, A. *et al.* (2016) 'A mathematical model for continuous crystallization', *Mathematical Methods in the Applied Sciences*, 39(5), pp. 1101–1120. doi: https://doi.org/10.1002/mma.3553.
20. Rawlings, J. B., Miller, S. M. and Witkowski, W. R. (1993) 'Model Identification and Control of Solution Crystallization Processes: A Review', *Industrial and Engineering Chemistry Research*, 32(7), pp. 1275–1296. doi: https://doi.org/10.1021/ie00019a002.
21. Szilagyi, B., Majumder, A. and Nagy, Z. K. (2020) 'Fundamentals of Population Balance Based Crystallization Process Modeling', in *The Handbook of Continuous Crystallization*. Cambridge: Royal Society of Chemistry, pp. 51–101. doi: https://doi.org/10.1039/9781788013581-00051.
22. Nagy, Z. K. *et al.* (2008) 'Determination of the kinetic parameters for the crystallization of paracetamol from water using metastable zone width experiments', *Industrial and Engineering Chemistry Research*, 47(4), pp. 1245–1252. doi: https://doi.org/10.1021/ie060637c.
23. Lee, T., Lin, H. Y. and Lee, H. L. (2013) 'Engineering reaction and crystallization and the impact on filtration, drying, and dissolution behaviors: The study of acetaminophen (paracetamol) by in-process controls', *Organic Process Research and Development*, 17(9), pp. 1168–1178. doi: https://doi.org/10.1021/op400129n.
24. Borsos, A., Majumder, A. and Nagy, Z. K. (2016) 'Multi-Impurity Adsorption Model for Modeling Crystal Purity and Shape Evolution during Crystallization Processes in Impure Media', *Crystal Growth & Design*, 16(2), pp. 555–568. doi: https://doi.org/10.1021/acs.cgd.5b00320.
25. Kubota, N. and Mullin, J. W. (1995) 'A kinetic model for crystal growth from aqueous solution in the presence of impurity', *Journal of Crystal Growth*, 152(3), pp. 203–208. doi: https://doi.org/10.1016/0022-0248(95)00128-X.
26. Yu, A. B., Zou, R. P. and Standish, N. (1996) 'Modifying the linear packing model for predicting the porosity of nonspherical particle mixtures', *Industrial and Engineering Chemistry Research*, 35(10), pp. 3730–3741. doi: https://doi.org/10.1021/ie950616a.
27. Zou, R. P. and Yu, A. B. (1996) 'Evaluation of the packing characteristics of mono-sized nonspherical particles', *Powder Technology*, 88(1), pp. 71–79. doi: https://doi.org/10.1016/0032-5910(96)03106-3.
28. Bourcier, D. *et al.* (2016) 'Influence of particle size and shape properties on cake resistance and compressibility during pressure filtration', *Chemical Engineering Science*. Elsevier, 144, pp. 176–187. doi: https://doi.org/10.1016/j.ces.2016.01.023.
29. Huggins, S., Cosbie, A. and Gaertner, J. (2019) 'Filtration case studies', *Chemical Engineering in the Pharmaceutical Industry: Active Pharmaceutical Ingredients*. Wiley Online Library, pp. 833–845.
30. Muskat, M. and Meres, M. W. (1936) 'The flow of heterogeneous fluids through porous media', *Physics*. American Institute of Physics, 7(9), pp. 346–363.
31. Wakeman, R. J. (1976) 'Vacuum dewatering and residual saturation of incompressible filter cakes', *International Journal of Mineral Processing*. Elsevier, 3(3), pp. 193–206.
32. Wakeman, R. J. (1979) 'Low-pressure dewatering kinetics of incompressible filter cakes, I. Variable total pressure loss or low-capacity systems', *International Journal of Mineral Processing*, 5(4), pp. 379–393. doi: https://doi.org/10.1016/0301-7516(79)90046-2.
33. Van Leer, B. (1974) 'Towards the ultimate conservative difference scheme. II. Monotonicity and conservation combined in a second-order scheme', *Journal of computational physics*. Academic Press, 14(4), pp. 361–370.
34. Burgschweiger, J. and Tsotsas, E. (2002) 'Experimental investigation and modelling of continuous fluidized bed drying under steady-state and dynamic conditions', *Chemical Engineering Science*, 57(24), pp. 5021–5038. doi: https://doi.org/10.1016/S0009-2509(02)00424-4.

35. Bird, R. B., Lightfoot, E. N. and Stewart, W. E. (1960) *Transport Phenomena*. John Wiley & Sons.
36. Ellis, F. (2002) 'Paracetamol – a curriculum resource' Royal Society of Chemistry
37. Bates, D. and Watts, D. G. (1988) *Nonlinear Regression Analysis and Its Applications*. New York: John Wiley & Sons.
38. Bilardello, P. *et al.* (1993) 'A general strategy for parameter estimation in differential—algebraic systems', *Computers & Chemical Engineering*, 17(5–6), pp. 517–525. doi: https://doi.org/10.1016/0098-1354(93)80040-T.
39. Bard, Y. (1974) *Nonlinear Parameter Estimation, Nonlinear Parameter Estimation*. London.: Academic Press.
40. Casas-Orozco, D. *et al.* (2018) 'Dynamic parameter estimation and identifiability analysis for heterogeneously-catalyzed reactions: Catalytic synthesis of nopol', *Chemical Engineering Research and Design*. Institution of Chemical Engineers, 134, pp. 226–237. doi: https://doi.org/10.1016/j.cherd.2018.04.002.
41. Wächter, A. and Biegler, L. T. (2006) 'On the implementation of an interior-point filter line-search algorithm for large-scale nonlinear programming', *Mathematical Programming*, 106(1), pp. 25–57. doi: https://doi.org/10.1007/s10107-004-0559-y.
42. Rapin, J. and Teytaud, O. (2018) 'Nevergrad - A gradient-free optimization platform', *GitHub repository*. GitHub.
43. Destro, F., I. Hur, V. Wang, M. Abdi, X. Feng, E. Wood, S. Coleman, P. Firth, A. Barton, M. Barolo, Z. K. Nagy (2021). Mathematical modeling and digital design of an intensified filtration-washing-drying unit for pharmaceutical continuous manufacturing. Chemical Engineering Science, 244, 116803
44. Liu, Y. C. *et al.* (2019) 'Development of Continuous Filtration in a Novel Continuous Filtration Carousel Integrated with Continuous Crystallization', *Organic Process Research and Development*, 23(12), pp. 2655–2665. doi: https://doi.org/10.1021/acs.oprd.9b00342.
45. Destro, F., I. Hur, V. Wang, M. Abdi, X. Feng, E. Wood, M. Barolo, Z. K. Nagy (2020). Digital design of an intensified filtration-drying unit for pharmaceutical upstream manufacturing. Presented at: the 2020 Virtual AIChE Annual Meeting, November 16-20.

Fast Model Predictive Control of Modular Systems for Continuous Manufacturing of Pharmaceuticals

Anastasia Nikolakopoulou, Matthias von Andrian, and Richard D. Braatz

1 Introduction

Pharmaceuticals have been traditionally manufactured using batch processing. The potential for reducing drug costs, production times, waste material, and product quality variations while providing the ability to respond to abrupt changes in demand has motivated research efforts in academia and industry over the last decade to develop continuous-flow processes for pharmaceutical manufacturing [1–3]. Of special interest is end-to-end synthesis in compact modular reconfigurable systems for on-demand continuous-flow manufacturing, which refers to the integration of multiple molecular synthesis and separation steps in series, starting with simple inexpensive molecules and continuously going through all of the manufacturing steps of the product. Such modular systems can substantially decrease manufacturing times, while reducing the potential for supply chain disruptions by enabling spatially localized on-demand production [4].

A compact modular continuous manufacturing platform has been developed at MIT where both synthesis and final drug formulation are combined [4]. This refrigerator-sized system allows for multistep synthesis, in-line purifications, semi-batch crystallization, and real-time process monitoring. It has lower level regulatory control systems that are designed to maintain local state variables at specified setpoint values. An in-line attenuated total reflection (ATR) Fourier transform infrared (FTIR) system was used to monitor the formation of the active pharmaceutical ingredients (APIs) in real-time. Other process parameters monitored through sensors, a data acquisition device (DAQ), and LabVIEW (National Instruments) were pressure, reactor temperature, and flowrates. More recently, artificial intelli-

A. Nikolakopoulou · M. von Andrian · R. D. Braatz (✉)
Massachusetts Institute of Technology, Cambridge, MA, USA
e-mail: anikol@mit.edu; matthias.von.andrian@gmail.com; braatz@mit.edu

© The Author(s), under exclusive license to Springer Nature Switzerland AG 2022
A. Fytopoulos et al. (eds.), *Optimization of Pharmaceutical Processes*, Springer
Optimization and Its Applications 189, https://doi.org/10.1007/978-3-030-90924-6_11

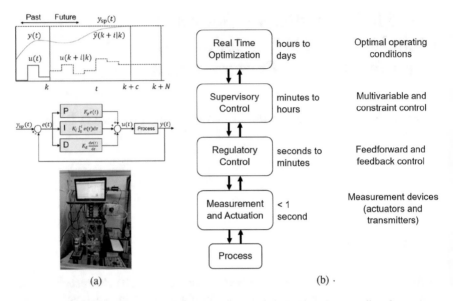

Fig. 1 Hierarchy of plant-wide optimization and control. In (**a**), bottom: a small-scale upstream atropine synthesis continuous manufacturing plant has sensors operating in the measurement level, middle: a PID control scheme is used at the regulatory level, top: MPC acts on the supervisory control level. In (**b**), optimization and control of processes follow a hierarchy based on information flow [6]

gence and robotics have been employed to design synthetic routes by generalizing previously published chemical reactions and consequently execute chemical recipe files in a robotically reconfigurable flow chemistry platform [5].

Traditionally, in the chemical industry, the regulatory control layer is part of a hierarchical scheme with higher level controllers and optimization layers above [6] (see Fig. 1). The regulatory layer involves proportional-integral-derivative (PID) controllers tuned using methods such as internal model control [7] and operating at fast time scales. The aim of the supervisory control level is to realize plant-wide objectives determined by a top level optimization. At the supervisory control level, more sophisticated control technologies such as model predictive control (MPC) that can handle input, state, and output constraints are often adopted [8]. MPC describes a class of algorithms that use a process model to predict the future plant behavior given past, present, and future control actions. The algorithm optimizes the future plant behavior subject to the sequence of future control actions at every control interval. The first control action of the sequence is implemented in the plant, and the optimization is solved again for the subsequent control interval.

MPC is the natural framework for the automation and control of continuous pharmaceutical processes. An advantage of using MPC is the ability to impose constraints in the manipulated variables (i.e., pump magnitudes and rate of change limitations) and the controlled variables (i.e., impurity content [9]). The inputs to the MPC layer are the continuous pharmaceutical plant's measured variables and overall plant-wide control objectives. Using plant-wide economic objectives such as the overall yield or production rate as the MPC controlled variables for pharmaceutical manufacturing plants has been previously explored [10]. The outputs of the MPC layer are the manipulated variables which are often mass flowrates. These flowrates constitute setpoints to lower level regulatory control systems. Together, the regulatory control layer and MPC layer form the plant-wide control system (e.g., [11]).

The MPC technology that is most widely used in the manufacturing industries is dynamic matrix control (DMC) [12], which is an algorithm that solves an online optimization at each control interval subject to operational constraints based on an input-output (IO) model for the process (e.g., [13–16]). DMC employs a finite step response model to make the predictions needed for computing the optimization objective. This approach has the advantage of making the online computational cost a function of the number of inputs of the manufacturing system as opposed to the number of states, which can easily be in the hundreds to thousands or more for an end-to-end manufacturing plant. Quadratic dynamic matrix control (QDMC) is a variation of the DMC algorithm that uses a quadratic rather than a linear control objective [17], is easier to tune and has been used in closed-loop simulation studies of continuous pharmaceutical manufacturing plants [9, 10, 18]. The wide usage of DMC in the chemical industry facilitates its use in the pharmaceutical industry, especially for small-molecule drugs, which are made by chemical synthesis.

A step response model can be constructed via system identification, specifically by perturbing the manipulated variables and recording the controlled variables (plant outputs) behavior. A plant-wide model can be used in place of the actual plant to enable step response model construction before experimental data is available, e.g., shortly after the manufacturing plant starts up. The parameters in the first-principles unit operations models can be identified in a much smaller scale system offline (e.g., a droplet-based system [19]). For the larger scale compact modular system, the same first-principles process model can be used but with larger geometric parameters and flowrates associated with the higher production rates. Using the same first-principles model equations for the different scales are enabled by the relatively small volumes at both scales; at these scales, the unit operations have fluid flows that are predictable and nearly ideal. Even with the simplified fluid flows, the first-principles model for the entire manufacturing plant has hundreds to thousands of states, due to the number of components and the numerics of unit operations (i.e., discretization of tubular reactors).

First-principles models for modular systems usually involve many tightly coupled partial and ordinary differential-algebraic equations (PDAEs/DAEs). For example, the widely applied numerical method of lines [20] involves spatial discretization of the PDAEs, resulting in a sparse system of DAEs with hundreds to tens of thousands of state variables. These models are commonly referred to as *singular systems* or *descriptor systems* in the control literature [21, 22]. Building first-principles plant-wide models introduces opportunities for optimizing the pharmaceutical plant operation. Many continuous pharmaceutical manufacturing processes are designed to operate over short operation times, which makes their operation more strongly impacted by unproductive dynamical plant operations (i.e., startup and shutdown). Therefore, methodologies that address the computation of optimal dynamical operations need to be explored.

Dynamic optimization (DO) is a widely known methodology for obtaining optimal trajectories for a dynamical system by optimizing a cost objective with respect to certain operating conditions (inputs, states) and constrained by equations that describe the dynamical operation (such as ODEs, DAEs, PDEs) [23]. This type of description is general enough to encompass a vast range of problem characteristics (integer-valued decision variables, multi-point constraints, uncertainty) and it is for the same reason that ubiquitous software solutions are difficult to implement [23]. The DOs are infinite-dimensional problems in their original formulation and there are many approaches for numerically solving these infinite-dimensional problems. *Dynamic programming* [24, 25] provides a mathematical formulation for computing the global optimum, but is very computationally expensive. Pontryagin's maximum principle [26] is a less expensive indirect approach, but may produce a solution that is only locally optimal. Limitations in these two approaches, related to treating problems with high state dimension for the former and treating inequality constraints for the latter, gave rise to the development of the so-called *direct methods*. In direct methods, the trajectory is parametrized and a nonlinear program (NLP) is formulated. Direct methods usually adopt one of three classes of numerical approaches: (1) the *sequential approach*, in which the time-varying input vector is parameterized in terms of a finite number of parameters to produce an optimization in which the process model appears as a constraint in the form of a DAE system, (2) the *simultaneous approach*, in which both the input and state variables are discretized to produce a nonlinear algebraic optimization [27], and (3) the *direct multiple shooting method* which is a hybrid approach where the state trajectory is partially eliminated from the NLP [28].

For the DO of startup of a continuous pharmaceutical manufacturing plant, the sequential method which deals with the DAE constraints by direct numerical simulation has been previously adopted resulting in a nonlinear program in which the only optimization variables are parameters that specify the input vector [18]. This approach is commonly used for this type of application [29–31].

When disturbances and model uncertainties are neglected, DO is a computationally tractable approach for DAE models with tens of thousands of states, since it can be solved offline and then have its optimal trajectory implemented online. During the first startup, the effects of model uncertainties can be significant when modeling modular systems for continuous-flow pharmaceutical manufacturing, as experimental data from the system are not yet available. In such a situation, feedback control is needed to reduce the effects of model uncertainties. Modular systems are highly nonlinear, which motivates the use of nonlinear model predictive control (NMPC) to suppress the effects of model uncertainties on operations and product quality by using nonlinear model predictions and real-time measurements to identify the optimal control inputs and then re-solving the arising nonlinear program at discrete time instances. NMPC has been implemented in some cases in fairly large scale systems [32].

The application of NMPC based on first-principles models during the startup of continuous-flow pharmaceutical manufacturing is challenging, however, as the models typically have highly nonlinear dynamics and thousands to tenths of thousands of states. Then the arising NLPs are usually nonconvex and have too high of a computational cost to be used in real-time implementation. On the other hand, implementing an optimal policy in an open-loop scheme has the disadvantage that the process disturbances and model uncertainties will result in a suboptimal operation and potentially off-spec product. As such, the closed-loop control of dynamical operations must be addressed, to suppress the effects of disturbances and model uncertainties on product quality. Government regulatory agencies are more likely to approve an industrial drug production facility that uses control software that has undergone extensive testing and implementation. This regulatory consideration results in a strong preference in the pharmaceutical industry to use linear MPC (LMPC) over NMPC. NMPC software solutions have so far been implemented in applications limited in size and scope compared to LMPC, partly due to the much higher computational complexity of NMPC and partly because LMPC provides adequate closed-loop performance in most supervisory control applications [8]. This chapter discusses how informed construction of IO models for QDMC can be leveraged to successfully control dynamical regions of the operation. LMPC such as QDMC can be combined with polynomial chaos theory to give fast stochastic MPC formulations to rigorously address parametric uncertainty [33, 34].

The rest of this chapter describes methodologies for dynamic optimization and QDMC implementation for modular systems with a high state dimension and significant nonlinear behavior. These methodologies are demonstrated in a computational case study for a compact modular plant for the continuous upstream manufacturing of atropine [35].

2 Modeling, Control, and Optimization of Modular Systems

This section describes a plant-wide model developed for a compact modular reconfigurable system for continuous-flow pharmaceutical manufacturing, discusses the supervisory control design methodology, and presents the dynamic optimization formulation to determine optimal dynamical operations such as startup.

2.1 Process Flowsheet

The plant-wide model is constructed in the context of a case study for the upstream synthesis of atropine, a central nervous system depressant, which can treat certain types of nerve agents, pesticide poisonings, certain types of slow heart rate conditions, and can decrease saliva production during surgery [35].

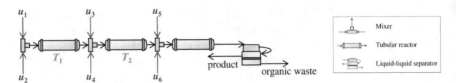

Fig. 2 Upstream atropine synthesis flowsheet showing three mixers, three tubular reactors, and one liquid-liquid separator. The mass flowrates of the six feed streams u_i are the manipulated variables, and the T_i are reactor temperatures controlled to a setpoint by resistive heating [18]

The process flowsheet in Fig. 2 shows the unit operations, which are three mixers, three tubular reactors, and a liquid-liquid separator, as well as the manipulated volumetric flowrates (u_i), and potential disturbances which are the temperatures in the first two reactors (T_i). The flowrates were manipulated through positive displacement pumps controlled in LabVIEW. The temperatures of the reactors 1 and 2 (Fig. 2) are held constant by keeping a jacket at a constant temperature using resistances.

The inputs to the atropine synthesis simulation are the volumetric flowrates of six feed streams:

- Tropine in dimethylformamide (u_1)
- Phenylacetyl chloride (u_2)
- Formaldehyde (u_3)
- Sodium hydroxide (u_4)
- Buffer solution (u_5)
- Organic solvent (u_6).

Each of the streams contains one or more of the fourteen species in the simulation.

Streams 1 and 2 are mixed in the first mixer, whose outlet flow connects to the first tubular reactor to produce a reaction intermediate in solution. That reactor outlet flow is then mixed with Streams 3 and 4 in the second mixer and directed to a second tubular reactor. The outlet flow of that chemical reactor is mixed with streams 5 and 6 in a third mixer, and subsequently sent to a packed bed. In the last unit operation a liquid-liquid separation is used to extract atropine in the aqueous phase.

A plug-and-play software module was developed for each unit operation. Modules can be automatically selected and interconnected to construct a dynamic model for the entire plant from the process flowsheet (Fig. 2). Each software module contains first-principles model equations for the associated unit operation, where "first-principles" refers to mass conservation equations, reaction stoichiometry, and reaction kinetics. Each tubular reactor was held at uniform, constant temperature by a heated jacked. Due to the high surface-to-volume ratio of the tubular reactors, the inlet flows to the reactors quickly reach the jacket temperature, so distributed parameter models for the energy balances were not needed and the temperature of each reactor was considered essentially equal to its jacket temperature. The temperature dynamics for the jackets were too slow to be used in the regulatory controls, so the temperature setpoints were determined by the higher level optimization.

2.2 Mathematical Description of Modules

Below is a description of the mathematical models for each module.

Mixer

Each mixer in the system is in-line, has very small volume, and is designed to have intensive mixing. The mixing of multiple streams is described by a mass conservation equation without accumulation for each chemical species,

$$\dot{m}_{\text{out},i} = \sum_{k=1}^{n_s} \dot{m}_{\text{in},i,k}, \text{ for } i = 1, \ldots, n_c, \tag{1}$$

where $\dot{m}_{\text{out},i}$ is the mixer outlet mass flowrate of species i, $\dot{m}_{\text{in},i,k}$ is the inlet mass flowrate of species i in the inlet flow k, n_s is the number of streams directed to the mixer, and n_c is the number of species. Some associated equations that describe variables of interest within each mixer unit are the total outlet mass flowrate,

$$\dot{m}_{\text{out, tot}} = \sum_{i=1}^{n_c} \dot{m}_{\text{out},i}, \tag{2}$$

and the molar concentration of species i,

$$c_{\text{out},i} = \frac{\dot{m}_{\text{out},i}\,\rho}{\dot{m}_{\text{out, tot}}\,M_i}, \text{ for } i = 1, \ldots, n_c, \tag{3}$$

where ρ is the solution volumetric mass density and M_i is the molar mass of species i. The solution volumetric mass density is calculated assuming additive volumes,

$$\rho = \left(\sum_{i=1}^{n_c} \frac{x_i}{\rho_i} \right)^{-1}, \tag{4}$$

where x_i is the mass fraction of species i in the stream of interest, and ρ_i the volumetric mass density of species i. This assumption is accurate for ideal solutions or for completely immiscible nonreacting mixtures. To simplify the nomenclature, the integer index that refers to each mixer is not shown. The above equations are replicated for every mixer, with the respective input and output variables.

Tubular Reactor

The tubular reactor is modeled by mass conservation equations formulated as partial differential equations (PDEs). The PDEs are discretized in space with n_d discretization points using a method of lines, and specifically backwards differences, resulting in an ODE system. The mass conservation equations in the tubular reactor are given by

$$
\frac{\partial c_{i,l}}{\partial t} = -Q_{tot} \frac{\partial c}{\partial V}\bigg|_{i,l} + r_{i,l}, \text{ for } i = 1, \ldots, n_c, \ l = 1, \ldots, n_d,
$$

$$
\frac{\partial c}{\partial V}\bigg|_{i,l} = \frac{c_{i,l} - c_{i,l-1}}{V_l - V_{l-1}},
$$

(5)

where $c_{i,l}$ is the molar concentration of species i at lth discretization point, Q_{tot} is the total volumetric flowrate inside the reactor, $r_{i,l}$ is the reaction rate of species i at lth discretization point, and V_l is the volume from the entrance of the reactor up to the lth discretization point. The last equation is the first-order spatial discretization of $\partial c/\partial V$. The inlet of the reactor is the 0th discretization point with a known concentration obtained from

$$
c_{in,i} = \frac{\dot{m}_{in,i}}{Q_{tot}M_i}, \text{ for } i = 1, \ldots, n_c,
$$

(6)

and the total volumetric flowrate in the reactor is

$$
Q_{tot} = \frac{\dot{m}_{in,\, tot}}{\rho},
$$

(7)

where $\dot{m}_{in,\, tot}$ is the total inlet mass flowrate. The density and hence the volumetric flowrate are assumed constant at every axial position in the tubular reactor.

The reaction rate matrix $r \in \mathbb{R}^{n_c \times n_d}$ with elements $r_{i,l}$ has rows that describe the reaction rate of each species i throughout the reactor and is given by

$$
r = SR,
$$

(8)

where $S \in \mathbb{R}^{n_c \times n_r}$ is the stoichiometry matrix, $R \in \mathbb{R}^{n_r \times n_d}$ is the reaction matrix, and n_r is the number of reactions. The reaction rates are modeled by an Arrhenius dependency on temperature. The kinetics can vary depending on the synthesis of the pharmaceutical of interest. The rate of the jth reaction at lth discretization point is

$$
R_{j,l} = k_j \exp\left(\frac{-E_{A,j}}{RT}\right) \prod_{m \in \mathcal{M}_j} c_{m,l}^{o_{m,j}}, \text{ for } j = 1, 2, \ldots, n_r, \ l = 1, 2, \ldots, n_d,
$$

(9)

where k_j is the constant prefactor for the jth reaction, $E_{A,j}$ is its activation energy, R is the ideal gas constant, T is the reactor temperature, M_j is the set containing the reactant species in the jth reaction, $c_{m,l}$ is the molar concentration of reactant species m at the lth discretization point, and $o_{m,j}$ is the reaction order of reactant species m in the jth reaction. A small-scale system can be used offline to acquire all the model-related parameters (e.g., a droplet-based system [19]).

For the synthesis of atropine, the activation energy and the prefactor for each reaction are obtained from linear regression on the experimental data from [35]. The reaction rates for the four reactions in the atropine synthesis process are modeled as being first order with respect to each of the reacting species

$$
R_{1,l} = k_1 \exp\left(\frac{-E_{A,1}}{RT}\right) c_{1,l} c_{3,l}, \quad R_{2,l} = k_2 \exp\left(\frac{-E_{A,2}}{RT}\right) c_{4,l} c_{7,l},
$$

$$
R_{3,l} = k_3 \exp\left(\frac{-E_{A,3}}{RT}\right) c_{5,l} c_{11,l}, \quad R_{4,l} = k_4 \exp\left(\frac{-E_{A,4}}{RT}\right) c_{5,l} c_{11,l}. \tag{10}
$$

Numbering of the species is based on their order of appearance in the chemical reaction network, obtained from [35]. All chemical reactions are modeled as homogeneous.

The species and total mass flowrates at the outlet of the tubular reactor are given by

$$
\dot{m}_{\text{out},i} = c_{i,n_d} Q_{\text{tot}} M_i, \quad \text{for } i = 1, \ldots, n_c,
$$

$$
\dot{m}_{\text{out, tot}} = \sum_{i=1}^{n_c} \dot{m}_{\text{out},i}. \tag{11}
$$

The tubular reactor ODEs (5) contribute the differential states $c_{i,l}$ ($n_c \times n_d$ in total) to the overall system. The algebraic equations (6)–(9) are inserted into (5) and do not contribute any algebraic states to the overall system of equations. Depending on the number of spatial discretization points n_d, a very large number of states can arise. The coarseness of the spatial discretization can be informed by order-of-magnitude analyses of the Péclet and Sherwood numbers to assess the relative contribution of dispersion on the mass transfer. A low dispersive transport rate would imply the need for a higher number of spatial discretization points to ensure that numerical diffusion in the numerical solution is smaller than the dispersion in the system. The selection of the number of spatial discretization points can also depend on the chemical reaction timescales, e.g., fast reaction rates require a high number of discretization points to accurately model the dynamics.

Liquid-Liquid Separator

The mass conservation equations for the liquid-liquid separator (LLS) assume an effective average uniform molar concentration $\bar{c}_i$ for each species i inside the unit, with dynamics modeled as

$$Q_{\text{tot}}\bar{c}_i = F_{\text{OR},i} + F_{\text{AQ},i}, \text{ for } i = 1, \dots, n_c, \tag{12}$$

$$V\frac{d\bar{c}_i}{dt} = Q_{\text{tot}}(c_{\text{in},i} - \bar{c}_i), \text{ for } i = 1, \dots, n_c, \tag{13}$$

where V is the volume of the liquid-liquid separator, F_i is the molar flowrate of species i, and the subscripts "OR" and "AQ" refer to the organic and aqueous phase, respectively. The constant density assumption inside the separator implies that

$$Q_{\text{tot}} = Q_{\text{OR}} + Q_{\text{AQ}}. \tag{14}$$

This assumption does not break during startup since the system at its starting state is filled with solvent. The solutes are assumed to exist in the organic stream in trace quantities, hence

$$\frac{x_{\text{in},s}}{x_{\text{in},s} + x_{\text{in},w}}Q_{\text{tot}} = Q_{\text{OR}}, \tag{15}$$

where $x_{\text{in},s}$ is the mass fraction of the solvent in the inlet of the liquid-liquid separator and $x_{\text{in},w}$ is the mass fraction of water in the inlet of the unit. The ratio describes the mass fraction of the organic solvent to the total amount of solvents (organic and water) in the feed stream of the liquid-liquid separator.

The phase equilibrium is modeled by

$$c_{\text{OR},i} = D_i c_{\text{AQ},i}, \text{ for } i = 1, \dots, n_c, \tag{16}$$

which assumes that the liquid-liquid equilibrium takes place instantaneously. The mass transfer kinetics can be modeled by a time delay, given enough data to characterize the mass transfer between the two liquid phases. The liquid-liquid separation partition coefficients D_i are assumed to have negligible variation with temperature and concentration, and they are approximated using the results from [35]. Direct use of (16) resulted in singularities when only one phase is present, which causes numerical problems during process simulation. To avoid such numerical problems, we used the alternative formulation

$$Q_{\text{AQ}}F_{\text{OR},i} = Q_{\text{OR}}D_i F_{\text{AQ},i}, \text{ for } i = 1, \dots, n_c, \tag{17}$$

which depends only on flowrates and does not carry the risk of having a null denominator. The LLS module is described by the differential and algebraic equations (12)–(15) and (17) which contribute to the system model the differential states $\bar{c}_i$ and the algebraic states $F_{OR,i}$, $F_{AQ,i}$, Q_{OR}, and Q_{AQ} ($3n_c + 2$ in total). These equations form an index-1 DAE.

Computational Considerations

In the atropine synthesis case study, to simplify the numerical solution of the plant-wide model, some algebraic manipulation was used to reduce the number of algebraic equations. For example, the variables associated with the mixer outlet were not introduced as algebraic states but were calculated and directed as inputs to the equations describing the downstream module. The equations that described the reactors and the separator were combined and the resulting DAE system was solved in MATLAB. Solvers that can handle stiff ODEs, such as `ode15s` in MATLAB, were used because the time scales of the reactions in the system vary significantly. Additionally, providing the Jacobian matrix or its sparsity pattern to the solver speeds up the calculations for systems of high state dimension. The computational time for a simulation of the operation of the plant from startup to steady state (~1 hr of operation) in a laptop with i7-5600U CPU at 2.60 GHz and 16.0 GB RAM was in the order of magnitude of 10 s for this system of approximately 10,000 states.

2.3   Control Design

The dynamics of the regulatory control loops are much faster than the open- and closed-loop dynamics at the MPC layer. This tight control at the lower level layer enables the simplification of the plant-wide model for the MPC design by excluding the closed-loop dynamics of the lower level control loops. For example, in the atropine synthesis case study, it is assumed that the pumps receive the flowrate setpoint instantaneously. The reactor temperatures are kept at setpoint which can be obtained from the optimization layer. The effectiveness of the separation of time scales between the regulatory and higher level control (supervisory) layers for the design of plant-wide control systems is well established in the literature (e.g., see the review by Ng and Stephanopoulos [36] and Larsson and Skogestad [37]).

Quadratic Dynamic Matrix Control

QDMC is heavily used in manufacturing largely because such processes often have very high state dimension, and the states of such models are typically not practically observable from the available measurements. QDMC is formulated as a quadratic program (QP) which can be solved by convex optimization algorithms

$$\min_{\Delta \mathbf{u}} \ \Delta \mathbf{u}^\top (\mathbf{G}^\top \mathbf{G} + \mathbf{W}_u) \Delta \mathbf{u} - 2\mathbf{e}^\top \mathbf{G} \Delta \mathbf{u} + \mathbf{e}^\top \mathbf{e},$$

subject to $\Delta \mathbf{u}_{\min} \leq \Delta \mathbf{u}(k) \leq \Delta \mathbf{u}_{\max},$ (18)

$$\mathbf{u}_{\min} \leq \mathbf{u}(k) \leq \mathbf{u}_{\max},$$

$$\mathbf{y}_{\min} \leq \hat{\mathbf{y}} \leq \mathbf{y}_{\max},$$

where $\Delta \mathbf{u}$ is the vector of future manipulated variable (MV) changes, $\mathbf{G}$ is the dynamic matrix which describes how present and future inputs affect the plant output and is constructed from the step response models, $\mathbf{e} = \mathbf{y}^{sp} - \mathbf{y}^p$ is the difference between the setpoint and the model prediction due to past and present terms, $\hat{\mathbf{y}}$ is the vector of the future plant output predictions, k denotes the current time instance, and $\mathbf{W}_u$ is a positive-definite matrix that penalizes changes in the manipulated variables in the cost function [16]. The execution time of the QP (18) depends on the control horizon c which determines the number of optimization variables and on the number of constraints. The prediction horizon p determines the future time window for which the plant behavior is simulated using the dynamical model. The tuning parameters of the QDMC are the $\mathbf{W}_u$, c, and p. Typically the matrix $\mathbf{W}_u$ is chosen to be diagonal, which was taken here. Higher values of the diagonal elements of $\mathbf{W}_u$ and/or c result in more conservative control. Detailed mathematical expressions, e.g., that define the elements of $\mathbf{G}$ in terms of step response coefficients, are described in any reference on QDMC [16, 17, 38].

QDMC requires a predictive model for the controlled variable (CV) as a function of the past and future values of the MVs. The predictive model can also include information regarding the effect of measured disturbances on the CV. For a plant with multiple inputs, step response models that describe how each MV affects the CV are created. These models should capture a wide and representative range of the operating regime. The step response models needed in QDMC can be automatically derived from the plant-wide simulation model by applying step changes for each MV. The CV response is recorded and then scaled to reflect how a unit change in the MV affects it. The overall multi-input model is built by combining the individual step responses for each MV. The same procedure is followed for each CV if the process has more than one control objective.

Step Response Models and Nonlinear Effects in a Modular System

In the atropine synthesis case study, the CVs were the mass production rate of atropine in the aqueous phase stream and the atropine yield which is defined as the ratio of the atropine mass flowrate over the theoretically possible atropine mass flowrate if all the reactants had completely reacted, based on the stoichiometrically limiting reactants. The MVs were the flowrates of the inlet streams $u_1 - u_6$. In a past study of the plant-wide control of continuous pharmaceutical manufacturing of a different pharmaceutical [9], API dosage and total impurity content were selected as the CVs.

Four consecutive steps of equal magnitude and a total deviation 20–80% from a nominal value both in increasing and decreasing directions were simulated starting from steady-state conditions for each MV. This type of step change program is also known as a staircase. The eight scaled step responses for each MV-CV pair were analyzed with one step response selected to construct the overall step response IO model which was used in QDMC, as described in Sections "Linear Input-Output Model Construction Methodology" and "Linear Input-Output Model Construction". The steps for each MV-CV pair are shown in Figs. 3 and 4.

The production rate and yield single-variable controllers were designed around different nominal steady-state operating conditions. Different sets of MV values were selected for each nominal operation in order to test the controllers against a wide range of nonlinearities that arise from differences in the chemistry depending on the operating region. Significant steady-state and dynamic nonlinearities were observed in the step responses (Figs. 3 and 4), especially for the mass production rate. Some observations are

- Many MV-CV pairs have nonlinear responses for their dynamics or steady-state values.
- All six MVs are mass flowrates that are inlets to the system, so positive steps in mass flowrates result in faster dynamics and shorter time delays than negative steps. The variation in plant dynamics can be about a factor of two for the output to reach steady state (e.g., u_1 in Fig. 3).
- Some of the steady-state gains are highly nonlinear, in some cases changing by a factor of ten or more (directional nonlinearities), or even changing sign (e.g., compare the responses for the positive and negative step changes for 80% in u_2 in Fig. 3). It is well-known that changing the size of the steady-state gain can result in unstable closed-loop systems when a feedback control system with integral action is applied [7].
- Under some conditions, the CV reaches a threshold so that further changes in the MV have small effects (e.g., -40% and -60% in u_2 in Fig. 4).
- The buffer solution and organic solvent mass flowrates (u_5 and u_6) have relatively small steady-state gains and so are not effective MVs.

The step response behavior of the CVs is dictated by the nonlinear dynamics of the process. Increasing the flowrate of an incoming stream may result in an excess of a reactant. Simultaneously, by increasing the total flowrate inside that unit operation, the concentration of other species can be diluted. These effects will influence the reaction rates. Additionally, changes in the flowrates affect the residence time which further impacts the extent of the reactions. These tradeoffs determine the overall increase or decrease of the production rate or yield for a given set of inputs. Lastly, operating the plant in nearly optimal values of a CV (that is, near its maximum or minimum achievable value) will result in a change in the sign of the steady-state process gain for some types of disturbances, which will cause instability or oscillations in the closed-loop dynamics [7].

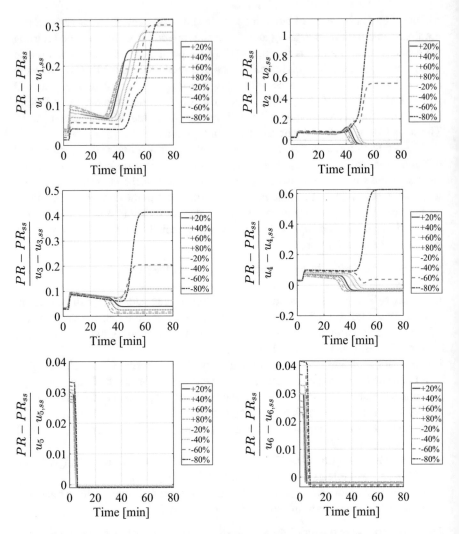

Fig. 3 Scaled transient responses of the production rate to step changes in the manipulated variables u_i, $i = 1, \ldots, 6$. Each step response is denoted by the step magnitude as a percentage of the nominal value of the corresponding manipulated variable. PR denotes the production rate and the subscript ss refers to the corresponding steady-state values of the operation prior to each step change [10]

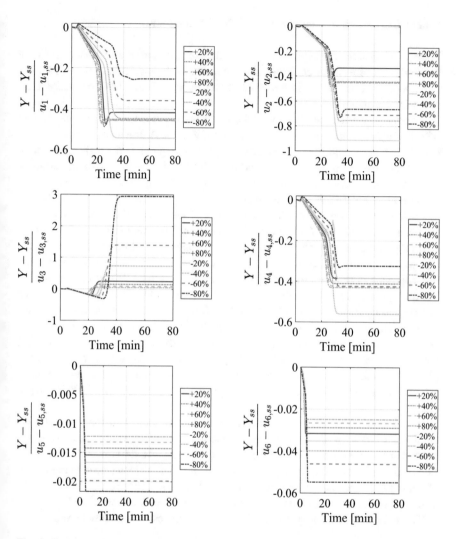

Fig. 4 Scaled transient responses of the atropine yield to step changes in the manipulated variables $u_i, i = 1, \ldots, 6$. Each step response is denoted by the step magnitude as a percentage of the nominal value of the corresponding manipulated variable. Y denotes the atropine yield and the subscript ss refers to the corresponding steady-state values of the operation prior to each step change [10]

Linear Input-Output Model Construction Methodology

There is no generally accepted method for the construction of a linear model to use in the design of a linear controller for a nonlinear process. This section discusses three approaches to selecting a step response model for each MV to construct the overall linear model for QDMC.

One strategy often used in industrial settings is to choose the step response model with the highest steady-state gain for all MV-CV pairs. A drawback of this strategy is that the plant would spend most time in operating regions with smaller gains than assumed by the controller, which would result in sluggish control. Also, this strategy does not address MV-CV pairs in which the steady-state gain can change sign.

Here an alternative strategy is taken that aims to address the linear model-plant mismatch which may arise when selecting a model for MV-CV pairs with gain sign changes. For an MV whose steady-state gain sign changes across the various step responses, its contribution to the overall model is eliminated. This means that the MV is treated as if it had no effect to the CV.[1] The motivation behind this approach is to avoid misdirecting the plant when the MV's effect on the CV has the opposite sign from what is assumed by the model. This approach reduces one degree of freedom per eliminated MV from the controller. Additionally, we account for the step response dynamics in the linear model construction by favoring step responses with fast dynamics. When the plant dynamics are slower than what the model predicts, the controller could be more conservative with respect to the plant. This conservatism could be offset by the potentially lower steady-state gains accompanying step responses with faster dynamics (e.g., -40% vs. -80% for u_1 in Fig. 3).

To address cases where removing degrees of freedom from the controller by eliminating MVs results in poor control, another alternative strategy is considered. Instead of completely eliminating the step response model exhibiting sign changes, a step response is selected that might reduce model-plant mismatch around the region of linearization for that MV. For the rest of the MVs, the same procedure is followed as in the previously mentioned approach (favoring somewhat faster dynamics).

These methods are compared for the atropine synthesis case study in Sect. 3.1.

2.4   Dynamic Optimization

Dynamic optimization (DO) is formulated as

$$\min_{\mathbf{u}} G(\mathbf{x}, \mathbf{z}, \mathbf{u}, \boldsymbol{\theta}) = \int_0^T g(t, \mathbf{x}, \mathbf{z}, \mathbf{u}, \boldsymbol{\theta}) \mathrm{d}t + h(\mathbf{x}, \mathbf{z}, \mathbf{u}, \boldsymbol{\theta}, t_f), \tag{19}$$

$$\text{subject to} \quad \mathbf{F}(t, \dot{\mathbf{x}}, \mathbf{x}, \mathbf{z}, \mathbf{u}, \boldsymbol{\theta}) = \mathbf{0}; \quad \mathbf{x}(0) = \mathbf{x}_0, \quad \mathbf{z}(0) = \mathbf{z}_0,$$

---

[1] For a control problem with a single output, this strategy will result in the MPC setting the MV associated with the zero step response coefficients to its steady-state value.

where $\mathbf{x} \in \mathbb{R}^{n_x}$ are the differential states, $\mathbf{z} \in \mathbb{R}^{n_z}$ are the algebraic states, $\mathbf{u} \in \mathbb{R}^{n_u}$ are the control variables or inputs of the process, $\boldsymbol{\theta} \in \mathbb{R}^{n_\theta}$ are time-invariant parameters of the model, t is time, $\mathbf{F}$ is a vector function that describes the system evolution involving differential and algebraic equations (DAEs), and g and h are algebraic functions. All $\mathbf{x}, \mathbf{z}, \mathbf{u}$ are functions of time. For distributed systems, where some states are continuous functions of spatial dimensions, the PDAEs can be discretized in space as described in Section "Tubular Reactor" resulting in (19).

Equation (19) describes an infinite-dimensional optimization, so a parametrization is needed for its numerical solution. The optimization horizon $[0, T]$ is discretized in n_t time stages such that $t \in [t_p, t_{p+1}]$, $p = 0, \ldots, n_t - 1$. The length of each of the n_t stages is allowed to vary, in order to more accurately determine switching times. Two commonly used control input parametrizations are the piecewise constant parametrization, in which the inputs are constant in each time stage, and the continuous piecewise affine parametrization, in which the inputs vary as an affine function of time in each time stage. These two control parametrizations are formulated as

$$\mathbf{u}(t) = \mathbf{u}_p, \ t \in [t_p, t_{p+1}], \ p = 0, \ldots, n_t - 1, \ \text{and}$$

$$\mathbf{u}(t) = \mathbf{u}_p + \frac{t - t_p}{t_{p+1} - t_p}(\mathbf{u}_{p+1} - \mathbf{u}_p), \ t \in [t_p, t_{p+1}], \ p = 0, \ldots, n_t - 1, \tag{20}$$

respectively.

For the atropine synthesis case study, the optimization objective focuses on waste minimization (excluding water) in the outlet streams from the LLS unit while maximizing the production of atropine. This formulation is tightly coupled to the concept of E-factor [39]. The algebraic functions referenced in the objective G are

$$g = \sum_{\substack{i=1 \\ i \neq n_w}}^{n_c} F_{OR,i} + \sum_{\substack{i=1 \\ i \neq n_w \\ i \neq n_a}}^{n_c} F_{AQ,i} - w_a F_{AQ,n_a}, \ h = \frac{t_{n_t} - t_0}{w_t}, \tag{21}$$

where n_w and n_a are indices that refer to water and atropine in the respective stream, $w_a = 100$ weighs the tradeoff between the two mass flow competing terms. This value is selected such that the term corresponding to the product flowrate is of similar magnitude as the waste term, and ensures that the optimization will not drift towards trivial solutions, e.g., nothing is produced and waste is minimized. The value of the weighting factor is informed by a series of optimizations for various values of T, $n_t = 1$, piecewise constant input parametrization, and values of $w_a = 50{-}10^3$ (Fig. 5). Similarly, $w_t = 100$ min is a scaling factor that ensures that h is in a similar order of magnitude as g for expected values of n_t. Other potential cost objectives such as reaching a target value for the production rate of atropine can be incorporated in the formulation as a terminal constraint or by appending a penalty term in the DO objective. The optimization variables are the volumetric

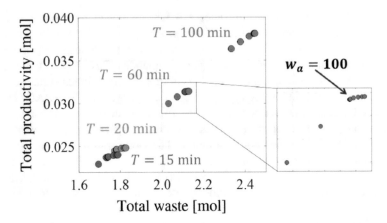

Fig. 5 A series of optimizations for the atropine synthesis startup for various values of T, $n_t = 1$, and for piecewise constant parametrizations indicate that the knee of pareto optimal solutions for the competing objectives of total productivity and total waste was obtained for a weighting factor of about $w_a = 100$ for all T

Table 1 Dynamic optimization constraints

Optimization variable	Minimum value	Maximum value
u_i [mL/min], $i = 1 - 4$	0	0.1
u_5 [mL/min]	0.1	1
u_6 [mL/min]	0	0.2
T_1, T_2 [K]	300	400
t_p / n_t [min]	20	500

flowrates $u_1 - u_6$, reactor temperatures T_1, T_2, and the length of each of the n_t stages $t_{p+1} - t_p$, $p = 0, \ldots, n_t - 1$. The input constraints are shown in Table 1.

After discretizing the optimization variables, (19) is an NLP that can be solved iteratively. In every iteration, the system is simulated by solving an initial value problem for a total time of $T = t_{n_t} - t_0 + 200$ min. After time t_{n_t}, the inputs $u_1 - u_6$, T_1, and T_2 are fixed to their last values and an additional 200 min of simulation ensures that the states and outputs have reached steady state, that is, that the process has transitioned from startup to its steady operation. The integral part of the objective function g is integrated alongside the DAE system and h is calculated at the end of each integration.

The nonlinear DAE system that simulates the upstream atropine synthesis in each iteration has 9114 differential states and 29 algebraic states, resulting in a very computationally intensive NLP unsuitable for real-time applications. The computational time of the simulated operation of the plant from startup to steady state in MATLAB is on the order of 10 s, when simulated on a laptop with Intel i7-5600U CPU at 2.60 GHz and 16.0 GB RAM. A DO is a nonconvex problem in general, hence converging to different local minima depending on the initial guesses for the optimal solution vector. To address this, the optimization was initialized with 100 random guesses, which were solved in parallel for a total time of 1–2 days in a system with two Intel Xeon Gold 6152 CPUs at 2.10 GHz and 262.0 GB RAM. The DOs were carried out in MATLAB using an adaptive mesh method. Reducing the computational time by using coarser spatial discretizations for the tubular reactors resulted in suboptimal startup. To control dynamical operations in real time, the DO problem can be solved offline and then the optimal trajectory can be provided as a setpoint to a fast linear MPC algorithm implementable in real time, thus suppressing the effects of disturbances and model uncertainties during the operation. Implementation of this approach on the atropine synthesis case study is presented in Sect. 3.2.

3 Control and Optimization Case Study Results

This section presents and discusses simulation results for the plant-wide control and dynamic optimization of the upstream atropine synthesis.

3.1 Quadratic Dynamic Matrix Control Simulation Study

For the atropine synthesis control case study, QDMC was implemented and $\mathbf{W}_u$, p, and c were tuned while simultaneously screening various linear models. Design parameters were selected to produce the most satisfactory closed-loop performance across all tests, which resulted in a prediction horizon of 300 min and a control horizon of 30 min. The prediction horizon was about 6–10 times the residence time of the nominal operation and 1.2 times the maximum residence time of the system (i.e., when all the flowrates are at their minimum possible value). This approach was followed to approximate an infinite-horizon control. The control horizon was chosen to be 1/10 of the prediction horizon. The weight matrix was $\mathbf{W}_u = \mathrm{diag}\{100\}$ for all MVs when controlling the production rate, and $\mathbf{W}_u = \mathrm{diag}\{50\}$ for all MVs when controlling the yield. The manipulated variables were constrained based on the pump specifications and the scale of the plant. The rate of change of the manipulated variables was set to 10% of their steady-state values to avoid aggressive control moves that might wear off the pumps or result in instabilities. The control simulation and the quadratic optimization were implemented in MATLAB. For a closed-loop plant operation of 8 h, the computational time of a closed-loop simulation was in the order of 6 min in a laptop with i7-5600U CPU at 2.60 GHz and 16.0 GB RAM. Sections "Production Rate Control", "Atropine Yield Control" and "Multivariable Control" show that this highly nonlinear dynamical system was successfully controlled using QDMC equipped with the selected step responses discussed in Section "Linear Input-Output Model Construction".

Linear Input-Output Model Construction

To control the upstream atropine synthesis plant with QDMC, multiple linear models were screened in closed-loop studies and the different linear IO model construction approaches discussed in Section "Linear Input-Output Model Construction Methodology" were tested. Three model construction approaches used in single-variable closed-loop studies are presented below. The corresponding step responses are shown in Figs. 3 and 4.

- Model 1 (M1) refers to the high steady-state gain model for the MVs. For the production rate as the CV, step responses that exhibit gain sign changes are excluded for these MVs. The resulting model denoted as M1-P is $[-80\%, 0, -80\%, 0, -80\%, -80\%]$ where the first element of the vector refers to u_1, the second element of the vector refers to u_2, etc. and -80% refers to the step response corresponding to a step change in the MV of -80% from its nominal value. For yield as the only CV, the high-gain model denoted as M1-Y is $[-20\%, -20\%, -80\%, -40\%, -80\%, -80\%]$.
- Model 2 (M2) refers to the high steady-state gain/fast-dynamics model with the contribution of MVs resulting in gain sign change eliminated. When the gain magnitude varies a lot, such as u_3 in Fig. 3, the low-gain model is selected. Then the models M2-P and M2-Y are $[-40\%, 0, +80\%, 0, -80\%, -80\%]$ and $[+80\%, -20\%, 0, -40\%, -80\%, -80\%]$ for the production rate and yield, respectively. The models that can be chosen are not unique, because there is a tradeoff between the fast dynamics and the high steady-state gain. The decision to eliminate the contributions of u_3 to the yield output is made due to big variations in the gain magnitude for that input.
- Model 3 (M3) refers to a similar model as M2 but does not eliminate the step responses for any MVs. Instead, linear models with a low steady-state gain are used, in cases where gain sign change occurs. These models are selected because of their fast dynamics and their ability to describe the behavior of the plant for most cases. Additionally, lower gains will maintain a not-too-sluggish control action. Hence the models $[-40\%, +80\%, +80\%, +80\%, -80\%, -80\%]$ and $[+80\%, -20\%, +80\%, -40\%, -80\%, -80\%]$ denoted as M3-P and M3-Y are selected for the production rate and yield, respectively.

For multivariable control, the linear model interactions should be taken into account when designing the QDMC model. For the atropine synthesis case study, results are presented for

- Model 1 (M1-M) with $[-80\%, 0, -80\%, 0, -80\%, -80\%]$ for the production rate and $[+80\%, -80\%, -80\%, +80\%, -80\%, -80\%]$ for the yield.
- Model 2 (M2-M) with $[-40\%, 0, +80\%, 0, -80\%, -80\%]$ and $[+80\%, +80\%, +80\%, +80\%, -80\%, -80\%]$ for the production rate and yield as CVs, respectively, and
- Model 3 (M3-M) $[-40\%, +80\%, +80\%, +80\%, -80\%, -80\%]$ and $[+80\%, +80\%, +80\%, +80\%, -80\%, -80\%]$ for the production rate and yield.

The step responses for the yield in multivariable control were obtained by linearizing the plant around the same operating conditions as those for the atropine production rate in Fig. 3. These operating conditions are not the same as for single-variable control of yield seen in Fig. 4. The resulting step responses for yield demonstrated mild directional nonlinearities, and time delays, but no steady-state sign changes, similarly to Fig. 4.

In the rest of this chapter, the same model notation is used to denote the QDMC designed with the corresponding linear model, e.g., M1-P refers to QDMC with M1-P as its predictive linear model for production rate as the CV, M1-Y refers to QDMC with the predictive linear model M1-Y for yield as the CV, etc.

Production Rate Control

The closed-loop responses for a setpoint tracking scenario for the production rate of atropine with up to $+40\%$ and -20% deviations from the nominal value, are shown in Fig. 6a. The QDMC with the predictive models M2-P and M3-P resulted in good closed-loop performance, reaching nearly zero steady-state error within 250–300 min after the setpoint change. The MPC provided very slow setpoint tracking for model M1-P, which is expected since using a high-gain linear model results in a very slow response when the plant is operating in a lower gain region.

The closed-loop responses were also tested for several disturbance scenarios. Some characteristic responses for temperature disturbances are shown in Fig. 6b. The temperatures of the reactors 1 and 2 (Fig. 2) are held constant by keeping a jacket at a constant temperature using resistances. However, a disturbance in that constant temperature will need to be rejected by manipulating the flowrates, since the physical system design does not allow for temperature manipulation on a short time scale. Small step disturbances $\pm 1\,°C$ and $\pm 5\,°C$ were applied to the temperatures T_1 and T_2. The controller successfully rejects each of the disturbances after about 250 min when the linear models M2-P and M3-P are used, while M1-P is very slow at rejecting the disturbances.

Step disturbances in the MVs were also examined. The disturbance rejection in one of the inputs, namely u_1, for a constant disturbance equal to $+40\%$ and -40% of the nominal value is shown in Fig. 6c. The results were similar for all other MV disturbances; M2-P and M3-P were observed to perform better than M1-P under the same circumstances. Finally, we examined scenarios where simultaneous MV disturbances occur. Two of the scenarios are shown in Fig. 6d, e. The time scale of the disturbance rejection as well as the model performance is similar to that of all the previously discussed cases.

Overall, the linear models M2-P and M3-P resulted in controllers that give significantly better closed-loop performance than M1-P. The controller using M1-P as a predictive model has slower, more sluggish dynamics across all tests, as expected. No significant difference in the closed-loop performance between models M2-P and M3-P was observed. M1-P differs from M2-P with respect to the step responses associated with u_1 and u_2, with higher steady-state gain step responses

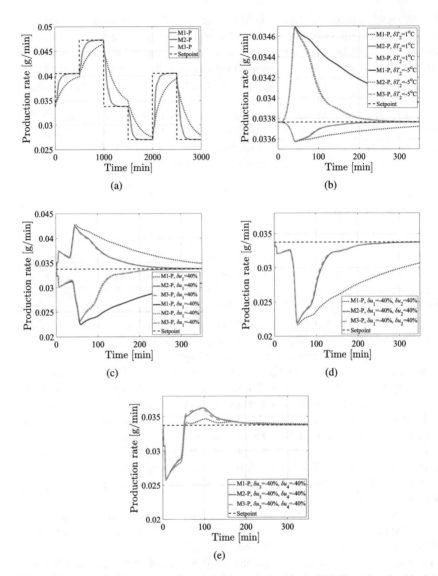

Fig. 6 Plant-wide control of atropine production rate based on QDMC equipped with three different linear models. The disturbances are steps introduced at the 2 min mark, starting from a steady-state operation. (**a**) Setpoint tracking of production rate. (**b**) Closed-loop response for a disturbance in the second reactor temperature T_2 of $+1\,°C$ and $-5\,°C$. (**c**) Closed-loop response for a disturbance in the input u_1, for $+40\%$ and -40% of the nominal value. (**d**) Closed-loop response to simultaneous disturbances in the inputs u_1 and u_2, for -40% and $+40\%$ of the nominal value respectively. (**e**) Closed-loop response to simultaneous disturbances in the inputs u_3 and u_4, for -40% of the nominal value for both inputs

having been selected for M1-P. M2-P and M3-P differ with respect to the step responses for u_2 and u_4, with no step responses being used for the former model and low-gain responses being selected for the latter model for both MVs. Eliminating the step responses does not seem to have a large effect on the closed-loop performance if the linear model selection corresponding to the remaining MVs is done carefully. Additionally, M3-P performs satisfactorily even without eliminating these two MVs. When opting to not exclude models with gain sign change, care must be taken to select models with the appropriate gain. Constructing a model with high steady-state gain that also exhibits gain sign change behavior will likely result in very poor closed-loop performance.

Atropine Yield Control

On-demand manufacturing can require operation in different conditions and/or control of different CVs depending on the utilization of the plant. To this end, this section evaluates the closed-loop performance of QDMC in an additional operating region of the plant while controlling a different CV, yield.

The closed-loop responses are shown in Fig. 7a for setpoint tracking of the yield of atropine of up to $+15\%$ and -35% deviation from the nominal value. All linear controllers provide good setpoint tracking control due to the similarities between the constructed linear models and the significantly reduced nonlinear effects observed for yield as a CV compared to the production rate (Fig. 4).

Step disturbances in the reactor temperatures T_1 and T_2 by ± 1 and $\pm 5\,°C$ were considered. Some characteristic closed-loop responses are shown in Fig. 7b. M2-Y and M3-Y provide a slightly slower closed-loop response in this case, by rejecting the disturbance at approximately 150 min and 200 min, respectively, whereas M1-Y rejects the disturbance at about 100 min.

Figure 7c is a representative closed-loop response for a disturbance in an MV, for $+40\%$ and -40% on the nominal value of u_4. Similarly to the response for a temperature disturbance, M1-Y provides a faster closed-loop response compared to M2-Y and M3-Y. Scenarios of simultaneous MV disturbances were also examined, with two of the scenarios shown in Fig. 7d, e. For a simultaneous disturbance in u_1 and u_3 shown in Fig. 7d, M3-Y provides the fastest closed-loop response, being able to reject the disturbance at about 100 min while M1-Y and M2-Y reject the disturbance at about 150 min. For the simultaneous disturbance in u_3 and u_4 shown in Fig. 7e, M3-Y provides again the fastest closed-loop response, being able to reject the disturbance at about 200 min while M2-Y rejects the disturbance at about 250 min. M1-Y is not able to reject the disturbance within 350 min.

M1-Y and M2-Y differ with respect to MVs u_1 and u_3. For u_1 a higher steady-state gain model is used in M1-Y while u_3 is eliminated in M2-Y since it exhibits a very large magnitude difference between the various gains. M2-Y and M3-Y differ only with respect to the model for u_3, with M3-Y using a model with a low gain. All of these models demonstrate good closed-loop performance for most cases. M1-Y is faster at rejecting disturbances in temperature and single MVs. M3-

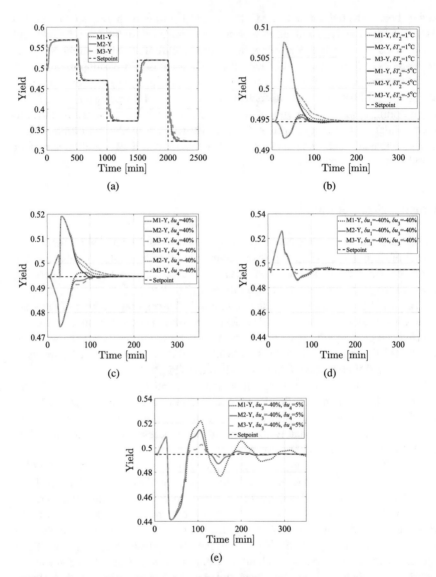

Fig. 7 Plant-wide control of atropine yield based on QDMC equipped with three different linear models. The disturbances are steps introduced at the 2 min mark, starting from a steady-state operation. (**a**) Setpoint tracking of yield. (**b**) Closed-loop response for a disturbance in the second reactor temperature T_2 of $+1\,^{\circ}$C and $-5\,^{\circ}$C. (**c**) Closed-loop response for a disturbance in the input u_4, for $+40\%$ and -40% of the nominal value. (**d**) Closed-loop response to simultaneous disturbances in the inputs u_1 and u_3, for -40% of the nominal value for both inputs. (**e**) Closed-loop response to simultaneous disturbances in the inputs u_3 and u_4, for -40% and $+5\%$ of the nominal value, respectively

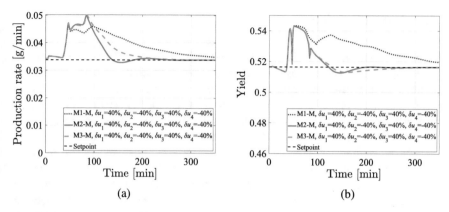

Fig. 8 Plant-wide multivariable control of (**a**) atropine production rate and (**b**) yield based on QDMC equipped with three different linear models. The simultaneous step disturbances in the MVs u_1–u_4, for $+40\%$, -40%, $+40\%$, and -40% of the nominal value, respectively, are introduced at the 2 min mark for a plant starting from steady-state operation

Y has the slowest response by a small margin for setpoint tracking and rejection of disturbances in temperature and single MVs, but offers the fastest closed-loop performance when there are multiple disturbances in the MVs. Overall, M2-Y has the most consistent closed-loop performance.

Multivariable Control

An advantage of advanced control methodologies such as QDMC is their ability to handle multivariable control. The production rate and yield of atropine were simultaneously controlled in some extreme operating scenarios to further test the linear model performance. The four MVs affecting the CVs the most were simultaneously disturbed by 5 and 40% in increasing and decreasing directions. One of these cases is shown in Fig. 8. Simultaneous disturbance rejection in both CVs is achieved by the controllers using models M2-M and M3-M at about 250 min.

M2-M and M3-M differ only with respect to the production rate model. Eliminating the contributions of the MVs with step responses demonstrating a gain sign change (u_2 and u_4) for the production rate in M2-M seems to result in faster closed-loop response. M1-M and M2-M have different models for both CVs. M1-M uses the high-gain model for production rate while M2-M adopts lower gain step responses for inputs u_1 and u_3. Regarding the yield predictive model, M1-M adopts a higher gain step response model compared to M2-M. Overall, M2-M outperforms the other controllers. M1-M provides a much slower disturbance rejection having a more sluggish, conservative control, compared to M2-M as expected, which is in agreement with the observations from the previously examined cases that the proposed models M2 (M2-P, M2-Y) and M3 (M3-P, M3-Y) provide an overall better control of the plant compared to M1 (M1-P, M1-Y).

3.2   Control of Startup

Offline computation of the NLP formulated in Sect. 2.4 resulted in optimal trajectories that were then used as a setpoint for QDMC to control the plant from the
point of no operation where the system is filled with the organic solvent to steady
state. The input-output formulation of QDMC was exploited to enable online control
implementation, since the associated QP is not a function of the state dimension.

Controlling startup which is a highly nonlinear region of operation with LMPC
can be challenging. Therefore, it is important to select a linear model that results in
good closed-loop performance when applied to a nonlinear system. The linear model
construction was informed by the insights gained from the analysis presented in
Sects. 2.3 and 3.1. The process was linearized around the final steady-state operating
conditions. QDMC was implemented for a prediction horizon of 300 min, a control
horizon of 30 min, and a weighting factor of $\mathbf{W}_u = \mathrm{diag}\{300\}$.

Dynamic Optimization Results

Dynamic optimization results using piecewise constant and continuous piecewise
affine input vector parametrizations are denoted as pwc and pwa, respectively,
followed by the number of stages n_t (Figs. 9 and 10). Results are presented for
$n_t = 1$ and $n_t = 2$. The resulting solutions were very similar, with the optimization
$\mathrm{pwc}_{n_t=2}$ returning a slightly better value for the objective function as seen in Fig. 9b.
The optimal values for the inputs seen in Fig. 10 vary the most between formulations
for u_3 and u_4. Both u_1 and u_3 operate at their maximum value most of the time. The
buffer solution and organic solvent flowrates u_5 and u_6 are realized in their trivial
value of 0, which results in minimal waste. This result is an artifact of the model,
which does not capture the phenomena related to varying pH in the LLS unit in great
detail due to limited experimental data. Interestingly, the optimal temperature T_1 is
significantly lower for $\mathrm{pwc}_{n_t=1}$ than for the other parameterizations, indicating that
the objective function is not very sensitive to T_1.

Quadratic Dynamic Matrix Control of Startup

Three MPC strategies for startup control were compared for each of the DO results
(Fig. 11). The first MPC strategy (labeled as "QDMC" in the plots) used the
dynamical trajectory obtained from the DO as a setpoint. Additionally, an approach
denoted as "QDMC+O" was investigated to examine if there is any significant
benefit from implementing the DO optimal inputs during the time period that there
is no product exiting from the system and hence no feedback to the MPC (this time
is from $t = 0$ to the residence time of the overall system). The third strategy labeled
as "QDMC SS" in the plots, was to use a steady-state setpoint to MPC (obtained as
the value of the DO solution at steady-state).

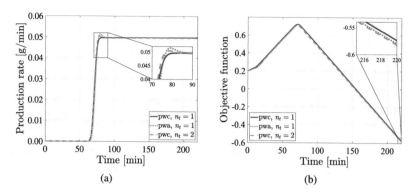

Fig. 9 Dynamic optimization results for $\text{pwc}_{n_t=1}$, $\text{pwa}_{n_t=1}$, and $\text{pwc}_{n_t=2}$ [18]. (**a**) Optimal production rate during startup. (**b**) Objective function value

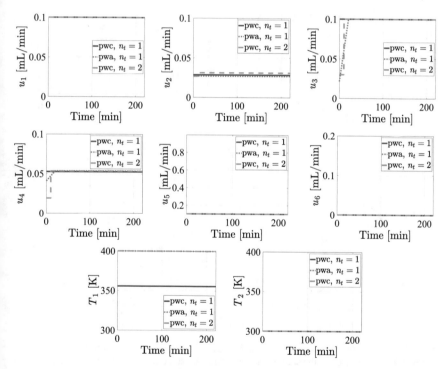

Fig. 10 Optimal inputs for the startup of upstream atropine synthesis for $\text{pwc}_{n_t=1}$, $\text{pwa}_{n_t=1}$, and $\text{pwc}_{n_t=2}$ [18]

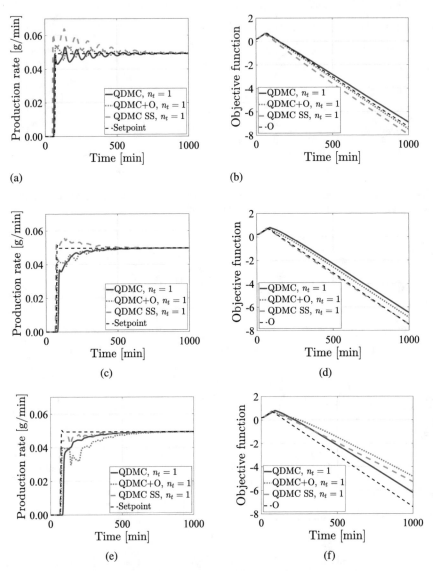

Fig. 11 QDMC performance for setpoint tracking of the production rate during startup. The optimal trajectories (setpoints) were obtained from dynamic optimization for various input vector parameterizations. The closed-loop responses are reported for different MPC strategies[18]. (**a**) Setpoint tracking for startup optimized with $pwc_{n_t=1}$. (**b**) Objective function values during startup controlled to a trajectory optimized with $pwc_{n_t=1}$ and objective function (O) obtained from optimization. (**c**) Setpoint tracking for startup optimized with $pwa_{n_t=1}$. (**d**) Objective function values during startup controlled to a trajectory optimized with $pwa_{n_t=1}$ and objective function (O) obtained from optimization. (**e**) Setpoint tracking for startup optimized with $pwc_{n_t=2}$. (**f**) Objective function values during startup controlled to a trajectory optimized with $pwc_{n_t=2}$ and objective function (O) obtained from optimization

Good closed-loop performance was achieved for the nominal plant startup operation (Fig. 11). For all input parameterizations, using the dynamical production rate setpoint trajectory from the DO to the MPC gave the best closed-loop performance (Fig. 11a, c and e). Using the optimal inputs during the no-feedback time period either gave similar or worse closed-loop performance. The objective function values for the closed-loop startup strategies were similar to the DO optimal solution, with the largest variation among MPC strategies being for the $pwc_{n_t=2}$ (Fig. 11b, d and f).

Quadratic Dynamic Matrix Control of Startup Under Parametric Uncertainty

The models for modular systems have significant parametric uncertainty. The closed-loop performance of QDMC in the presence of parametric uncertainty and significant nonlinear phenomena during the plant startup was studied. For the atropine synthesis case study, the parameter with the largest effect on the production rate as identified by sensitivity analysis is k_3 (with a nominal value of 24 mol/(mL min)), which is the prefactor of the chemical reaction that uses tropine ester and formaldehyde to produce atropine [35]. The closed-loop responses for different values of k_3 for dynamical or steady-state production rate setpoint trajectories in Fig. 12a, b show good robustness for most parameter realizations. As the value of the kinetic parameter is reduced, the convergence to the setpoint slows. As expected, the closed-loop MPC strategies outperform the open-loop implementation of the optimal inputs under the presence of model uncertainty which results in significant production rate variation (Fig. 12a, b and c).

In Fig. 12a and b which use the same QDMC tuning parameters, the dynamical setpoint from the DO results in better closed-loop performance than using the steady-state setpoint. Namely, the closed-loop trajectories in Fig. 12a, b have significant oscillations for large values of the uncertain parameter k_3. The oscillations can be reduced by detuning the QDMC, albeit with slower closed-loop response.

4 Conclusions

This chapter describes formulational, methodological, and computational aspects of plant-wide control and optimization of modular, reconfigurable systems for continuous-flow pharmaceutical manufacturing. One of the main computational challenges for such systems is the high number of states that arise from the first-principles mathematical descriptions of such systems. For state-space models of high dimension, nonlinear MPC can only be implemented offline due to the associated high computational costs.

These costs can be reduced by replacing state-space models by input-output models. QDMC is a control methodology that uses linear input-output models and has been used for decades in the chemical industry, and is a promising approach

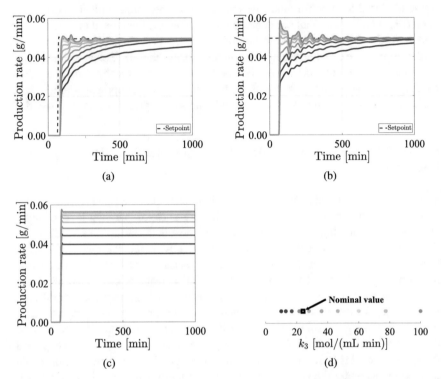

Fig. 12 Closed- and open-loop startup operations under time-invariant parametric uncertainty in k_3. The optimal setpoints are obtained from pwc$_{n_t=2}$. The optimal control inputs obtained from the same nonlinear dynamic optimization are used to simulate the open-loop responses in (**c**). Plot (**d**) defines the color coding for the three plots at the top [18]. (**a**) Setpoint tracking of production rate following a dynamical trajectory (QDMC), under parametric uncertainty. (**b**) Setpoint tracking of production rate for a steady-state setpoint trajectory (QDMC SS) under parametric uncertainty. (**c**) Open-loop startup operation under parametric uncertainty, showing a strong sensitivity to the value of k_3. (**d**) Uncertain parameter k_3 value realizations

for plant-wide control in the pharmaceutical industry. However, linear models can result in poor closed-loop performance when applied to nonlinear operations. For modular systems, strong steady-state and dynamic nonlinearities were observed between the manipulated and controlled variables associated with plant-wide control in a computational case study for the upstream atropine synthesis. We demonstrated two strategies for constructing linear models with improved closed-loop performance: (1) among multiple step responses obtained for different sized steps in the manipulated variables, use the step response models that have larger steady-state gains while maintaining fast dynamics, (2) when the steady-state gain for a step response for an MV-CV pair changes sign, eliminate that step response, or select a model that reduces linear model-plant mismatch. These strategies provided high-performance closed-loop control compared to a commonly used strategy in a simulation case study for the continuous-flow manufacturing of atropine under disturbances for single-variable and multivariable control. The reasoning behind the improved closed-loop performance achieved by these strategies is that they are designed to reduce the sensitivity of the control actions to model-plant mismatch. Although these strategies are design guidelines rather than proofs, the case study demonstrated that they should be considered when trying to design a linear model predictive controller to control a highly nonlinear dynamical system.

This chapter also discussed the formulation of dynamic optimization of dynamical operating regions of continuous pharmaceutical manufacturing plants with a focus on startup. Dynamic optimization is formulated as a nonlinear program by employing an input vector parametrization resulting in a direct sequential approach. Time-varying production rate profiles determined by the dynamic optimization solution were provided as setpoint trajectories to QDMC equipped with carefully constructed linear models. Good closed-loop performance was observed for startup control simulations for the atropine synthesis case study even under the presence of parametric uncertainty.

An alternative to first-principles and linear models discussed in this chapter is the construction of data-driven nonlinear models such as dynamic artificial neural networks (DANNs), whose online simulation cost is very low. System identification to build such nonlinear models requires a large quantity of data, which can result in significant wasted material if obtained by running experiments on the physical system. An approach to deal with the limited data available during startup, while exploiting the low computational cost of DANNs, is to build the DANN based on a large quantity of simulation data produced by a first-principles model. Then the DANN would be used in a nonlinear model predictive control (NMPC) algorithm that is runnable in real time. An alternative DANN-based approach is to design approximate MPC strategies in which the control law is learned by data. Such strategies have been shown to give good closed-loop performance in simulations, and guarantees of their theoretical properties have been recently derived [40, 41]. Another alternative DANN-based approach employs the mathematical framework of matrix inequalities, and theoretical results for analyzing stability and performance and for control design have been derived (e.g., see [42, 43] and citations therein). Given that DANNs have been used in the control of nonlinear dynamical systems in industrial practice for decades, it is conceivable that such approaches could someday become sufficiently accepted that they could be applied in the control of modular pharmaceutical manufacturing.

Acknowledgments The Klavs F. Jensen group at MIT is acknowledged for providing input on the models and for access to their lab spaces.

This work was supported by the DARPA Make-It program under contract ARO W911NF-16-2-0023. Any opinions, findings, and conclusions or recommendations expressed in this material are those of the authors and do not necessarily reflect the views of the financial sponsor.

References

1. S. Mascia, P. L. Heider, H. Zhang, R. Lakerveld, B. Benyahia, P. I. Barton, R. D. Braatz, C. L. Cooney, J. M. B. Evans, T. F. Jamison, K. F. Jensen, A. S. Myerson, and B. L. Trout, "End-to-end continuous manufacturing of pharmaceuticals: Integrated synthesis, purification, and final dosage formation," *Angewandte Chemie International Edition*, vol. 52, no. 47, pp. 12359–12363, 2013.
2. I. R. Baxendale, R. D. Braatz, B. K. Hodnett, K. F. Jensen, M. D. Johnson, P. Sharratt, J.-P. Sherlock, and A. J. Florence, "Achieving continuous manufacturing: Technologies and approaches for synthesis, workup and isolation of drug substance," *Journal of Pharmaceutical Sciences*, vol. 104, no. 3, pp. 781–791, 2015.
3. A. S. Myerson, M. Krumme, M. Nasr, H. Thomas, and R. D. Braatz, "Control systems engineering in continuous pharmaceutical manufacturing," *Journal of Pharmaceutical Sciences*, vol. 104, no. 3, pp. 832–839, 2015.
4. A. Adamo, R. L. Beingessner, M. Behnam, J. Chen, T. F. Jamison, K. F. Jensen, J.-C. M. Monbaliu, A. S. Myerson, E. M. Revalor, D. R. Snead, T. Stelzer, N. Weeranoppanant, S. Y. Wong, and P. Zhang, "On-demand continuous-flow production of pharmaceuticals in a compact, reconfigurable system," *Science*, vol. 352, no. 6281, pp. 61–67, 2016.
5. C. W. Coley, D. A. Thomas III, J. A. M. Lummiss, J. N. Jaworski, C. P. Breen, V. Schultz, T. Hart, J. S. Fishman, L. Rogers, H. Gao, R. W. Hicklin, P. P. Plehiers, J. Byington, J. S. Piotti, W. H. Green, A. J. Hart, T. F. Jamison, and K. F. Jensen, "A robotic platform for flow synthesis of organic compounds informed by AI planning," *Science*, vol. 365, no. 6453, 2019.
6. D. E. Seborg, T. F. Edgar, D. A. Mellichamp, and F. J. Doyle III, *Process Dynamics and Control*. Wiley, 2011.
7. M. Morari and E. Zafiriou, *Robust Process Control*. Piscataway, NJ: Prentice Hall, 1989.
8. S. J. Qin and T. A. Badgwell, "A survey of industrial model predictive control technology," *Control Engineering Practice*, vol. 11, pp. 733–764, 2003.
9. A. Mesbah, J. A. Paulson, R. Lakerveld, and R. D. Braatz, "Model predictive control of an integrated continuous pharmaceutical manufacturing pilot plant," *Organic Process Research & Development*, vol. 21, pp. 844–854, 2017.
10. A. Nikolakopoulou, M. von Andrian, and R. D. Braatz, "Plantwide control of a compact modular reconfigurable system for continuous-flow pharmaceutical manufacturing," in *Proc. American Control Conference*, pp. 2158–2163, 2019.
11. R. Lakerveld, B. Benyahia, P. L. Heider, H. Zhang, A. Wolfe, C. J. Testa, S. Ogden, D. R. Hersey, S. Mascia, J. M. B. Evans, R. D. Braatz, and P. I. Barton, "The application of an automated control strategy for an integrated continuous pharmaceutical pilot plant," *Organic Process Research & Development*, vol. 19, no. 9, pp. 1088–1100, 2015.
12. C. R. Cutler and B. L. Ramaker, "Dynamic Matrix Control – A computer control algorithm," in *AIChE National Meeting*, (Houston, Texas), 1979.
13. K. R. Muske and J. B. Rawlings, "Model predictive control with linear models," *AIChE Journal*, vol. 39, no. 2, pp. 262–287, 1993.
14. M. Morari and J. H. Lee, "Model predictive control: Past, present and future," *Computers & Chemical Engineering*, vol. 23, pp. 667–682, 1999.
15. J. B. Rawlings, D. Q. Mayne, and M. M. Diehl, *Model Predictive Control: Theory, Computation and Design*. Wisconsin: Nob Hill Publishing, 2017.
16. E. Ikonen, "Model Predictive Control and State Estimation," tech. rep., University of Oulu, Finland, 2017.
17. C. E. Garcia and A. M. Morshedi, "Quadratic programming solution of dynamic matrix control (QDMC)," *Chemical Engineering Communications*, vol. 46, no. 1–3, pp. 73–87, 1986.
18. A. Nikolakopoulou, M. von Andrian, and R. D. Braatz, "Fast model predictive control of startup of a compact modular reconfigurable system for continuous-flow pharmaceutical manufacturing," in *Proc. American Control Conference*, pp. 2778–2783, 2020.

19. Y.-J. Hwang, C. W. Coley, M. Abolhasani, A. L. Marzinzik, G. Koch, C. Spanka, H. Lehmann, and K. F. Jensen, "Segmented flow platform for on-demand medicinal chemistry and compound synthesis in oscillating droplets," *Chemical Communications*, vol. 53, no. 49, pp. 6649–6652, 2017.
20. W. E. Schiesser, *The Numerical Method of Lines: Integration of Partial Differential Equations*. San Diego, CA: Academic Press, Inc., 1991.
21. U. M. Ascher and L. R. Petzold, *Computer Methods for Ordinary Differential Equations and Differential-Algebraic Equations*. Philadelphia, PA: SIAM, 1998.
22. K. E. Brenan, S. L. Campbell, and L. R. Petzold, *Numerical Solution of Initial-Value Problems in Differential Algebraic Equations*. Philadelphia, PA: SIAM, 1996.
23. J. Andersson, *A General-Purpose Software Framework for Dynamic Optimization*. PhD thesis, KU Leuven, Leuven, Belgium, October 2013.
24. R. E. Bellman, *Dynamic Programming*. New Jersey: Princeton University Press, 1957.
25. D. P. Bertsekas, *Dynamic Programming and Optimal Control*, vol. II. Athena Scientific, 3rd ed., 2007.
26. L. Pontryagin, V. Boltyanski, R. Gamkrelidze, and E. Miscenko, *The Mathematical Theory of Optimal Processes*. Chichester: Wiley, 1962.
27. L. T. Biegler, "Solution of dynamic optimization problems by successive quadratic programming and orthogonal collocation," *Computers & Chemical Engineering*, vol. 8, no. 3/4, pp. 243–247, 1984.
28. H. G. Bock and K. J. Plitt, "A multiple shooting algorithm for direct solution of optimal control problems," in *Proc. IFAC World Congress*, pp. 1603–1608, 1984.
29. A. M. Sahlodin and P. I. Barton, "Optimal campaign continuous manufacturing," *Industrial & Engineering Chemistry Research*, vol. 54, pp. 11344–11359, 2015.
30. M. Patrascu and P. I. Barton, "Optimal campaigns in end-to-end continuous pharmaceuticals manufacturing. Part 2: Dynamic optimization," *Chemical Engineering and Processing – Process Intensification*, vol. 125, pp. 124–132, 2018.
31. M. Patrascu and P. I. Barton, "Optimal dynamic continuous manufacturing of pharmaceuticals with recycle," *Industrial & Engineering Chemistry Research*, vol. 58, pp. 13423–13436, 2019.
32. Z. Nagy, R. Findeisen, M. Diehl, F. Allgöwer, H. G. Bock, S. Agachi, J. P. Schlöder, and D. Leineweber, "Real-time feasibility of nonlinear predictive control for large scale processes – A case study," in *Proc. American Control Conference*, pp. 4249–4253, 2000.
33. M. von Andrian and R. D. Braatz, "Offset-free input-output formulations of stochastic model predictive control based on polynomial chaos theory," in *Proc. American Control Conference*, pp. 360–365, 2019.
34. M. von Andrian and R. D. Braatz, "Stochastic dynamic optimization and model predictive control based on polynomial chaos theory and symbolic arithmetic," in *Proc. American Control Conference*, pp. 3399–3404, 2020.
35. A.-C. Bédard, A. R. Longstreet, J. Britton, Y. Wang, H. Moriguchi, R. W. Hicklin, W. H. Green, and T. F. Jamison, "Minimizing E-factor in the continuous-flow synthesis of diazepam and atropine," *Bioorganic & Medicinal Chemistry*, vol. 25, no. 23, pp. 6233–6241, 2017.
36. C. Ng and G. Stephanopoulos, "Plant-wide control structures and strategies," *IFAC Proceedings Volumes*, vol. 31, no. 11, pp. 1–16, 1998.
37. T. Larsson and S. Skogestad, "Plantwide control – A review and a new design procedure," *Modeling, Identification and Control*, vol. 21, no. 4, pp. 209–240, 2000.
38. B. W. Bequette, *Process Control: Modeling, Design and Simulation*. Piscataway, NJ: Prentice Hall, 2003.
39. R. A. Sheldon, "The E-factor: Fifteen years on," *Green Chemistry*, vol. 9, no. 2, pp. 1261–1384, 2007.
40. A. D. Bonzanini, J. A. Paulson, D. B. Graves, and A. Mesbah, "Toward safe dose delivery in plasma medicine using projected neural network-based fast approximate NMPC," in *Proc. IFAC World Congress*, pp. 5353–5359, 2020.

41. H. H. Nguyen, T. Zieger, S. C. Wells, A. Nikolakopoulou, R. D. Braatz, and R. Findeisen, "Stability certificates for neural network learning-based controllers using robust control theory," in *Proc. American Control Conference*, in press, 2021.
42. A. Nikolakopoulou, M. S. Hong, and R. D. Braatz, "Feedback control of dynamic artificial neural networks using linear matrix inequalities," in *Proc. IEEE Conference on Decision and Control*, pp. 2210–2215, 2020.
43. A. Nikolakopoulou, M. S. Hong, and R. D. Braatz, "Output feedback control and estimation of dynamic neural networks using linear matrix inequalities," in *Proc. American Control Conference*, in press, 2021.

Dynamic Modeling and Control of a Continuous Biopharmaceutical Manufacturing Plant

Mohammad Amin Boojari, Simone Perra, Giorgio Colombo, Matteo Grossi,
Mark Nicholas Jones, Isuru Udugama, Morteza Nikkhah Nasab,
Mohammad Fakroleslam, Ali M. Sahlodin, Seyed Abbas Shojaosadati,
Krist V. Gernaey, and Seyed Soheil Mansouri

1 Introduction

With an annual growth rate estimated at more than 7% by 2024, biopharmaceuticals are an expanding industrial sector that delivers an increasingly heterogeneous range of products. The estimated market value is predicted to exceed $1100 billion in 2021 [1]. In this context, half of the global drug development is projected to be bio based within the next decade [2]. Biopharmaceutical manufacturing traditionally involves a similar sequence of unit operations that are divided into two main parts: upstream and downstream. The upstream processes typically comprise cell culture and harvest steps. Downstream processing includes all steps required to purify a biological product from cell culture broth to the final purified product. It typically involves multiple steps of centrifugation for biomass cell separation from the broth, filtration to obtain a higher biomolecule concentration stream, and a purification treatment, usually through chromatography [3]. Batch/fed-batch bioprocessing is currently the state of the art in the biopharmaceutical industry; each unit operation is completed

M. A. Boojari · S. A. Shojaosadati
Biotechnology Group, Faculty of Chemical Engineering, Tarbiat Modares University, Tehran, Iran

S. Perra · G. Colombo · M. Grossi · M. N. Jones · I. Udugama · K. V. Gernaey
S. S. Mansouri (✉)
Process and Systems Engineering Centre (PROSYS), Department of Chemical and Biochemical Engineering, Technical University of Denmark, Kgs. Lyngby, Denmark
e-mail: seso@kt.dtu.dk

M. N. Nasab · A. M. Sahlodin
Process Systems Engineering Laboratory, Department of Chemical Engineering, AmirKabir University of Technology (Tehran Polytechnic), Tehran, Iran

M. Fakroleslam
Process Engineering Department, Faculty of Chemical Engineering, Tarbiat Modares University, Tehran, Iran

© The Author(s), under exclusive license to Springer Nature Switzerland AG 2022   323
A. Fytopoulos et al. (eds.), *Optimization of Pharmaceutical Processes*, Springer
Optimization and Its Applications 189, https://doi.org/10.1007/978-3-030-90924-6_12

in sequence. The product outflow from one unit is typically collected in a large holding tank before being processed in the next step [4, 5]. This type of operation enables the design and optimization of the individual unit operations and facilitates off-line evaluation of key product quality attributes prior to subsequent processing steps. Improving product quality is especially crucial for biopharmaceuticals. Some studies have shown that protein aggregation and denaturation may occur if proteins are long-lastingly bound to chromatographic resins as a result of protein unfolding and interactions with other proteins on the resin surface [6–8]. Therefore, batch operation of a packed chromatography column could result in a wide variation in product quality; the proteins that are initially loaded on the column remain in the bound state over an hour, while proteins near the end of the load only stay bounded for a short period of time [5].

The final product must comply with the strict quality constraints of local and international regulatory agencies; it is easier to implement quality monitoring if each step is separated. Currently, a strong constraint of biopharmaceutical production is the strict time frame in which the process can be optimized. Regulators approve the drug and the related production process together, and after the approval, the process design is fixed. Considering that the major companies compete to release new active pharmaceutical ingredients (APIs) in the shortest time window possible, in order to exploit the drug product patents for a more extended period, the resources dedicated to process synthesis and optimization are relatively limited. However, due to the ever-increasing global competition, the industrial scenario is gradually shifting toward a continuous manufacturing standard.

Continuous processes require smaller operative volumes, reducing the complexity and the costs of controlling the key parameters of a large bioreactor. A smaller reactor size also reduces the chance of safety and quality hazards such as mutations, necrosis, and high concentration of by-products. These events lead to discarding entire production batches and halt the production, making up for major economic losses. An economic study by Walthe et al. [9] indicated that an integrated continuous biomanufacturing platform could reduce costs (net present value) by 55% compared to traditional batch processing. Much greater benefits have been reported for non-monoclonal antibody products in a continuous process, with more than a threefold decrease in capital costs [10]. In another study, the bioprocessing trend over the last 20 years was investigated. In the 1990s, the prevalent design for stable protein production was developed using 10–20 kL stainless steel bioreactors and large volume purification columns. A decade later, biotechnology companies switched to smaller bioreactors (e.g., 2 kL) and columns with smaller processing lots at a higher frequency. The continuous integrated operation is seen in this sense as a transitional phase in the process progression, moving toward high intensification, smaller equipment, smaller processing lots, and maximum capacity utilization [4].

Major pharmaceutical companies (e.g., Bayer, Lilly, GSK, Pfizer) are proceeding with major investments with the aim of developing the first integrated continuous processes [11]. In 2019, GSK launched the first continuous biopharmaceutical plant in Singapore to produce Daprodustat [12]. The declared benefit is a high production capacity, with a 50% reduction of the environmental impact. The FDA has officially embraced continuous processing applied to drug production and encourages the companies to exploit the new technologies and modeling tools to design more flexible and modular continuous plants.

Continuous processing also has the potential to bring about substantial changes in product quality through improved monitoring and accuracy of the microenvironment in the manufacturing process. Current batch processes generate biotherapeutics with wide variability [10]. For example, recombinant proteins, which are secreted by Chinese Hamster Ovary (CHO) cells at the start of a cell culture in a nutrient-rich environment, will remain in the bioreactor for several days before subsequent downstream processing.

According to several studies, a wide range of residence times in batch processes results in variations in the glycosylation profile, the extent of deamidation, and the level of degradation/aggregation [13–15].

The FDA's latest Regulatory Science Strategic Plan centered primarily on the use of quality by design (QbD) to enhance the manufacturing process to ensure and improve product quality. With this in mind, the FDA has established three new fields that would improve manufacturing quality, one of which is the use of "continuous processing" [16]. Janet Woodcock, Director of the Center for Drug Evaluation and Research, recently recognized continuous manufacturing as a crucial tool in modernizing pharmaceutical production [17].

While regulatory challenges are often recognized as a concern in adopting continuous bioprocessing, the FDA approved the first biopharmaceutical product manufactured via continuous perfusion in 1993, and today approximately 20 marketed biologic products from several companies use different elements of continuous bioprocessing [18, 19].

Development in biopharmaceutical manufacturing has increased interest in the application of process analytical technology (PAT), which ensures the final product quality through designing, analyzing, and controlling manufacturing through timely measurement of critical quality and performance attributes [20]. On-line measurement of critical quality attributes (CQAs) gives much more data on multivariable interactions and dynamics, with the potential for increased understanding of the process [2]. Depending on the process understanding, the data have been used to make first-principles models for each biopharmaceutical unit operation. The constructed models and real-time process monitoring facilitate the implementation of advanced control algorithms for producing higher-quality products [2]. The consistent product quality obtained by the real-time measurements and control strategy enables PAT to be recognized as a tool for applying the quality by design (QbD) approach advocated by regulatory agencies [21, 22]. The biological molecules' complexity and processes pose difficulties for the application of PAT to biopharmaceuticals, but the number and variety of high-tech instruments being built means that PAT is increasingly applied to biopharmaceuticals, where the variety of high-tech tools being developed ensures effective application [23, 24].

The increased data provided by PAT and associated feedforward and feedback control systems would be crucial to ensuring efficient long-term continuous operation.

2 Continuous Bioprocessing

2.1 Recent Developments in Upstream Processing

Batch, fed-batch, and continuous or perfusion are common cultivation modes employed for biopharmaceutical production. In batch cultivation, all essential nutrients are.

provided in the initial base medium. In the fed-batch process, nutrients are continuously fed into the bioreactor, while products remain in the bioreactor until the end of the cultivation. Perfusion culture involves the constant feeding of fresh media and removing spent media and products while retaining cells inside the bioreactor. A short product retention time in perfusion culture preserves product quality. This processing mode is more challenging regarding technique and sterility [25]. In a continuous or chemostat cultivation, fresh medium is continuously fed, and liquid culture containing products and microorganisms is continually removed at the same rate to keep the culture volume constant.

A perfusion culture is a favored option for the production of therapeutic monoclonal antibodies (mAbs) using mammalian cells since this cultivation mode reduces the residence time of the mAbs in the bioreactor. The cell retention devices (spin filter, tangential filters of flow, and alternating tangential flow filtration systems) in perfusion cultivation are crucial for recovering the culture medium, which contains the bioreactor's desired product [26].

Recent advances in upstream manufacturing have led to cost-effective, high-yield, and speedy biopharmaceutical production.

High-throughput devices (HTPDs) have been developed for the upstream process, such as mini-bioreactors and multi-well plates. These HTPDs now make it very simple to carry out all the screening experiments, including process optimization, to save time and cost before proceeding to scale up the biopharmaceutical production [26]. Continuous bioprocessing needs to be optimized for perfusion cell culture. Therefore, equipment manufacturers are motivated to develop appropriate HTP perfusion microbioreactors for perfusion culture optimization [19, 26].

Recent advances in single-use (SU) cultivation systems, including single-use probes/sensors and fluid components, have resulted in rapid upstream processing developments. Implementing single-use upstream processing led to less capital and operating costs with greater flexibility [26, 27]. A study on integrated continuous processing reported that about 30% of cost savings could be accomplished using disposable technologies concerning the stainless steel (SS) batch process [28]. The different types of single-use disposable systems include wave, stirred tank (ST), orbitally shaken (OS), and pneumatically mixed bioreactors [26, 29, 30].

Process Analytical Technology (PAT) for Upstream Processes

PAT enables the consistent generation of products with predetermined quality through real-time monitoring and process control. Process parameters that influence CQAs are called critical process parameters and must be observed or controlled to ensure that the process ends up with the desired quality [26]. Contrary to the principles of continuous processing, some of the existing testing methods involve long off-line protocols (e.g., bioburden). This leads to increasing cycle times, delays timely go/no-go decisions, and impairs the chance of real-time release testing [19]. There is a necessity for innovation in sensor technology, its configuration, and its robustness such that PAT can be applied for the advancement of continuous cultures [26]. The development of analytical process tools for perfusion bioreactor performance analysis has substantially contributed to regulatory issues regarding biopharmaceutical manufacturing [31]. The PAT tools are based on spectroscopy, which is used on-line (integrated into the bioreactor system), in-line (directly connected to the bioreactor), and at-line (manual sampling and analysis) and includes near-infrared (NIR), fluorescence, IR, and Raman [19, 26]. NIR spectroscopy has been widely implemented to determine the concentration of individual components in cell culture broth [32]. Raman spectroscopy can be applied in the pharmaceutical industry to monitor structural/chemical changes in proteins [19, 33, 34]. Examples of direct on-line quality attribute measurements include glycoform patterns such as sialylation [35]. The challenge would be to develop sensors for easier integration into continuous bioprocesses including the implementation of fiber-optic technology [36], noninvasive process monitoring [37], and the incorporation of advanced sensors into automated process control strategies [19].

2.2 Recent Progress in Downstream Processing

While continuous upstream bioprocessing is relatively well developed, the integration of continuous downstream processing remains an area of further development. In a typical bioprocess, an upstream bioreactor is followed by batch unit operations, which include clarification, hold steps, capture, and polishing [19]. The use of cell separation devices such as an alternating tangential flow (ATF) cell separation device typically addresses the clarification aspect of a continuous bioprocess. Periodic countercurrent chromatography (PCC) and simulated moving bed (SMB) chromatography are the two main options for continuous capture and polishing chromatography [19]. A chromatographic column unit operation typically includes load, wash, elution, and regeneration step. In both PCC and SMB chromatography, multiple columns in series run these steps in a cyclic manner. Continuous purification has progressed from SMB with six columns [38], to PCC with three columns [39], to twin-column chromatography with two columns [40]. Each method has its advantages and disadvantages. Basically, the balance between yield, capacity utilization, and productivity should be considered, and the optimum process would depend on several variables, including operating conditions. In multicolumn systems, elution streams from each column are typically pooled. In order to make sure that low-quality eluent material from a defective column is not pooled with material that has been processed properly, it would be helpful for individual columns to be monitored real time combined with feedback control to divert material from a malfunctioning column [19].

Process Analytical Technology (PAT) for Downstream Processing

There has been limited deployment of downstream PAT in bioprocessing. The restricted application can be attributed to the limited number of sensor options in downstream operations and systems [19]. PAT tools are used in the downstream processing to analyze protein concentrations, protein purity, host cell DNA, endotoxins, host cell proteins, and process-related impurities [26]. For these purposes, high-performance liquid chromatography (HPLC), spectroscopy, spectrometry, circular dichroism, and other tools have been used to monitor in-process CQAs in chromatography processes [41, 42]. In a study by Tiwari et al., an on-line HPLC was used as a PAT tool for an automated sampling of a product stream eluting from a chromatography column [43]. Fourier transform infrared (FTIR) spectroscopy has also been used in-line as a PAT tool for near real-time PEGylation degree estimation in chromatography [44].

Quick upstream testing of bioreactor samples has potential downstream benefits, in particular with regard to bulk harvest disposal. Decisions taken before the downstream processing will make it possible to confine contaminated cultures to the bioreactor, sparing cleanup of tanks and chromatography units [19]. It would be possible to apply advanced techniques such as next-generation sequencing toward viral screening; however, these technologies would require rigorous approaches for data analysis.

3 Modeling Approaches

The purpose of modeling is to represent physical phenomena through mathematical means. This quantitative understanding of the process reflects a high level of process understanding and is crucial to an effective control strategy design for quality. Models can be mostly divided into data-driven models and first-principles models. Data-driven models are intended to explain the process behavior using the input-output data collected [45]. Data-driven methods like principal component analysis (PCA) [46], partial least squares (PLS) [47], multiple linear regression [48], and artificial neural networks (ANN) [49] have been used to monitor and model biomanufacturing processes. The main advantages of data-driven models are that less fundamental and mechanistic information is required in comparison to first-principles models, and accordingly, the models can be more straightforwardly developed [45]. However, such models perform poorly on extrapolation and do not contain any mechanistic knowledge of the underlying processes, which limits their application to a predictive design and optimization [45]. A first-principles model, on the other hand, aims at both explaining and defining the process behavior. The models involve incorporating mathematical descriptions of the mass, energy, and momentum conservation laws, chemical and biological kinetics thermodynamics, and transport phenomena dynamics into a model that describes the unit operation [2, 45]. Mechanistic considerations within the model make it possible to use them for process synthesis, optimization, and scale-up.

Among various bioprocess modeling strategies, first-principles dynamic models are important as they predict temporal changes in the relevant bioprocess variables [50].

Dynamic models for the fermentation process can be classified into unstructured and structured models and as nonsegregated or segregated [45]. In unstructured models, only the extracellular concentrations in a bioreactor are considered, and intracellular dynamics of the cells are ignored, while in structured models, both intracellular information and extracellular conditions are considered [45, 50]. In nonsegregated models, all microorganisms are taken to be similar, while in segregated models, there could be several populations of microorganisms with different characteristics.

Complex interactions between the extracellular environment and intracellular enzymes and metabolites require the use of complex models. Genome-scale stoichiometric models currently have the best approximation of cell metabolic capabilities [50].

Metabolic and mechanistic model combinations result in a more comprehensive knowledge of the cellular organization. However, unstructured models provide acceptable results in many cases such as when the balanced growth condition is satisfied [51]. Therefore, using a bioreactor and a macrokinetic model in combination can be an effective compromise between simplifying the comprehensive process description usually provided by highly complex alternatives such as metabolic models.

Most of the work in the bioprocessing industry has revolved around modeling unit operations [45]. Models for bioreactor and chromatography are mature [46, 52–54]. However, unit operations do not operate individually, and changing a unit's operating conditions will affect downstream processing. This is what motivates integrated plant models. Despite the studies on the dynamic modeling and designing plant-wide control strategy for continuous pharmaceutical manufacturing (CM) [55–57], the researches on developing a benchmark process model in the domain of continuous biopharmaceutical manufacturing (CBM) are very limited [58].

In this study, an end-to-end biopharmaceutical production process of the API lovastatin is developed through a systematic process synthesis and design approach and then simulated. The developed simulation is intended to be used as a benchmark process model. It captures the generic process dynamics of a biopharmaceutical process. As such, it is well suited to use as a test problem to evaluate different processing scenarios in continuous and semicontinuous fermentation processes.

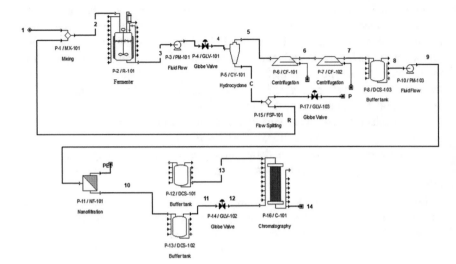

Fig. 1 End-to-end plant diagram

4   Reference Plant Introduction

The adopted case study is based on a steady-state design of an integrated biomanufacturing process to produce lovastatin [59] through fermentation of the fun-
gus*Aspergillus terreus*. It is fundamental at this point to state that the goal of the
adopted model is not to be developed as a study on a specific biomolecule; lovastatin
production has been selected as a case study for convenience and data availability.
However, this model is proposed as a generic pathway for upstream production and
downstream purification of a biomolecule produced by fermentation [60].

In the upstream section, lovastatin is produced by the biomass (*Aspergillus
terreus*) in a CSTR (continuous stirred tank reactor) fermenter. The fermenter is
constantly fed fresh medium from a mixing unit that outputs a homogeneous solution. The fermentation broth coming from the CSTR fermenter is processed through
a hydro-cyclone (HC-01) separator. The hydro-cyclone outputs two streams: the
stream rich (R) in biomass is recycled back into the CSTR and partially purged;
the stream poor in biomass (5) is sent to the downstream section. The downstream
section consists of a sequence of separation steps. The centrifugation steps remove
the remaining biomass and other heavy contaminants; the nanofiltration section
is designed to concentrate the solution before the final purification step. The
chromatography section is designed to obtain a solution of purified API; the
technology of reversed-phase chromatography is adopted in this case (Fig. 1).

5   Introduction to Lovastatin

Lovastatin, mainly produced through fermentation, was the first statin to be approved by the Food and Drug Administration in 1987 and made available on the pharmaceutical market as an anticholesterolemic drug. Although lovastatin production is outdated, its collocation in the reacting mixture as an extracellular product, which typically requires the use of fewer unit operations in the downstream purification train than that of intracellular products, along with the availability of an unstructured kinetic model, is intended to be an essential factor for the choice of the API lovastatin as a suitable case for the development of a benchmark process model [59].

Lovastatin is a secondary metabolite belonging to the group of organic compounds. The main known organisms to produce it are *Penicillium citrinum*, *Monascus ruber*, and *Aspergillus terreus*. Considering *Aspergillus terreus*, it releases lovastatin as a secondary metabolite, with an extracellular expression, in the form of β-hydroxy acid–mevinolinic acid [61]. The highest lovastatin titer, achieved with an optimized fed-batch process, fluctuates around 1 g/l with productivity around 6 mg/l/h [62].

6   Upstream Process Design and Kinetic Model Selection

6.1   Kinetic Model

The first step requires selecting an unstructured kinetic model to describe the underlying physical and chemical phenomena occurring during the biochemical reaction of interest. This type of model is so conceived that they enable the prediction of the specific growth/consumption rate by means of a single black box stoichiometry, which is a function of one or a few independent variables. As proposed by Bizukojc et al. [62], rates of consumption or production of reactants and products in lovastatin biosynthesis are based on an empirical relation using yield coefficients instead of stoichiometric coefficients that would be difficult to evaluate owing to the complex stoichiometry of fermentation reactions. The implemented model [62] is based on studies on the strain *Aspergillus terreus* ATCC 20542 in aqueous liquid suspension. The reference work aims to retrieve a microkinetic model for lovastatin production, based on a set of batch and fed-batch runs over different reaction volumes. The model is here adapted to be integrated into a continuous process model. Considering the high amount of biomass required for production, a Contois' type kinetic is selected for substrate consumption, in which the medium principal components are lactose, considered as the exclusive carbon source, and yeast extract, as the nitrogen source. The excess of organic nitrogen exerts inhibition of lovastatin biosynthesis and lactose uptake. Lactose is utilized both for the biomass growth and for the lovastatin synthesis, and therefore, two separate terms are required in the specific mass balance. In this case, product inhibition is neglected as it becomes relevant only for product titers higher than 200 mg l^{-1}. Lovastatin production begins in the exponential growth phase and stabilizes during the stationary phase; this is accounted for in the model with two distinct production rates relative to the two metabolic steps.

The nomenclature—in an appendix to this chapter—includes the meaning of the various parameters used in the equations below. The formulas refer to the substrates lactose (LAC) and nitrogen (N), the fungal biomass (X), and the product lovastatin (LOV).

Other solid by-products are found in the fermentation broth, but their presence is neglected in the present model as they do not apparently influence the target API's production. The same reasoning is applied to the low concentration salts dissolved in the broth, which have a negligible effect on the production. Water production related to the organism metabolism is neglected in the kinetic equations, and the molecule is neglected in the species balance. In any case, water is present in excess by orders of magnitude; therefore, it is convenient to avoid complexity in the model. The resulting model is given in Eqs. (1)–(4).

$$r_{LA} = -\frac{1}{Y_{X/LA}} \cdot \mu_{max} \frac{C_{LA}}{C_{LA} + K_{LA} + C_X} \cdot \frac{C_N}{C_N + K_N + C_X} \cdot \frac{K_{I,N}}{K_{I,N} + C_X}$$
$$-\frac{1}{Y_{LO/LA}} \cdot q_{max}^{LO} \cdot \frac{C_{LA}}{C_{LA} + K_{LA}^{LO} + C_X} \cdot \frac{K_{I,N}^{LO}}{K_{I,N}^{LO} + C_X} \tag{1}$$

$$r_N = -\frac{1}{Y_{X/N}} \cdot \mu_{max} \cdot \frac{C_{LA}}{C_{LA} + K_{LA} + C_X} \cdot \frac{C_N}{C_N + K_N + C_X} \tag{2}$$

$$r_X = \frac{C_{LA}}{C_{LA} + K_{LA} + C_X} \cdot \frac{C_N}{C_N + K_N + C_X} \tag{3}$$

$$r_{LO} = q_{max}^{LO} \cdot \frac{C_{LA}}{C_{LA} + K_{LA}^{LO} + C_X} \cdot \frac{K_{I,N}^{LO}}{K_{I,N}^{LO} + C_X} + K_{LO} \cdot C_{LA} \tag{4}$$

The terms r_{LAC} and r_N represent the volumetric substrate uptake rates, while r_X and r_{LOV} are the volumetric production rates of biomass and lovastatin.

6.2   Mixer – P1/MX10

The mixing unit implemented in the current work is a static mixer, a precision device for the continuous mixing of materials without moving parts. The recycle stream and the fresh feed are mixed in this unit before entering the reactor. For the sake of this simulation, it is assumed perfect and instantaneous mixing, and the following total and species balance equations are implemented into the block P1/MX10.

$$Q_1 + Q_R - Q_2 = 0 \tag{5}$$

$$C_{X,1} \cdot Q_1 + C_{X,R} \cdot Q_R - C_{X,2} \cdot Q_2 = 0 \tag{6}$$

$$C_{LA,1} \cdot Q_1 + C_{LA,R} \cdot Q_R - C_{LA,2} \cdot Q_2 = 0 \tag{7}$$

$$C_{LO,1} \cdot Q_1 + C_{LO,R} \cdot Q_R - C_{LO,2} \cdot Q_2 = 0 \tag{8}$$

$$C_{N,1} \cdot Q_1 + C_{N,R} \cdot Q_R - C_{N,2} \cdot Q_2 = 0 \tag{9}$$

6.3 Bioreactor: P2/R10

The entire production is considered to happen inside a continuous stirred tank reactor (CSTR), with the assumption of constant liquid density over time and no liquid accumulation. The primary assumption introduced by the CSTR model is to consider an instantaneous and perfect mixing inside the bioreactor: this means that the output stream composition is identical to the composition of the material inside the reactor, which is a function of residence time and kinetic rates of reaction. As claimed by Bizukojc et al. [62], the thermal effects of lovastatin generation are negligible for the present reaction; therefore, in the current work, the temperature inside the bioreactor is assumed as constant. The conditions such as pH, temperature, stirring speed, etc., of the bioreactor processing are assumed equal to those of the experimental tests [62]. The current values of the kinetic rates have been evaluated. Considering the previous assumptions, the model for a transient state analysis is developed. The total and species mass balances are as provided in Eqs. (10)–(14).

$$\frac{dV}{dt} = Q_2 - Q_3 \tag{10}$$

$$\frac{d(C_{LA} \cdot V)}{dt} = C_{LA,2} \cdot Q_2 - C_{LA,3} \cdot Q_3 + r_{lA} \cdot C_{X,3} \cdot V \tag{11}$$

$$\frac{d(C_N \cdot V)}{dt} = C_{N,2} \cdot Q_2 - C_{N,3} \cdot Q_3 + r_N \cdot C_{X,3} \cdot V \tag{12}$$

$$\frac{d(C_{LO} \cdot V)}{dt} = C_{LO,2} \cdot Q_2 - C_{LO,3} \cdot Q_3 + r_{LO} \cdot C_{X,3} \cdot V \tag{13}$$

$$\frac{d(C_X \cdot V)}{dt} = C_{X,2} \cdot Q_2 - C_{X,3} \cdot Q_3 + r_X \cdot C_{X,3} \cdot V \tag{14}$$

6.4 Hydro-Cyclone Separator: P5/CY10

The implementation of the hydro-cyclone in the recirculation loop is based on the theory of Villadsen et al. [3], introducing the benefits of increased productivity and easier downstream treatment, with the downside of increasing operative costs due to additional pumping. Hydro-cyclones are density-based separators that allow separating solid particles—in this case, biomass—from a liquid suspension by means of centripetal forces within a vortex. Assuming an optimized design for the process flow rate, the proposed model [23] is based on the split ratio $\alpha = Q_C/Q_5$. The second parameter to be introduced is the separation efficiency β defined as $\beta = C_{X,C}/C_{X,4}$. In the case study, $\alpha = 0.6$ and $\beta = 1.6$ have been selected for the current hydro-cyclone model. It is assumed that the cyclone affects exclusively the cell concentration, so the mass balances are given as follows:

$$Q_5 + Q_4 - Q_C = 0 \tag{15}$$

$$C_{X,4} \cdot Q_4 + C_{X,5} \cdot Q_5 - C_{X,C} \cdot Q_C = 0 \tag{16}$$

$$C_{LA,4} \cdot Q_4 + C_{LA,5} \cdot Q_5 - C_{LA,C} \cdot Q_C = 0 \tag{17}$$

$$C_{N,4} \cdot Q_4 + C_{N,5} \cdot Q_5 - C_{N,C} \cdot Q_C = 0 \tag{18}$$

$$C_{LO,4} \cdot Q_4 + C_{LO,5} \cdot Q_5 - C_{LO,C} \cdot Q_C = 0 \tag{19}$$

6.5 Purge – P15/FSP10

The purge is present in order to control the amount of biomass that is recycled; it is a necessary element to avoid the accumulation of by-products and nonviable biomass in the recycle loop. As seen in the mass balance (Eq. 20), the purge introduces two streams into the system; the purge stream (Q_P) is removed, while the recycle stream (Q_R) is sent back to the mixing section.

$$Q_C - Q_R - Q_P = 0 \tag{20}$$

6.6 Operating Parameters

Herein, **the critical design parameters** are introduced for the continuous fermentation system with biomass recycle. The volumetric recirculation factor RF (Eq. 21) is an important parameter for the recycle loop performance, representing the ratio between the recirculation stream flow rate Q_R and the medium inlet flow rate Q_1. Therefore, this value regulates the biomass concentration in the bioreactor.

Then the selection of the recirculation factor is based on the value that grants the highest production peak. The optimal retrieved value is RF = 0.8 [36]. The cell recirculation ratio (Eq. 22) relates the biomass concentration in the recycle stream to the concentration leaving the bioreactor. Increasing the β ratio at a constant dilution rate brings an increase in overall API productivity and final titer. The dilution rate D is the ratio between the CSTR inlet flow rate Q_2 and its volume V. A high dilution rate implies a low residence time for the liquid phase inside the bioreactor vessel, so the biomass cells have lesser time to produce lovastatin. As the kinetic rates for lovastatin production are particularly slow, it is necessary to reduce the rate as much as possible; therefore, considering the smaller scale of continuous processing equipment, a relatively large bioreactor volume of 5000 L has been selected. The purge ratio P_R is directly proportional to the amount of material removed from the system through the purge. In fact, the use of a high purge ratio would mean in general, a lower amount of biomass is recycled and thus a drop in product yield; on the other hand, the amount of impurities in the recirculation loop would decrease.

$$RF = \frac{Q_R}{Q_1} \tag{21}$$

$$D = \frac{Q_2}{V} \tag{22}$$

$$P_R = \frac{Q_P}{Q_C} \tag{23}$$

7 Downstream Process Design and Modeling

7.1 Centrifugation System: P6/CF10

The selection of centrifugation as a first step is widespread in the pharmaceutical industry and allows the removal of the solid bulk that would completely impair all the following separation steps. In this case, considering the objective to create an end-to-end benchmark, a continuous centrifugation system is implemented. The selected equipment is a tubular bowl centrifuge, which is a common choice for biomass removal.

The main parameter in selecting a centrifuge is the radial force, generally expressed in relation to the gravitational force. For the adopted model, the force (F) is related to the distance from the center of rotation and the rotational speed through Eq. 24 [63].

$$F = 11.18 \cdot r \cdot \left(\frac{N}{1000}\right)^2 \tag{24}$$

where F is the relative centrifugal radial force, r is the distance from the center of rotation [cm], and N is the rotational speed [rpm]. In order to estimate the amount of separated cells in a simplified procedure, a separation efficiency factor (X) is implemented. This factor represents the mass fraction of biomass that is removed from the feed. This method is effectively adopted in multiple industrial cases [64]. The selection of the separation efficiency factor is guided by literature research. The value ranges from $X = 90\%$ to $X = 98\%$; for the present case, the selected factor is $X = 95\%$. Considering that it is required to obtain a biomass concentration below the threshold of 30 mg/l, a single centrifuge is not sufficient. It has been assumed that the centrifugation process influences only the biomass concentration; moreover, consistent with the other process units, mixture density is considered as constant. For simplicity, only the balances of the first centrifuge are reported below; the balances of the second one are similar.

$$Q_6 - Q_5 = 0 \qquad (25)$$

$$(1 - X) \cdot Q_6 \cdot C_{X,6} - Q_5 \cdot C_{X,5} = 0 \qquad (26)$$

$$Q_T \cdot C_{LO,6} - Q_5 \cdot C_{LO,5} = 0 \qquad (27)$$

$$Q_T \cdot C_{LA,6} - Q_5 \cdot C_{LA,5} = 0 \qquad (28)$$

$$Q_T \cdot C_{N,6} - Q_5 \cdot C_{N,5} = 0 \qquad (29)$$

7.2 Buffer Tank: P8/DCS10

Buffer tanks are the most straightforward solution in continuous manufacturing if it is required to reduce the flow rate and concentration fluctuations. The capacity of the tank is proportional to the degree of smoothing it can offer. Installation of the tank before the nanofiltration process has been necessary also to allow the membrane cleaning or replacement without shutting down the entire process. The buffer tank volume capacity has to be large enough in order to smoothen flow rate and concentration deviations, but on the other hand, the residence time is constrained by the biological degradation of the product molecules. Lovastatin biological degradation time is correlated to pH, temperature, by-products, and other parameters [61] that in the current work have not been examined. In the absence of experimental data, a reference liquid volume of 1000 L has been considered. The total volumetric flow rate and component mass balances are expressed in Eqs. (30)–(33).

$$\frac{dV}{dt} = Q_8 - Q_7 \qquad (30)$$

Fig. 2 Generic concentration profile of the solute in nanofiltration membrane processing

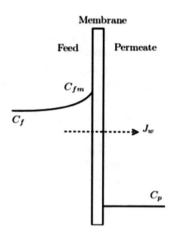

$$\frac{d\,(C_{LA}.V)}{dt} = C_{LA,8} \cdot Q_8 - C_{LA,7} \cdot Q_N \tag{31}$$

$$\frac{d\,(C_{LO}.V)}{dt} = C_{LO,8} \cdot Q_8 - C_{L0,7} \cdot Q_N \tag{32}$$

$$\frac{d\,(C_N.V)}{dt} = C_{N,8} \cdot Q_8 - C_{N,7} \cdot Q_N \tag{33}$$

7.3 Nanofiltration: P11/NF10

It is necessary to concentrate as much as possible the API solution in order to reduce the costs and the required capacity of the chromatography section. The API is a minor constituent dissolved in a large water volume. Nanofiltration is the general choice to concentrate the fermentation broth, especially in the pharmaceutical industry [65]. The typical operating pressure is between 5 and 40 bar, and the membrane pore size varies between 0.5 and 2 nm for a molecular weight cutoff value of approximately 300–500 g/mol (lovastatin molecular weight is around 404.5 g/mol) [59]. The mass transfer process plays a key role in understanding the mechanism of filtration, and two parameters characterize this process: the rejection factor (Rej) of the solute and the permeance (Perm) of the solvent. The rejection factor for a specific compound is given by

$$Rej_i = 1 - \frac{C_{i,PE}}{C_{i,f}} \tag{34}$$

where $C_{i,p}$ is the concentration of the solute in the permeate stream and $C_{i,f}$ is the concentration of the solute on the retentive side of the membrane, as reported in Fig. 2.

Considering that the separation of components in this application is caused by a steric exclusion mechanism, the model is based on a set of experimental Rej values of comparable components on a commercial membrane—DOW NF90—with a molecular weight cutoff of 300–500 g/mol. A strong assumption adopted in the refence work is to maintain constant rejection factors in different operating conditions; for a more specific implementation, it would be necessary to retrieve different Rej values depending on inlet stream concentration and operating conditions. In this case, a pressure-dependent rejection factor is implemented for lovastatin, based on experimental performance curves from literature [66, 67]. It is useful to introduce the permeate volumetric flux Jw, which is generally estimated through the Hagen-Poiseuille equation adapted for membrane parameters [67]:

$$J_W = \frac{1}{\mu \cdot (R_m + R_{CP})} \cdot \Delta P \qquad (35)$$

where μ is the feed's dynamic viscosity, Rm is the membrane resistance, and RCP is the concentration polarization boundary resistance. The membrane resistance Rm is dependent on the effective pore radius, the effective membrane thickness, and the effective porosity of the membrane.

In this case, the membrane selection is based on the work of Košutić et al. [68] in which an analogous case of filtration for a similar component is developed with a DOW NF90 membrane. From the same study, an experimental value for the permeate volumetric flux Jw = 57.90 L/m²/h has been adopted as the steady-state reference value, corresponding to a pressure gradient of ΔP = 8 bar. The retentive flow rate is typically 10–15% of the incoming flux [31]; with this target value, the membrane surface (AM) is set to 0.398 m². Assuming a constant feed dynamic viscosity μ and a membrane resistance R_m not dependent on a pressure gradient, it is possible to define a resistance factor RF:

$$RF = (\mu.Rm)^{-1} \qquad (36)$$

Peeva et al. formulated a model for continuous nanofiltration operations based on a set of linear algebraic equations (pore flow mechanism) [69]. The model is applied to the present study to simulate the behavior of lactose, nitrogen, and lovastatin concentrations in the retentive and permeate streams.

The nanofiltration model equations reported below consist of an overall volumetric balance (Eq. 37), three mass component balances (Eqs. 38–40), the membrane permeate equation (Eq. 41), and three concentration balances derived from the rejection factor definition:

$$Q_9 - Q_{PE} - Q_{10} = 0 \qquad (37)$$

$$Q_9 \cdot C_{LO,9} - Q_{PE} \cdot C_{LO,PE} - Q_{10} \cdot C_{LO,10} = 0 \qquad (38)$$

$$Q_9 \cdot C_{LA,9} - Q_{PE} \cdot C_{LA,PE} - Q_{10} \cdot C_{LA,10} = 0 \qquad (39)$$

$$Q_9 \cdot C_{N,9} - Q_{PE} \cdot C_{N,PE} - Q_{10} \cdot C_{N,10} = 0 \tag{40}$$

$$Q_{PE} = A_M \cdot J_W \tag{41}$$

$$C_{LA,PE} = C_{LA,10} \cdot \left(1 - Rej_{LA}\right) \tag{42}$$

$$C_{N,PE} = C_{N,10} \cdot \left(1 - Rej_N\right) \tag{43}$$

$$C_{LO,PE} = C_{LO,10} \cdot \left(1 - Rej_{LO}\right) \tag{44}$$

7.4 Buffer Tank: PC13/DCS10

This tank accumulates the volume that is the fed in a discontinuous operation to the chromatography section. It fills up constantly and it discharges a specific liquid volume at regular intervals. It is a crucial element considering the high residence time of the chromatography operation. The tank also allows to mitigate small variations in the concentration of the feed, before the injection. The precautions described for the T-01 tank are still valid. The total volumetric flow rate and component mass balances for the tank are expressed as follows:

$$\frac{dV}{dt} = Q_{10} - Q_{11} \tag{45}$$

$$\frac{d\left(C_{LA}.V\right)}{dt} = C_{LA,10} \cdot Q_{10} - C_{LA,11} \cdot Q_H \tag{46}$$

$$\frac{d\left(C_{LO}.V\right)}{dt} = C_{LO,10} \cdot Q_{10} - C_{LO,11} \cdot Q_H \tag{47}$$

$$\frac{d\left(C_N.V\right)}{dt} = C_{N,10} \cdot Q_{10} - C_{N10} \cdot Q_H \tag{48}$$

7.5 Chromatography Columns – P16/C10

The concentrated stream produced from nanofiltration is stored in a buffer tank, ready to be processed by chromatographic columns. This represents the last stage of downstream processing and is referred to as the purification step, in which lovastatin is separated from the other compounds. As lovastatin is a non-polar compound, the reversed-phase HPLC (RP-HPLC) method was adopted for the present case study. In order to obtain industrial-scale production, it is required to use multiple RP-HPLC columns in parallel.

The implemented species mass balance is

$$\frac{\partial}{\partial t}m_{acc,i}(x,t) = \dot{m}^x_{conv,i}(x,t) - \dot{m}^{x+dx}_{conv,i}(x,t) + \dot{m}^x_{disp,i}(x,t) + \dot{m}^{x+dx}_{disp,i}(x,t) - \dot{m}^x_{mt,i}(x,t)$$
$$(49)$$

where m_{acc} is a mass accumulation term, $m_{conv,i}$ is convective mass flow rate, and $m_{mt,i}$ is mass transfer rate into particles. It is assumed that the total mass transfer into the particle surface is equal to the accumulation of the ith component.

$$\frac{\partial}{\partial t}m_{acc,ads,i} = \dot{m}_{mt,i} \qquad (50)$$

where $m\bar{m}_{acc,ads,i}$ is the overall accumulation of the ith component in the stationary phase.

The design and the count of the columns were developed with the following constraints. It is assumed that the injected solvent flow rate is pumped at constant $Q_S=20l/h$, and the solvent injection time is retrieved as

$$t_{inj} = \frac{V_{inj}}{Q_S} \qquad (51)$$

where t_{inj} [h] is injection time and V_{inj} [l] is injected solvent volume. Considering a column with a volume capacity of 15 L, the working time of the developed chromatography model takes around 12 h to achieve compound separation. Thus, the aim of the sizing process is that the columns process the amount of liquid that is expected to enter the buffer tank in 12 h. Each injection provides an overall volume of 30.8 L that has to be distributed equally among the chromatography columns. Utilizing columns with a capacity volume of 15 L, at least six HPLC columns are required to process the injected liquid volume. Therefore, considering six HPLC columns working in parallel, the steady-state injection time is around 0.26 h for each column, and the overall injection time lasts around 1.54 h. The mobile phase flow velocity u is given by the ratio between the solvent flow rate and the cross-section area A of the column:

$$u = \frac{Q_S}{A_{HPLC}} \qquad (52)$$

where A_{HPLC} [m^2] is the section area of HPLC column and u[m/h] is the mobile phase flow velocity.

8 Control Strategy

Every chemical process is a dynamic system that changes over time. To handle such variations, the study and application of an effective control system is crucial. A well-functioning control strategy is vital for the automated operation and monitoring of complex technical processes. An effective process control strategy can improve process safety and profitability.

In this section, a plant-wide control strategy has been developed for a continuous biopharmaceutical manufacturing case. Continuous processing is gaining significant ground in pharmaceutical drug development, as the cost benefits in many cases outweigh the practical challenges. Moving to continuous manufacturing generally requires more process knowledge, advanced monitoring, and control technologies than batch processes. On the other hand, the potential benefits are increased productivity, higher time efficiency, and a reduction of both energy needs and overall amount of waste.

As already stated, the basis of the current work is a steady-state model taken from the literature of a pharmaceutical bioprocess designed for the production of lovastatin [52], in which a plant-wide process synthesis has been undertaken and a computer simulation has been developed in the MATLAB/Simulink programming environment (Fig. 3). The challenge now is to design and implement an effective multivariable feedback control strategy in this reference model, which should optimize the performance of the plant as a whole instead of isolated unit operations. The questions to be answered concern what are the variables to measure, manipulate, or regulate and how to achieve a robust control system for the pharmaceutical process that correctly copes with external disturbances, uncertainties, and implementation errors. A comprehensive control structure has been developed and implemented into a computational testing model at a later stage in the next section. The control structure strategy adopted in the current study relies on feedback control principles.

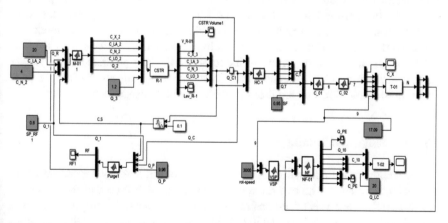

Fig. 3 Continuous open-loop benchmark simulation in Simulink

Table 1 The values of the stationary base case scenario for the upstream process (concentrations and bioreactor volume)

Concentration	Biomass	Lactose	Adenine	Lovastatin
C_1 [g/l]	0	20	4	0
C_2 [g/l]	36.71	7.35	1.49	0.1
C_3 [g/l]	106.35	14.81	2.52	1.2
C_5 [g/l]	10.64	14.81	2.52	1.2
C_R [g/l]	170.16	14.81	2.52	1.2
C_{PE} [g/l]	0	7.79	1.83	0.11
C_{00} [g/l]	0	77.91	8.7	11
CSTR volume, L				5000

Table 2 The values of the stationary base case scenario for the upstream process (flow rates)

Q_1 [l/h]	35.60
Q_2 [l/h]	64.02
Q_5 [l/h]	25.63
Q_C [l/h]	38.42
Q_R [l/h]	9.96
Q_P [l/h]	28.50
Q_{PE} [l/h]	23.07
Q_{10} [l/h]	2.56

8.1 Upstream Control Structure

Based on the values of the key parameters suggested in the optimal design parameters evaluation carried out in the literature reference study [52], which represents the starting point of the current work, an optimal steady-state base case for the upstream process has been determined using the computational model. In other words, a steady-state base case scenario has been achieved by setting the flow rates Q_1, Q_4, and Q_P to the proper value to obtain the best possible key parameter values, according to the reference study. The stationary values obtained for each concentration and flow rate are listed in Tables 1 and 2, respectively.

Control Design and Tuning

The selection and implementation of a suitable control strategy for the upstream process was pursued. The control system design has been preceded by degrees of freedom (DOF) analysis of the upstream process in order to identify the variables suitable to be manipulated. The DOF is defined as the number of controlled variables that can be regulated by the control system [70]. In this framework, the number of degrees of freedom thus corresponds strictly to the number of manipulated variables that may be utilized in control loops. The DOF quantity is evaluated as the difference between the total number of variables and the number of chemical and physical equations:

Table 3 Independent
variables of the continuous
section

Stream	Variables
1	Q_1
2	$Q_2, C_{X,2}, C_{LA,2}, C_{N,2}, C_{LO,2}$
3	$Q_3, C_{LA,3}, C_{N,3}, C_{N,2}, C_{LO,3}$
5	$Q_5, C_{X,5}$
C	$C_{X,3}$
P	Q_P
R	Q_R

DOF = number of variables of the system–number of equations of the system.

All the upstream process units such as mixer, bioreactor, and hydro-cyclone rely on one overall volumetric balance and four species balance equations. When these equations are added together with the purge volumetric balance (Eq. 20), the total number of equations results in 16 (from Eq. 5 to Eq. 20). Considering hydro-cyclone dynamics – hydro-cyclone split ratio $a=0.6$ and hydro-cyclone separation factor $\beta=1.9$ – two degrees of freedom are saturated. β value is proportional to the amount of biomass that is present in the reactor at any time, therefore increasing the total production of the molecule. Another effect is that increasing β reduces the amount of biomass sent to the downstream section, easing the separation procedure.

Rearranging and modifying the equations by applying all the simplifications, three hydro-cyclone balances turn into null identities. The number of equations is therefore reduced to 13.

The total number of **independent** variables (reported in Table 3) considering the bioreactor volume V is 16. Ultimately, the final DOF count is three, meaning that there are three variables suitable to be manipulated (Q_4, Q_P, and Q_1) and as many controlled variables (V, $C_{LOV,4}$, and RF) to be selected.

The bioreactor has been equipped with a level controller, whose aim is to maintain a stable amount of liquid in the vessel by manipulating the outgoing flow rate. A Relative Gain Array (RGA) and the Niederlinski index (NI) [71] have then been computed to obtain an appropriate pairing of the controlled and manipulated variables for the design of two other control loops. Given the process transfer functions, the RGA is used to obtain a tentative loop pairing for the decentralized control system. For a 2×2 control system, the RGA reads

$$RGA = \begin{pmatrix} \lambda_{11} & \lambda_{12} \\ \lambda_{21} & \lambda_{22} \end{pmatrix},$$

where the columns and the rows correspond to the manipulated and controlled variables, respectively. Pairing of a controlled variable with a manipulated variable must be avoided if their corresponding relative gain λ_{ij} is negative. The RGA criterion favors pairing of a controlled and a manipulated variable with the relative gain as close to 1 as possible in order to minimize the effects of loop interactions

Table 4 Index notation for the upstream manipulated and controlled variables

Manipulated variables		Controlled variables	
Q_1	Q_P	$C_{LOV,4}$	RF
u_1	u_2	y_1	y_2

Table 5 RGA and NI results of the control loop pairing configurations

Pairing	RGA	NI
Diagonal (u_1-y_1, u_2-y_2)	$\lambda_{11} = \lambda_{22} = -0.57$	-1.75
Off-diagonal (u_1-y_2, u_2-y_1)	$\lambda_{12} = \lambda_{21} = 1.57$	0.64

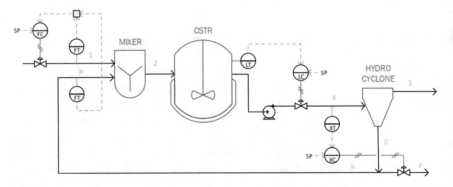

Fig. 4 Complete control system design of the upstream process

on the control performance. The NI is then used to ascertain the stability of the closed-loop system using the recommended RGA pairing. A positive NI provides a sufficient condition for stability. The index notation used for these manipulated and controlled variables is shown in Table 4, and the results of the two pairing combinations are reported in Table 5.

Thus, off-diagonal pairing (u_1-y_2, u_2-y_1) has been selected to be implemented in the upstream process. This means that product concentration $C_{LOV,4}$ is controlled by manipulating the purge flow rate Q_P and the recirculation factor RF is controlled by manipulating the mixer inlet flow rate Q_1. The comprehensive control structure is represented in Fig. 4.

The parameters of each controller have been selected by relying on analytical tuning rules (the SIMC rule [65] is used here) and through an integrated Simulink tuning tool named "PID Tuner." The devised process units and control structure have been implemented into a computational simulation model, developed in the MATLAB/Simulink environment. For implementing "PID Controller" blocks in the computational model, controller parameters are specified as shown in Table 6.

Table 6 Upstream controllers' tuned parameters

Controlled variable	Manipulated variable	Tuning method	Controller parameters		
			K_c	τ_I [h]	τ_D [h]
Bioreactor level, V	Bioreactor effluent rate, Q_4	SIMC	−12.5	0.8	–
Lovastatin concentration, $C_{LOV,4}$	Purge flow rate, Q_P	PID tuner	−8.211	406.08	$92.72(\tau_D = 2.41)$
Recirculation factor, RF	Mixer inlet flow rate, Q_1	PID tuner	0.047	0.1546	–

Table 7 The values of the stationary base case scenario for the downstream process (concentrations and volume capacities of buffer tanks)

Concentration	Cells	Lactose	Nitrogen	Lovastatin
C_5 [g/l]	10.64	14.81	2.52	1.2
C_6 [g/l]	0.53	14.81	2.52	1.2
C_7 [g/l]	0.03	14.81	2.52	1.2
C_9 [g/l]	–	14.81	2.52	1.2
C_{10} [g/l]	–	14.81	8.70	11
C_{PE} [g/l]	–	7.79	1.83	0.11
C_{11} [g/l]	–	77.91	8.7	11
Buffer tank "A" volume, L				1000
Buffer tank "B" volume, L				100

Table 8 The values of the stationary base case scenario for the downstream process (flow rates)

Q_5 [l/h]	25.63
Q_6 [l/h]	25.63
Q_7 [l/h]	25.63
Q_8 [l/h]	25.63
Q_{10} [l/h]	2.57
Q_{PE} [l/h]	23.07
Q_{11} [l/h]	20 for $t \leq t_{inj}$

8.2 Downstream Control Structure

Starting from the upstream inputs, an optimal steady-state base case for the downstream process has been determined based on the considerations and assumptions made throughout the downstream equipment's modeling. The steady-state values for the concentrations, flow rates, and buffer tank volumes are listed in Tables 7 and 8.

Control Design and Tuning

The design and implementation of a suitable control strategy for downstream processing have been dealt with differently compared to the upstream process. Due

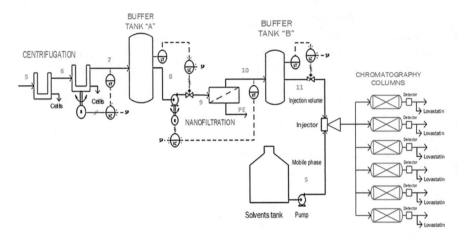

Fig. 5 Overview of the complete control system design of the downstream process

to the higher intrinsic complexity of downstream process units, a comprehensive analysis of the system degrees of freedom and control loop interactions has not been carried out. On the other hand, a trial and error strategy has been adopted, whose methodology is to select manipulated and controlled variables based on process control experience and literature examples and then simulate the effect of external disturbances in the designed computational model to prove their effectiveness and stability.

The upper limit for residual biomass concentration in the centrifuge outlet stream has been observed introducing a PI controller that enhances the centrifuge's separation efficiency by increasing its rotational speed. The first buffer tank has been provided with a sluggish PI level controller that smooths the inlet flow rate oscillations to the outlet stream, which is then pumped by a variable speed pump to pass through the nanofiltration membrane. To achieve a stable lovastatin concentration in the retentate stream, a PI controller regulates the pump's rotational speed needed to provide the correct pressure gradient to the nanofiltration process. For the second buffer tank, a different type of level control has been designed, which is not operating continuously and has a discrete-time nature. This discrete-time P controller follows the discontinuous nature of chromatography columns, actuating its corrective action every time right before each injection run of the chromatography columns. The control purpose is to increase or reduce the sample volumes injected in the chromatography columns in order to keep a fixed amount of liquid volume of the tank. The complete control structure of the downstream process is reported in Fig. 5.

As for the upstream process, the implemented controllers' settings have been tuned by applying analytical tuning rules or using an integrated Simulink tuning tool with the designed controller parameters specified as shown in Table 9.

Table 9 Downstream controllers and tuned parameter values

Controlled variable	Manipulated variable	Tuning method	Controller parameters		
			K_c	τ_I [h]	τ_D [h]
Residual biomass concentration, $C_{X,7}$	Centrifuge rotational speed	PID tuner	-4.8×10^{-4}	0.1	–
Buffer tank "A" level, V	Buffer tank "A" outlet flow rate, Q_9	SIMC	-71×10^{-4}	560	–
Buffer tank "B" level, V	Buffer tank "A" outlet flow rate, Q_{11}	PID tuner	0.17	–	–
Produced lovastatin concentration, $C_{LOV,10}$	Rotational speed of the pump	PID tuner	0.23	1	–

9 Unification of the Computational Models and Final Simulation

In this section, the upstream and downstream computational models are finalized and ready to be unified in a single comprehensive Simulink model, which will be further tested for several disturbances. The comprehensive Simulink computational model is represented in Fig. 6.

In this context, the medium stream nitrogen concentration $C_{N,1}$ as a simulation case for testing the designed control system is subjected to a permanent -15% step change at time $t = 200$ h, as reported in Fig. 7.

The whole control system performs a coordinated response, in which each controller adjusts the manipulated variables to take action against the disturbance, thus moving the controlled variables back to their set points. The plots of the upstream and downstream manipulated and controlled variables are summarized in Figs. 8 and 9, respectively.

The lack of the nitrogen substrate has an inhibitory effect on lovastatin production, as can be appreciated from the drop of CSTR lovastatin concentration in the bottom center graph of Fig. 8. The concentration controller closes the purge stream valve to enhance biomass recirculation, increasing recirculation flow rate Q_R and then recirculation factor RF. This generates an increment in the CSTR volume, not appreciable from the bottom left graph of Fig. 8 because of the tight level controller that closes the CSTR outlet stream valve, reducing the flow rate Q_4. This implies a longer residence time of biomass cells in the reactor, which have more time to produce lovastatin. To reestablish the RF to its set point, the third controller closes the medium stream valve to reduce the mixer's feed flow rate Q_1, as shown in the top-right graph of Fig. 8. Eventually, after a prolonged time due to the slow kinetics

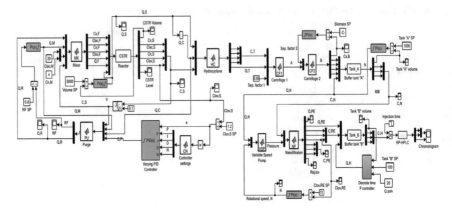

Fig. 6 Unified Simulink model of upstream and downstream processes

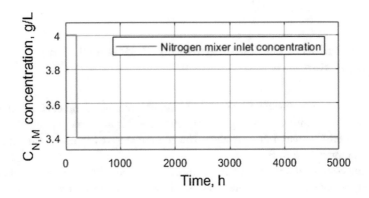

Fig. 7 Step change disturbance in medium nitrogen concentration $C_{N,1}$

of the biological production of lovastatin, a new steady-state operating point is reached in which all the controlled variables are settled back to their set point values.

Due to the simulated disturbance, the stream entering the centrifuges contains a reduced amount of biomass, and its flow rate Q_5 is lower. The first effect is visible from the bottom left biomass concentration graph of Fig. 9. The residual biomass concentration set point is already at an acceptable value; instead of keeping the rotational speed of the centrifuge (and thus the separation factor X_2) at a higher value than required, a reduction of the rotational speed contributes to saving electric power. The reduced flow rate from the upstream makes the buffer tank volume V_A decrease, as shown in the bottom center graph of Fig. 9. The level controller closes the tank outlet stream valve to achieve a reduction in the outlet flow rate Q_9, which smoothly settles to a new steady-state value. The reduction of Q_9 implies a reduction of permeate Q_{PE} and retentate Q_{10} flow rates; at the same time, the retentate stream is more concentrated, meaning that its lovastatin concentration rises. As reported in the top-right graph of Fig. 9, the pump head pressure ΔP initially rises slightly

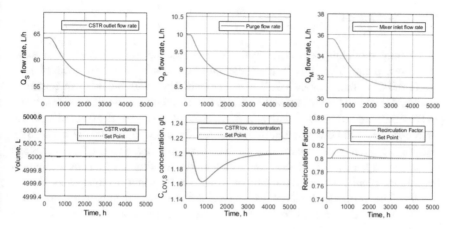

Fig. 8 Upstream process manipulated variables (above) and respective controlled variables (below) following the introduction of a step change in the medium nitrogen concentration

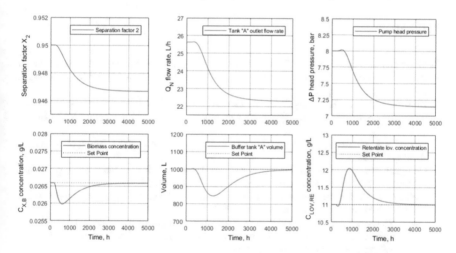

Fig. 9 Downstream process manipulated variables (above) and respective controlled variables (below)

because of the reduced Q_9 but afterward drops because of the motor pump rotational speed N reduction (also in this case, with the purpose of saving electric power) induced by the lovastatin concentration controller. As stated in Sect. 8.2, the level controller of buffer tank "A" is sluggish and is not affecting the correct functionality of the lovastatin concentration controller, which is tuned with settings that are more aggressive.

10   Conclusion

A dynamic modeling was developed for a continuous biopharmaceutical manufacturing plant. The modeling of the unit operations was implemented in a MATLAB/Simulink framework. The benchmark simulator includes an upstream section, in which a CSTR bioreactor is implemented with a biomass recycle system, and a downstream section, which is composed of a sequence of centrifugation, nanofiltration, and chromatography operations for the isolation of the target API. Various regulatory and supervisory control strategies can be used for the control of the developed dynamic model. As a case study, we simulated a semicontinuous benchmark plant for the production of lovastatin by using a multiple PI control system. The introduced model can be used for dynamic simulation of CBM processes and as a testbed for confirming the effectiveness of optimization and control.

References

1. Moorkens E, Meuwissen N, Huys I, Declerck P, Vulto AG, Simoens S: The market of biopharmaceutical medicines: a snapshot of a diverse industrial landscape. Frontiers in pharmacology 2017, 8:314.
2. Hong MS, Severson KA, Jiang M, Lu AE, Love JC, Braatz RD: Challenges and opportunities in biopharmaceutical manufacturing control. Computers & Chemical Engineering 2018,**110**:106-114.
3. Villadsen J, Nielsen J, Lidén G: Bioreaction engineering principles. Springer Science & Business Media; 2011.
4. Croughan MS, Konstantinov KB, Cooney C: The future of industrial bioprocessing: batch or continuous? Biotechnology and bioengineering 2015,**112**:648-651.
5. Zydney AL: Continuous downstream processing for high value biological products: a review. Biotechnology and bioengineering 2016,**113**:465-475.
6. Guo J, Zhang S, Carta G: Unfolding and aggregation of a glycosylated monoclonal antibody on a cation exchange column. Part I. Chromatographic elution and batch adsorption behavior. Journal of Chromatography A 2014,**1356**:117-128.
7. Gospodarek AM, Hiser DE, O'Connell JP, Fernandez EJ: Unfolding of a model protein on ion exchange and mixed mode chromatography surfaces. Journal of Chromatography A 2014,**1355**:238-252.
8. Gillespie R, Nguyen T, Macneil S, Jones L, Crampton S, Vunnum S: Cation exchange surface-mediated denaturation of an aglycosylated immunoglobulin (IgG1). Journal of Chromatography A 2012,**1251**:101-110.
9. Walther J, Godawat R, Hwang C, Abe Y, Sinclair A, Konstantinov K: The business impact of an integrated continuous biomanufacturing platform for recombinant protein production. Journal of biotechnology 2015,**213**:3-12.
10. Zydney AL: Perspectives on integrated continuous bioprocessing—opportunities and challenges. Current Opinion in Chemical Engineering 2015,**10**:8-13.
11. Cole KP, Johnson MD: Continuous flow technology vs. the batch-by-batch approach to produce pharmaceutical compounds. Expert Rev Clin Pharmacol 2018,**11**:5-13.
12. Bailey CK, Caltabiano S, Cobitz AR, Huang C, Mahar KM, Patel VV: A randomized, 29-day, dose-ranging, efficacy and safety study of daprodustat, administered three times weekly in patients with anemia on hemodialysis. BMC nephrology 2019,**20**:1-12.

13. Pacis E, Yu M, Autsen J, Bayer R, Li F: Effects of cell culture conditions on antibody N-linked glycosylation—what affects high mannose 5 glycoform. Biotechnology and bioengineering 2011,**108**:2348-2358.

14. Liu H, Gaza-Bulseco G, Faldu D, Chumsae C, Sun J: Heterogeneity of monoclonal antibodies. Journal of pharmaceutical sciences 2008,**97**:2426-2447.

15. Joshi V, Shivach T, Kumar V, Yadav N, Rathore A: Avoiding antibody aggregation during processing: establishing hold times. Biotechnology journal 2014,**9**:1195-1205.

16. Food U, Administration D: Advancing regulatory science at FDA: a strategic plan. Washington DC 2011.

17. Woodcock J: Modernizing pharmaceutical manufacturing–continuous manufacturing as a key enabler. In International Symposium on Continuous Manufacturing of Pharmaceuticals, Cambridge, MA; 2014.

18. Langer ES, Rader RA: Continuous bioprocessing and perfusion: wider adoption coming as bioprocessing matures. BioProcessing Journal 2014,**13**:43-49.

19. Fisher AC, Kamga M-H, Agarabi C, Brorson K, Lee SL, Yoon S: The current scientific and regulatory landscape in advancing integrated continuous biopharmaceutical manufacturing. Trends in biotechnology 2019,**37**:253-267.

20. Health UDo, Services H: Guidance for industry: PAT—A framework for innovative pharmaceutical development, manufacturing, and quality assurance. Food and Drug Administration, Rockville, MD 2004.

21. FDA U: Guidance for Industry. Q8 (R2) Pharmaceutical Development. Maryland: Food and Drug Administration 2009.

22. Rathore AS, Winkle H: Quality by design for biopharmaceuticals. Nature biotechnology 2009,**27**:26-34.

23. Read E, Park J, Shah R, Riley B, Brorson K, Rathore A: Process analytical technology (PAT) for biopharmaceutical products: Part I. Concepts and applications. Biotechnology and Bioengineering 2010,**105**:276-284.

24. Glassey J, Gernaey K, Clemens C, Schulz TW, Oliveira R, Striedner G, Mandenius C-F: Process analytical technology (PAT) for biopharmaceuticals. Biotechnology Journal 2011,**6**:369-377.

25. Gronemeyer P, Ditz R, Strube J: Trends in upstream and downstream process development for antibody manufacturing. Bioengineering 2014,**1**:188-212.

26. Tripathi NK, Shrivastava A: Recent developments in bioprocessing of recombinant proteins: expression hosts and process development. Frontiers in Bioengineering and Biotechnology 2019,**7**.

27. Boedeker B, Goldstein A, Mahajan E: Fully disposable manufacturing concepts for clinical and commercial manufacturing and ballroom concepts. In New Bioprocessing Strategies: Development and Manufacturing of Recombinant Antibodies and Proteins. Springer; 2017:179-210.

28. Jacquemart R, Vandersluis M, Zhao M, Sukhija K, Sidhu N, Stout J: A single-use strategy to enable manufacturing of affordable biologics. Computational and Structural Biotechnology Journal 2016,**14**:309-318.

29. Raven N, Rasche S, Kuehn C, Anderlei T, Klöckner W, Schuster F, Henquet M, Bosch D, Büchs J, Fischer R: Scaled-up manufacturing of recombinant antibodies produced by plant cells in a 200-L orbitally-shaken disposable bioreactor. Biotechnology and Bioengineering 2015,**112**:308-321.

30. Ghasemi A, Bozorg A, Rahmati F, Mirhassani R, Hosseininasab S: Comprehensive study on Wave bioreactor system to scale up the cultivation of and recombinant protein expression in baculovirus-infected insect cells. Biochemical Engineering Journal 2019,**143**:121-130.

31. Somasundaram B, Pleitt K, Shave E, Baker K, Lua LH: Progression of continuous downstream processing of monoclonal antibodies: Current trends and challenges. Biotechnology and Bioengineering 2018,**115**:2893-2907.

32. Triadaphillou S, Martin E, Montague G, Norden A, Jeffkins P, Stimpson S: Fermentation process tracking through enhanced spectral calibration modeling. Biotechnology and Bioengineering 2007,**97**:554-567.

33. Gryniewicz CM, Kauffman JF: Multivariate calibration of covalent aggregate fraction to the Raman spectrum of regular human insulin. Journal of pharmaceutical sciences 2008,**97**:3727-3734.
34. Hédoux A, Willart J, Ionov R, Affouard F, Guinet Y, Paccou L, Lerbret A, Descamps M: Analysis of sugar bioprotective mechanisms on the thermal denaturation of lysozyme from Raman scattering and differential scanning calorimetry investigations. The Journal of Physical Chemistry B 2006,**110**:22886-22893.
35. Markely LRA, Ong BT, Hoi KM, Teo G, Lu MY, Wang DI: A high-throughput method for quantification of glycoprotein sialylation. Analytical biochemistry 2010,**407**:128-133.
36. Zibaii MI, Kazemi A, Latifi H, Azar MK, Hosseini SM, Ghezelaiagh MH: Measuring bacterial growth by refractive index tapered fiber optic biosensor. Journal of Photochemistry and Photobiology B: Biology 2010,**101**:313-320.
37. Ge X, Kostov Y, Rao G: High-stability non-invasive autoclavable naked optical CO2 sensor. Biosensors and Bioelectronics 2003,**18**:857-865.
38. Keβler LC, Gueorguieva L, Rinas U, Seidel-Morgenstern A: Step gradients in 3-zone simulated moving bed chromatography: application to the purification of antibodies and bone morphogenetic protein-2. Journal of Chromatography A 2007,**1176**:69-78.
39. Warikoo V, Godawat R, Brower K, Jain S, Cummings D, Simons E, Johnson T, Walther J, Yu M, Wright B: Integrated continuous production of recombinant therapeutic proteins. Biotechnology and bioengineering 2012,**109**:3018-3029.
40. Angarita M, Müller-Späth T, Baur D, Lievrouw R, Lissens G, Morbidelli M: Twin-column CaptureSMB: a novel cyclic process for protein A affinity chromatography. Journal of Chromatography A 2015,**1389**:85-95.
41. Rathore AS, Parr L, Dermawan S, Lawson K, Lu Y: Large scale demonstration of a process analytical technology application in bioprocessing: Use of on-line high performance liquid chromatography for making real time pooling decisions for process chromatography. Biotechnology progress 2010,**26**:448-457.
42. Joshi VS, Kumar V: A rapid HPLC method for enabling PAT application for processing of GCSF. 2013.
43. Tiwari A, Kateja N, Chanana S, Rathore AS: Use of HPLC as an enabler of process analytical technology in process chromatography. Analytical chemistry 2018,**90**:7824-7829.
44. Sanden A, Suhm S, Rüdt M, Hubbuch J: Fourier-transform infrared spectroscopy as a process analytical technology for near real time in-line estimation of the degree of PEGylation in chromatography. Journal of Chromatography A 2019,**1608**:460410.
45. Lu AE, Paulson JA, Mozdzierz NJ, Stockdale A, Versypt ANF, Love KR, Love JC, Braatz RD: Control systems technology in the advanced manufacturing of biologic drugs. In 2015 IEEE Conference on Control Applications (CCA). IEEE; 2015:1505-1515.
46. Gunther JC, Seborg DE, Conner JS: Fault detection and diagnosis in industrial fed-batch cell culture. IFAC Proceedings Volumes 2006,**39**:203-208.
47. Zhang H, Lennox B: Integrated condition monitoring and control of fed-batch fermentation processes. Journal of Process Control 2004,**14**:41-50.
48. Gordon SH, Whatel SC, Wheeler BC, James C: Multivariate FTIR analysis of substrates for protein, polysaccharide, lipid and microbe content: Potential for solid-state fermentations. Biotechnology Advances 1993,**11**:665-675.
49. Rosa SM, Soria MA, Vélez CG, Galvagno MA: Improvement of a two-stage fermentation process for docosahexaenoic acid production by Aurantiochytrium limacinum SR21 applying statistical experimental designs and data analysis. Bioresource Technology 2010,**101**:2367-2374.
50. Emenike VN, Schenkendorf R, Krewer U: Model-based optimization of biopharmaceutical manufacturing in Pichia pastoris based on dynamic flux balance analysis. Computers & Chemical Engineering 2018,**118**:1-13.
51. Barrigon JM, Valero F, Montesinos JL: A macrokinetic model-based comparative meta-analysis of recombinant protein production by Pichia pastoris under AOX1 promoter. Biotechnology and Bioengineering 2015,**112**:1132-1145.

52. Guiochon G, Lin B: Modeling for preparative chromatography. Academic press; 2003.
53. Karst DJ, Scibona E, Serra E, Bielser JM, Souquet J, Stettler M, Broly H, Soos M, Morbidelli M, Villiger TK: Modulation and modeling of monoclonal antibody N-linked glycosylation in mammalian cell perfusion reactors. Biotechnology and Bioengineering 2017,114:1978-1990.
54. Cinar A, Parulekar SJ, Undey C, Birol G: Batch fermentation: modeling: monitoring, and control. CRC press; 2003.
55. Benyahia B, Lakerveld R, Barton PI: A Plant-Wide Dynamic Model of a Continuous Pharmaceutical Process. Industrial & Engineering Chemistry Research 2012,51:15393-15412.
56. Sahlodin AM, Barton PI: Optimal Campaign Continuous Manufacturing. Industrial & Engineering Chemistry Research 2015,54:11344-11359.
57. Lakerveld R, Benyahia B, Braatz RD, Barton PI: Model-based design of a plant-wide control strategy for a continuous pharmaceutical plant. AIChE Journal 2013,59:3671-3685.
58. Kumar A, Udugama IA, Gargalo CL, Gernaey KV: Why Is Batch Processing Still Dominating the Biologics Landscape? Towards an Integrated Continuous Bioprocessing Alternative. Processes 2020,8.
59. Colombo G: Development of bio-based production process: process synthesis, design and simulation. 2018.
60. Perra S: The study of lovastatin production as a benchmark simulation model for bio-manufacturing processes. 2019.
61. Yoshida M, Oliveira M, Gomes E, Mussel W, Castro W, Soares C: Thermal characterization of lovastatin in pharmaceutical formulations. Journal of thermal analysis and calorimetry 2011,106:657-664.
62. Bizukojc M, Ledakowicz S: A macrokinetic modelling of the biosynthesis of lovastatin by Aspergillus terreus. Journal of biotechnology 2007,130:422-435.
63. Rickwood D: Centrifugation: a practical approach; 1984.
64. Flickinger MC, Drew SW: Encyclopedia of bioprocess technology. John Wiley; 1999.
65. Jozala AF, Geraldes DC, Tundisi LL, Feitosa VdA, Breyer CA, Cardoso SL, Mazzola PG, Oliveira-Nascimento Ld, Rangel-Yagui CdO, Magalhães PdO: Biopharmaceuticals from microorganisms: from production to purification. Brazilian Journal of Microbiology 2016,47:51-63.
66. Van der Horst H, Timmer J, Robbertsen T, Leenders J: Use of nanofiltration for concentration and demineralization in the dairy industry: Model for mass transport. Journal of membrane science 1995,104:205-218.
67. Wang R, Li Y, Wang J, You G, Cai C, Chen BH: Modeling the permeate flux and rejection of nanofiltration membrane separation with high concentration uncharged aqueous solutions. Desalination 2012,299:44-49.
68. Košutić K, Dolar D, Ašperger D, Kunst B: Removal of antibiotics from a model wastewater by RO/NF membranes. Separation and purification technology 2007,53:244-249.
69. Peeva L, da Silva Burgal J, Valtcheva I, Livingston AG: Continuous purification of active pharmaceutical ingredients using multistage organic solvent nanofiltration membrane cascade. Chemical Engineering Science 2014,116:183-194.
70. Ponton JW: Degrees of freedom analysis in process control. Chemical Engineering Science 1994,49:2089-2095.
71. Seborg DE, Edgar, T, Mellichamp DA, Doyle FJ III. Process dynamics and control, 4th ed. Hoboken. John Wiley & Sons; 2016.

Overview of Scheduling Methods for Pharmaceutical Production

Shamik Misra and Christos T. Maravelias

1 Introduction

Increasing competition and strong government regulations compel the pharmaceutical industry to adopt improved decision-making practices to develop efficient manufacturing processes. Pharmaceutical products are generally produced on a small scale and required to meet high purity standards [1]. Though continuous pharmaceutical manufacturing processes are investigated [2], the majority of the facilities in a pharmaceutical plant still operate in batch mode due to product variability and strict quality requirement [3]. As manufacturing is riddled with complexities involving shared resources, cleaning requirements, and unit setups, production scheduling plays an important role in maintaining efficient time-to-market performance.

Scheduling is a decision-making process which concerned with the allocation of limited shared resources to different competing activities over time while aiming to optimize single or multiple objectives. Despite several exact and approximate solution methods proposed over the last three decades, production scheduling remains one of the most active topics of research in the process systems engineering (PSE) community [4–9]. Exact scheduling methods based on mixed-integer programming models can be classified into two categories: (1) precedence-based models [10–16] and (2) time grid-based models. The latter can further be categorized based on the

S. Misra
Department of Chemical and Biological Engineering, University of Wisconsin, Madison, WI, USA
e-mail: misra7@wisc.edu

C. T. Maravelias (✉)
Andlinger Center for Energy and the Environment and Department of Chemical and Biological Engineering, Princeton University, Princeton, NJ, USA
e-mail: maravelias@princeton.edu

© The Author(s), under exclusive license to Springer Nature Switzerland AG 2022
A. Fytopoulos et al. (eds.), *Optimization of Pharmaceutical Processes*, Springer
Optimization and Its Applications 189, https://doi.org/10.1007/978-3-030-90924-6_13

time representation techniques used, viz., discrete time [17–22], continuous time [23–29], and mixed time [30–32] representation.

In the following, we restrict our review to some specific scheduling frameworks proposed in the literature that have direct application toward the pharmaceutical industry. Castro et al. studied a pharmaceutical batch plant and proposed a decomposition-based solution strategy to tackle the complexity of the large production facilities [33]. The same problem was further investigated by Kopanos et al., who proposed two precedence-based MILP models to address complexities related to changeover costs and due times [34]. Stefansson et al. investigated a multistage, multiproduct pharmaceutical production problem and proposed both discrete and continuous time grid-based scheduling frameworks [35]. Kabra et al. proposed a continuous time grid-based model to solve the problem introduced by Lakhdar et al. [36] and include specific features related to the handling of shelf life, waste disposal, and changeovers in a biopharmaceutical plant [37]. Liu et al. proposed a discrete time-based MIP model to simultaneously optimize production and maintenance decisions of a biopharmaceutical plant under performance decay [38]. Motivated by the real-world scheduling problem in the chemical-pharmaceutical industry, Moniz et al. proposed a discrete time-based scheduling model that solves multiple instances of the problem and produces optimal schedules and also helps to evaluate the process alternatives and their associated costs [39]. Eberle et al. proposed an immediate precedence-based scheduling model for a single-unit, single-stage, multiple product sterile drug manufacturing facility while incorporating complexities regarding sterile holding times [40].

One of the major advantages of models based on discrete-time grid(s) is that the common time grid provides a reference grid of time to all the shred resources such as materials and utilities. Discrete-time grid is also advantageous in monitoring and modeling consumption/inventory profiles of utilities/inventories without introducing nonlinear constraints [41, 42]. Furthermore, the discrete-time models are easily scalable and can be extended to incorporate multiple units/stages, with minimal structural changes. In the following, we present an overview of discrete time grid-based production scheduling models starting from single-unit single-stage problems to multiunit multistage problems. We also present concepts and modeling techniques to incorporate complexities related to changeover times and costs, batching decisions, shared resources, and storage.

2 Single-Unit Scheduling

Though scarce in chemical engineering applications, a single-unit scheduling environment can be considered a building block toward formulating models for more complex scheduling environments. In the single-unit environment, multiple batches need to be scheduled on a single unit. As all the production is met by one unit, the number of batches required to complete the production need can be precalculated, so the batching decisions can be made independently. We assume that we are given a set of batches $i \in \mathbf{I}$, with processing time τ_i, which are needed to be scheduled on a single unit. If we do not specify additional limitations related to task due time, the time required to finish all the batches can simply be calculated as $\sum_i \tau_i$. However, the problem gets complicated when the batches need to be scheduled, respecting the release time (ρ_i) and due time (ε_i) of each batch. Furthermore, there can be sequence-dependent changeover times ($\sigma_{ii'}$) and costs ($\gamma_{ii'}^{CH}$) that also need to be considered.

2.1 Discrete-Time Grid Model

Index $n \in \mathbf{N} = \{0, 1, 2, \ldots, N\}$ is used to denote the time points between the minimum release time and the maximum due time. The scheduling horizon is divided into $|\mathbf{N}| - 1$ time periods of equal length δ, where period n runs between time points $n - 1$ and n. Generally, the greatest common factor among all time-related data is chosen as the length of the time periods (δ); however, small δ might lead to large size problems which can be computationally intractable. In such cases, a coarser discretization might be necessary, and to ensure the feasibility of the solution, all the time-related parameters (i.e., processing times, due, release, and changeover times) should be represented on the discrete-time grid in the following manner:

$$\overline{\tau}_i = \lceil \tau_i/\delta \rceil, \overline{\rho}_i = \lceil \rho_i/\delta \rceil, \overline{\varepsilon}_i = \lfloor \varepsilon_i/\delta \rfloor, \overline{\sigma}_{ii'} = \lceil \sigma_{ii'}/\delta \rceil$$

A binary variable X_{in} is introduced to represent the allocation of task i at time point n. Each batch should be executed once.

$$\sum_n X_{in} = 1, \qquad i \qquad (1)$$

Now the unit can process only one task at any point in time, and no other tasks can be allocated to that unit until and unless the previous task is finished. This no-overlap restriction is enforced as follows:

$$\sum_i \sum_{n' \geq n - \overline{\tau}_i + 1}^{n} X_{in'} \leq 1, \qquad n \qquad (2)$$

Release and due time constraints are enforced via fixing the binary variables that are outside the available window to zero:

$$X_{in} = 0, \quad i, n < \overline{\rho}_i, n > \overline{\varepsilon}_i - \overline{\tau}_i \qquad (3)$$

The start or end time of a batch can be calculated by multiplying the time points with the corresponding binary variables. Using this idea, we can write the constraint to calculate makespan as follows:

$$MS \geq \sum_n (n + \overline{\tau}_i) X_{in}, \qquad i \qquad\qquad (4)$$

In a similar way, we can also calculate the earliness $(\overline{\varepsilon}_i - \sum_n (n + \overline{\tau}_i) X_{in})$ or lateness of a batch $(\sum_n (n + \overline{\tau}_i) X_{in} - \overline{\varepsilon}_i)$ and write the following objective functions:

$$\min MS \qquad\qquad (5)$$

$$\min \sum_i \omega_i \left(\overline{\varepsilon}_i - \sum_n (n + \overline{\tau}_i) X_{in} \right) \qquad\qquad (6)$$

$$\min \sum_i \omega_i \left(\sum_n (n + \overline{\tau}_i) X_{in} - \overline{\varepsilon}_i \right) \qquad\qquad (7)$$

To denote tardiness, a variable $L_i \in \mathbb{R}_+$ is defined that captures the nonnegative tardiness for each batch, as shown in Eq. (8). The objective function to minimize total tardiness is described in Eq. (9).

$$L_i \geq \sum_n (n + \overline{\tau}_i) X_{in} - \overline{\varepsilon}_i, \qquad i \qquad\qquad (8)$$

$$\min \sum_i \omega_i L_i \qquad\qquad (9)$$

2.2 Changeover Time

If changeovers do not incur any additional costs, then changeover times can be enforced using binary variable X_{in}. The additional constraints that can be added to the abovementioned model to represent the changeover times are described in Eqs. (10) and (11).

$$\sum_{i' \neq i} \sum_{n' = n - \overline{\tau}_{i'} - \overline{\sigma}_{i'i} + 1}^{n - \overline{\tau}_{i'}} X_{i'n'} \leq M_i (1 - X_{in}), \qquad i, n \qquad\qquad (10)$$

Equation (10) ensures sufficient separation between batches by enforcing that if a batch i starts at a time point n, then no other batch i' can start between time points ranging from $n - \overline{\tau}_{i'} - \overline{\sigma}_{i'i} + 1$ to $n - \overline{\tau}_{i'}$. A valid value for the big-M parameter (M_i) is

$$M_i = \sum_{i' \neq i} \overline{\sigma}_{i'i}, \qquad i \qquad\qquad (11)$$

2.3 Changeover Cost

Though Eqs. (10) and (11) suffice to incorporate the effects of changeover times in the model, to account for changeover costs, new binary variables need to be introduced. Though multiple approaches are available, we hereby describe two methods that require the introduction of the following two binary variables:

- $\overline{X}_{in} = 1$ if during time period n, the unit is set up to carry out batch i.
- $Z_{ii'n} = 1$ if the unit setup switches from batch i to batch i' at time point n.

The first method is only applicable when we want to calculate the changeover costs; however, no changeover time is needed to be accounted for. Note that the variable $\overline{X}_{in}$ does not only indicate the processing of batch i but rather denotes whether unit setup supports processing of batch i. The variable $\overline{X}_{in}$ can assume value 1, when the batch i is executed in the unit and also during idle time. The set of constraints required to activate $Z_{ii'n}$ variables, which are then required to calculate the changeover costs, is given in Eqs. (12)–(16).

$$\sum_i \overline{X}_{in} = 1, \qquad n \tag{12}$$

$$\sum_{n'=n-\tau_i}^{n-1} X_{in'} = \overline{X}_{in}, \qquad i, n \tag{13}$$

$$\sum_{i' \neq i} Z_{ii'n} \leq \overline{X}_{i,n-1}, \qquad i, n \tag{14}$$

$$\sum_{i \neq i'} Z_{ii'n} \leq \overline{X}_{i'n}, \qquad i', n \tag{15}$$

$$Z_{ii'n} \geq \overline{X}_{i,n-1} + \overline{X}_{i'n} - 1, \qquad i, i \neq i', n \tag{16}$$

To incorporate both changeover costs and time, we adopt the second method, which introduces the following constraint to replace Eqs. (12) and (14)–(16):

$$\overline{X}_{in} = \overline{X}_{i,n-1} + \sum_{i' \neq i} Z_{i'i,n-\overline{\sigma}_{i'i}} - \sum_{i' \neq i} Z_{ii'n}, \qquad i, n \tag{17}$$

The changeover cost minimization objective is

$$\min \sum_{ii'n} \gamma_{ii'}^{CH} Z_{ii'n} \tag{18}$$

3   Single Stage Scheduling

In this section, we discuss problems in the single stage (parallel unit) environment and demonstrate how the model discussed in the previous section can be extended to incorporate the characteristics of single stage environment. In single stage problem, one task can be carried out in multiple units with different capacities; hence, the problem of batching also arises. However, at the onset, we assume that the batching decisions have already been taken. So we aim to schedule a set of batches ($\mathbf{I}$) on a set of units ($\mathbf{J}$). Each batch $i \in \mathbf{I}$ has its own release (ρ_i) and due (ε_i) time and is carried out only once in the horizon on exactly one compatible unit ($j \in \mathbf{J}_i \in \mathbf{J}$). The set of batches that can be processed in unit j is denoted by $\mathbf{I}_j$. The processing cost of batch i in unit j is γ_{ij}^P, and the processing time is τ_{ij}. The changeover time/costs are denoted by $\tau_{ii'j}/\gamma_{ii'j}^{CH}$.

3.1   Discrete-Time Grid Model

We use a similar method as described in the previous section to calculate the time points used in discrete-time grid. All time-related parameters are converted as follows:

$$\bar{\tau}_{ij} = \lceil \tau_{ij}/\delta \rceil , \bar{\rho}_i = \lceil \rho_i/\delta \rceil , \bar{\varepsilon}_i = \lfloor \varepsilon_i/\delta \rfloor , \bar{\sigma}_{ii'j} = \lceil \sigma_{ii'j}/\delta \rceil$$

We introduce the binary variable X_{ijn} that assumes value 1 if batch i starts on unit j at time point n. As mentioned earlier, each batch is executed only once, which is enforced as follows:

$$\sum_{j,n} X_{ijn} = 1, \qquad i \qquad (19)$$

Note that $\sum_j X_{ijn}$ is equivalent to the variable X_{in}, which is used in the single-unit model to describe that the batch i starts at time point n in some unit. Similarly, the no-overlap restriction can also be expressed in a very similar manner in the parallel unit environment as follows:

$$\sum_i \sum_{n' \geq n - \bar{\tau}_{ij} + 1}^{n} X_{ijn'} \leq 1, \qquad j, n \qquad (20)$$

The release and due time constraints are enforced by fixing the variables outside the available windows to zero:

$$X_{ijn} = 0, \quad i, j, n < \bar{\rho}_i, n > \bar{\varepsilon}_i - \bar{\tau}_{ij} \qquad (21)$$

The makespan can be calculated as

$$MS \geq \sum_{j,n} \left(n + \overline{\tau}_{ij}\right) X_{ijn}, \qquad i \qquad (22)$$

Next, we present the objective functions for the minimization of makespan (Eq. 23), weighted earliness (Eq. 24), lateness (Eq. 25), and tardiness (Eqs. 26 and 27).

$$\min MS \qquad (23)$$

$$\min \sum_i \omega_i \left(\overline{\varepsilon}_i - \sum_{j,n} \left(n + \overline{\tau}_{ij}\right) X_{ijn}\right) \qquad (24)$$

$$\min \sum_i \omega_i \left(\sum_{j,n} \left(n + \overline{\tau}_{ij}\right) X_{ijn} - \overline{\varepsilon}_i\right) \qquad (25)$$

$$L_i \geq \sum_{j,n} \left(n + \overline{\tau}_{ij}\right) X_{ijn} - \overline{\varepsilon}_i, \qquad i \qquad (26)$$

$$\min \sum_i \omega_i L_i \qquad (27)$$

A nonnegative variable L_i is used to indicate the tardiness of each batch in Eqs. (26) and (27).

3.2 Changeover Time and Costs

The ideas to model changeover times presented in the earlier section can be extended for single stage scheduling models using binary variable X_{ijn}:

$$\sum_{i' \neq i} \sum_{n'=n-\overline{\tau}_{i'j}-\overline{\sigma}_{i'ij}+1}^{n-\overline{\tau}_{i'j}} X_{i'jn'} \leq M_{ij} \left(1 - X_{ijn}\right), \qquad i, j, n \qquad (28)$$

To incorporate both changeover times and costs, we introduce the following two binary variables:

- $\overline{X}_{ijn} = 1$ if during time period n, unit j is set up to carry out batch i.
- $Z_{ii'jn} = 1$ if there is a changeover in unit j set up from batch i to batch i' at time point n.

Batch i can only be carried out if the unit j is set up to carry out that batch:

$$\sum_{n' \geq n-\overline{\tau}_{ij}}^{n-1} X_{ijn'} \leq \overline{X}_{ijn}, \qquad i, j, n \qquad (29)$$

The transition between unit setups, through the activation of the transition binary variable $Z_{ii'jn}$, is described in Eq. (30), while the total cost minimization objective function is given in Eq. (31), where the first term represents the processing cost and the second term denotes the changeover cost.

$$\overline{X}_{ijn} = \overline{X}_{ij,n-1} + \sum_{i'\neq i} Z_{i'ij,n-\overline{\sigma}_{i'i}-1} - \sum_{i'\neq i} Z_{ii'j,n-1}, \qquad i, j, n \qquad (30)$$

$$\min \sum_{ij}\left(\gamma_{ij}^{P}\sum_{n}X_{ijn}\right) + \sum_{ii'j}\left(\gamma_{ii'j}^{CH}\sum_{n}Z_{ii'jn}\right) \qquad (31)$$

3.3 Batching Decisions

If the units have different capacities (β_j), then the number of batches required to meet demand becomes a decision variable; that is, batching, assignment, and timing decisions have to be made simultaneously. As the number and size of the batches need to be calculated, we use index i to denote orders. A set of orders **I**, for which demand (ξ_i) is specified, need to be carried out in a set of units **J**. Multiple batches are required to fulfill the specified order demands, and these batches can be carried out in compatible units $(j \in \mathbf{J}_i \in \mathbf{J})$. The necessary number of batches to fulfill certain order can be calculated as

$$\sum_{j\in\mathbf{J}_i,n}\beta_j X_{ijn} \geq \xi_i, \qquad i \qquad (32)$$

To model batches with variable sizes, Eqs. (33) and (34) can be used replacing Eq. (32).

$$\sum_{j\in\mathbf{J}_i,n}B_{ijn} \geq \xi_i, \qquad i \qquad (33)$$

$$\beta_{ij}^{MIN}X_{ijn} \leq B_{ijn} \leq \beta_{ij}^{MAX}X_{ijn}, \qquad i, j, n \qquad (34)$$

3.4 Shared Resources

In the above discussion, we have assumed only one type of shared resources, and that is the unit in which a batch is processed. However, in reality, there might be a number of resources required to carry out a batch (e.g., labor, heating/cooling medium, electricity, etc.). These resources can be classified into two categories: renewable and nonrenewable resources. For example, one personnel needs to be *engaged* at the starting of each batch, and once the batch is completed, that personnel gets *freed*. For example, in case renewable resources (e.g. man power), one personnel needs to be *engaged* at the starting of each batch and once the batch is completed that personnel gets *freed*. On the contrary, the non-renewable resources (e.g., coloring agent) get consumed during the processing of a batch. The resources can further be classified based on their utilization pattern. For example, engagement of some resources only depends on the execution of batch (e.g., a unit required to process a batch), whereas consumption of some resources varies with the batch sizes (e.g., cooling water). Based on these ideas, we classify resources in three types: (1) Type A: resource engagement/consumption only depends on the execution of batch; (2) Type B: resource engagement/consumption depends on the size of the batch; and (3) Type C: both batch execution and size decisions affect the resource engagement/consumption.

If φ_{im} denotes the fixed consumption of resource m during the processing of batch i and ψ_{im} represents the variable consumption, then the total resource consumption (R_{im}) during the execution of batch i can be calculated as $R_{im} = \varphi_{im} + \psi_{im} B_i$, where B_i denotes the batch size. It is to note that for Type A resources, $\psi_{im} = 0$ and for Type B resources, $\varphi_{im} = 0$. Both parameters will have nonzero values for Type C resources. To simplify, we ignore changeovers in the following model.

The quantity of resource (m) engaged/freed at the starting/end of a batch i is captured through two nonnegative continuous variables, R_{imn}^I / R_{imn}^o, calculated as follows:

$$R_{imn}^I = \varphi_{im} \sum_j X_{ijn} + \psi_{im} \sum_j B_{ijn}, \qquad i, m, n \qquad (35)$$

$$R_{imn}^o = \varphi_{im} \sum_j X_{ij,n-\bar{\tau}_{ij}} + \psi_{im} \sum_j B_{ij,n-\bar{\tau}_{ij}}, \qquad i, m, n \qquad (36)$$

The total consumption of resource m, due to the execution of all tasks during time period n, can be calculated and constrained by the maximum availability of that resource (χ_m) as follows:

$$R_{mn} = R_{m,n-1} + \sum_i R_{im,n-1}^I - \sum_i R_{im,n-1}^o \leq \chi_m, \qquad m, n \qquad (37)$$

If batch sizes are fixed, then $\psi_{im} \sum_j B_{ijn} = \psi_{im} \beta_i \sum_j X_{ijn}$ and $\psi_{im} \sum_j B_{ij,n-\bar{\tau}_{ij}} = \psi_{im} \beta_i \sum_j X_{ij,n-\bar{\tau}_{ij}}$, which leads to the following equation (with $\psi_{im}^T = \varphi_{im} + \psi_{im} \beta_i$):

$$R_{mn} = R_{m,n-1} + \psi_{im}^T \sum_j X_{ij,n-1} - \psi_{im}^T \sum_j X_{ij,n-\bar{\tau}_{ij}-1} \leq \chi_m, \qquad m, n \qquad (38)$$

Alternative to Eqs. (35)–(37), we can write the resource consumption constraint based on the no-overlap constraints described in Eq. (20). The consumption of resources m at time point n can be expressed as

$$\sum_{ij} \sum_{n' \geq n-\tau_{ij}}^{n-1} \varphi_{im} \sum_{j} X_{ijn'} + \psi_{im} \sum_{j} B_{ijn'} \leq \chi_m, \qquad m, n \qquad (39)$$

It should be noted that for unary resources (e.g., units), $\varphi_{im} = 1$ and $\psi_{im} = 0$. Setting these values in Eq. (39), we get Eq. (20), which essentially indicates that maximum one unit can be engaged during the execution of a batch.

So the discrete-time model to simultaneously compute assignment, sequencing, batching, and resource consumption decisions should include Eqs. (19)–(21), (32)–(34), and (35)–(37) or (39).

In addition to the type of resources consumption discussed above, batch transitions can also trigger resource consumptions; for example, in a pharmaceutical process, transition from one batch to another might warrant cleaning in between, which requires resources related to the cleaning activity. We can easily formulate such constraints by replacing X_{ijn} variables with the changeover variables $Z_{ii'jn}$.

The total cost minimization objective function includes batch processing, changeover, and resource consumption costs. It can be expressed as follows where γ_m^{RES} represents the resource unit cost:

$$\min \sum_{ij} \left(\gamma_{ij}^{P} \sum_{n} X_{ijn} \right) + \sum_{ii'j} \left(\gamma_{ii'j}^{CH} \sum_{n} Z_{ii'jn} \right) + \sum_{m} \left(\gamma_m^{RES} \delta \sum_{n} R_{mn} \right)$$
$$(40)$$

4 Multistage Scheduling

In this section, the modes for the multistage production environment are discussed (Fig. 1). We consider problems with fixed batching decisions. Each stage has multiple units $j \in \mathbf{J}_k$ with $\bigcup_k \mathbf{J}_k = \mathbf{J}$ and $\mathbf{J}_k \cap \mathbf{J}_{k'} = \varnothing$, which means that each stage has its own set of units. A set of batches ($\mathbf{I}$) are processed at each stage exactly once, and each batch should be processed in only one unit. The precedence relation among different stages of the same batch needs to be maintained, which means stage $k + 1$ of batch i can only start after its processing at stage k is finished. Set $\mathbf{I}_j$ includes the batches that can be carried out in unit j, whereas $\mathbf{J}_{ik}$ includes the units at every stage k in which batch i can be processed. Each batch $i \in \mathbf{I}$ has its own release (ρ_i) and due (ε_i) time, and the processing cost/time of batch i in unit j is $\gamma_{ij}^{P}/\tau_{ij}$. The changeover time/costs are denoted by $\tau_{ii'j}/\gamma_{ii'j}^{CH}$. The modelling for problem classes involving changeover costs and times can be achieved following the techniques shown in Sect. "Single Stage Scheduling".

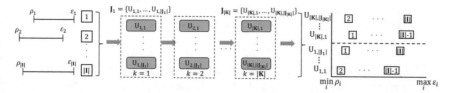

Fig. 1 Representation of multistage batch production scheduling problem and the resultant optimal solution

4.1 Discrete-Time Grid Model

The time discretization techniques are the same as described in the previous sections. We introduce binary variable X_{ijn}, which assumes value 1 if batch i starts on unit j at time point n. Each batch must be processed on only one unit and exactly once:

$$\sum_{j \in J_{ik}} \sum_n X_{ijn} = 1, \qquad i, k \qquad (41)$$

The no-overlap restriction is enforced through a constraint similar to the one described in Sect. "Single Stage Scheduling":

$$\sum_i \sum_{n' \geq n - \overline{\tau}_{ij} + 1}^{n} X_{ijn'} \leq 1, \qquad j, n \qquad (42)$$

The release and due time constraints are enforced by fixing the early and late binaries to zero:

$$X_{ijn} = 0, \quad i, j, n < \overline{\rho}_i; \qquad X_{ijn} = 0, i, j, n > \overline{\varepsilon}_i - \overline{\tau}_{ij} \qquad (43)$$

As mentioned earlier, we need to enforce that stage k of a batch needs to be finished before the next stage of that batch starts. We present two different formulations to enforce this precedence relation.

Aggregated start and finish batch-stage time: The precedence relation is directly enforced through the X_{ijn} variables. The processing of batch i starts at $\sum_{j \in J_{ik}} \sum_n n X_{ijn}$ and ends at $\sum_{j \in J_{ik}} \sum_n (n + \overline{\tau}_{ij}) X_{ijn}$, so we have

$$\sum_{j \in J_{ik}} \sum_n n X_{ijn} \geq \sum_{j \in J_{i,k-1}} \sum_n (n + \overline{\tau}_{ij}) X_{ijn}, \qquad i, k > 1 \qquad (44)$$

Disaggregated start and finish batch-stage time: The first approach is written for every batch and every stage. In the second approach, we only use X_{ijn} variables to ensure that if the processing of stage k of batch i starts at time n, then the stage $k + 1$ of that batch cannot start at any time point n.

$$\sum_{j\in \mathbf{J}_{ik}}\sum_{n'\geq n} X_{ijn'-\bar{\tau}_{ij}} + \sum_{j\in \mathbf{J}_{i,k+1}}\sum_{n'<n} X_{ijn'} \leq 1, \qquad i,k \geq 1, n \tag{45}$$

The precedence constraints are written for each batch, stage, and time period, so the problem size increases, but compared to the first approach, the model becomes tighter. Objective functions are independent of the approaches used to enforce the precedence relations. The objective functions to minimize makespan (Eqs. 46 and 47), weighted earliness (Eq. 48), and weighted lateness (Eq. 49) are described in the following:

$$MS \geq \sum_{j\in \mathbf{J}_{i,|\mathbf{K}|}}\sum_{n}(n+\bar{\tau}_{ij}) X_{ijn}, \qquad i \tag{46}$$

$$\min MS \tag{47}$$

$$\min \sum_{i}\omega_i \left(\bar{\varepsilon}_i - \sum_{j\in \mathbf{J}_{i,|\mathbf{K}|}}\sum_{n}(n+\bar{\tau}_{ij}) X_{ijn}\right) \tag{48}$$

$$\min \sum_{i}\omega_i \left(\sum_{j\in \mathbf{J}_{i,|\mathbf{K}|}}\sum_{n}(n+\bar{\tau}_{ij}) X_{ijn} - \bar{\varepsilon}_i\right) \tag{49}$$

Similar to the single stage environment, we define a variable $L_i \in \mathbb{R}_+$ to represent the tardiness.

$$L_i \geq \sum_{j\in \mathbf{J}_{i,|\mathbf{K}|}}\sum_{n}(n+\bar{\tau}_{ij}) X_{ijn} - \bar{\varepsilon}_i, \qquad i \tag{50}$$

The minimization of tardiness objective function is expressed as follows:

$$\min \sum_{i}\omega_i L_i \tag{51}$$

The cost minimization objective function is

$$\min \sum_{i,j}\left(\gamma_{ij}^{P}\sum_{n}X_{ijn}\right) + \sum_{ii'j}\left(\gamma_{ii'j}^{CH}\sum_{n}Z_{ii'jn}\right) \tag{52}$$

4.2 Storage Constraints

In the discussion so far, we have assumed that enough storage vessels are available to store all the intermediates and products produced by the batches in all stages. We also assumed that there are no time limitations on the storage of these materials between two consecutive stages. However, in reality, limited storage capacity and time might constrain the production, and incorporating these constraints is essential to generate an implementable schedule. In some chemical or biopharmaceutical production, products are generated in batches, and different batches of the same products/intermediates cannot be mixed, which demands multiple storage vessels for storing these batches. Furthermore, if batching decisions are considered, the size of the storage vessels will influence batch sizes. If enough vessels of sufficient sizes are available, then we can assume unlimited storage policy; else, the storage policy is limited, and the multistage production schedule is influenced by both the number and size of the available storage vessels. Another important factor is storage time, which is often important for pharmaceutical processes due to the low shelf life of the intermediate products. Accounting for the waiting time in the processing units is also important and might be used instead of an actual storage vessel in case of limited availability. For further information on modelling of the storage constraints in a multistage facility, the interested reader can refer to Sundaramoorthy et al. [19]

5   Illustrative Example

In this section, we demonstrate the applicability of the abovementioned discrete-time scheduling models through some case studies. The instances are designed to demonstrate the modelling of changeovers and utility (resource) constraints and the efficacy of discrete-time models. We have solved all the instances using the FICO Xpress Optimization Suite and the "mmxprs" module version 2.8.1 on an Intel Core i7 (2.3 GHz) unit with 32GB RAM [43], and the model characteristics for each of these instances are provided in Table 1.

For the first two instances, we consider a production facility involving two production stages and four units: two units per stage. Ten batches need to be processed in this facility, and unlimited storage policy is assumed. Data for this example is taken from Sundaramoorthy et al. [19] and modified accordingly (Figs. 2 and 3).

Two different instances of this example are considered. In the first instance, we do not consider changeover times, while in the second, we find the optimum schedule incorporating changeover times. The objective is to minimize the makespan. The resultant optimal schedules for these two instances are shown in Fig. 2a and b.

Table 1   Model statistics for the instances

	Instance 1	Instance 2	Instance 3
Objective	Makespan minimization	Makespan minimization	Cost minimization
Constraints	604	10,659	51,831
Continuous variables	1	1	99
Binary variables	890	890	80,661
Computational time (s)	0.1	3	2309

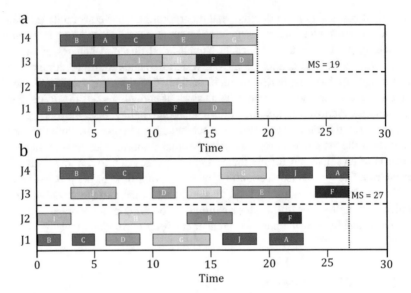

Fig. 2 Gantt chart of optimal solutions for Instances 1 and 2

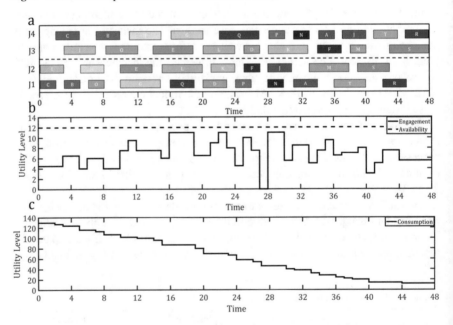

Fig. 3 Gantt chart and utility profiles of optimal solutions for Instance 3. (**a**) Optimum schedule; (**b**) consumption and availability of utility (EL) required for batch execution; (**c**) consumption of utility (CW) required for changeover

We next present a large size instance, in which 20 batches are to be scheduled. Each batch is to be processed in two stages, and each stage has two dedicated units in which the batches can be processed. We also consider utility requirements and illustrate the effect of limited utility on the optimum schedule. We assume that the processing of each batch requires electricity (EL) in both stages. Furthermore, it is assumed that each changeover among batches incurs cost and requires the consumption of cleaning water (CW), which is assumed to be a nonrenewable utility with initial inventory of 130 tons. The cost of CW is assumed to be included in the changeover cost. The objective is to minimize the total (processing + changeover + utility) cost.

Figure 3 shows the Gantt chart and utility profiles of the optimum solution for the third instance. Figure 3b depicts the engagements of EL utility that coincide with the processing of batches, whereas Fig. 3c illustrates the consumption profile of CW utility, which is triggered by the changeovers. This example demonstrates how the intricacies related to changeover time cost and utility requirements can be modeled. Nevertheless, as the computational requirements increase with problem size, advanced solution methods may be necessary to solve large industrial-scale instances. A set of such solution methods, including tightening methodologies and reformulation techniques applicable to multistage, multiproduct production environment, are described in Merchan et al. [20] and Lee and Maravelias [21, 22].

6 Conclusion

This chapter provides an overview of discrete-time batch scheduling models that can be used to schedule chemical and biopharmaceutical manufacturing environments. Concepts and techniques regarding the formulation of such models are discussed, starting from the single-unit problem and building up to problems in multiproduct multistage facilities. The structure of the discrete-time models remains almost the same from a single-unit to multiunit multistage problems, and complex decisions related to batching, changeover, and shared resources can be easily modeled. Furthermore, as the time grid is explicit, time-sensitive nuances such as time varying resource availability, intermediate orders can also be easily incorporated into the model. We showed, through a medium-size case study of a multiproduct multistage facility, how the aforementioned features can be incorporated.

References

1. Marques, C. M., Moniz, S., de Sousa, J. P., Barbosa-Povoa, A. P. & Reklaitis, G. Decision-support challenges in the chemical-pharmaceutical industry: Findings and future research directions. *Comput. Chem. Eng.* **134**, 106672 (2020).

2. Lee, S. L. *et al.* Modernizing Pharmaceutical Manufacturing: from Batch to Continuous Production. *J. Pharm. Innov.***10**, 191–199 (2015).

3. Georgiadis, G. P., Elekidis, A. P. & Georgiadis, M. C. Optimization-Based Scheduling for the Process Industries: From Theory to Real-Life Industrial Applications. *Processes* vol. 7 (2019).

4. Reklaitis, G. V. Overview of Scheduling and Planning of Batch Process Operations BT - Batch Processing Systems Engineering. in (eds. Reklaitis, G. V, Sunol, A. K., Rippin, D. W. T. & Hortaçsu, Ö.) 660–705 (Springer Berlin Heidelberg, 1996).

5. Kallrath, J. Planning and scheduling in the process industry. *OR Spectr.***24**, 219–250 (2002).

6. Floudas, C. a. & Lin, X. Continuous-time versus discrete-time approaches for scheduling of chemical processes: A review. *Comput. Chem. Eng.***28**, 2109–2129 (2004).

7. Méndez, C. a., Cerdá, J., Grossmann, I. E., Harjunkoski, I. & Fahl, M. State-of-the-art review of optimization methods for short-term scheduling of batch processes. *Comput. Chem. Eng.***30**, 913–946 (2006).

8. Maravelias, C. T. General framework and modeling approach classification for chemical production scheduling. *AIChE J.***58**, 1812–1828 (2012).

9. Harjunkoski, I. *et al.* Scope for industrial applications of production scheduling models and solution methods. *Comput. Chem. Eng.***62**, 161–193 (2014).

10. Méndez, C. A., Henning, G. P. & Cerdá, J. Optimal scheduling of batch plants satisfying multiple product orders with different due-dates. *Comput. Chem. Eng.***24**, 2223–2245 (2000).

11. Méndez, C. A., Henning, G. P. & Cerdá, J. An MILP continuous-time approach to short-term scheduling of resource-constrained multistage flowshop batch facilities. *Comput. Chem. Eng.***25**, 701–711 (2001).

12. Gupta, S. & Karimi, I. A. An Improved MILP Formulation for Scheduling Multiproduct, Multistage Batch Plants. *Ind. Eng. Chem. Res.***42**, 2365–2380 (2003).

13. Sundaramoorthy, A. & Maravelias, C. T. Modeling of Storage in Batching and Scheduling of Multistage Processes. *Ind. Eng. Chem. Res.***47**, 6648–6660 (2008).

14. Sundaramoorthy, A. & Maravelias, C. T. Simultaneous Batching and Scheduling in Multistage Multiproduct Processes. *Ind. Eng. Chem. Res.***47**, 1546–1555 (2008).

15. Kopanos, G. M., Laínez, J. M. & Puigjaner, L. An Efficient Mixed-Integer Linear Programming Scheduling Framework for Addressing Sequence-Dependent Setup Issues in Batch Plants. *Ind. Eng. Chem. Res.***48**, 6346–6357 (2009).

16. Cerdá, J., Henning, G. P. & Grossmann, I. E. A Mixed-Integer Linear Programming Model for Short-Term Scheduling of Single-Stage Multiproduct Batch Plants with Parallel Lines. *Ind. Eng. Chem. Res.***36**, 1695–1707 (1997).

17. Kondili, E., Pantelides, C. C. & Sargent, R. W. H. A general algorithm for short-term scheduling of batch operations—I. MILP formulation. *Comput. Chem. Eng.***17**, 211–227 (1993).

18. Shah, N., Pantelides, C. C. & Sargent, R. W. H. A general algorithm for short-term scheduling of batch operations—II. Computational issues. *Comput. Chem. Eng.***17**, 229–244 (1993).

19. Sundaramoorthy, A., Maravelias, C. T. & Prasad, P. Scheduling of Multistage Batch Processes under Utility Constraints. *Ind. Eng. Chem. Res.***48**, 6050–6058 (2009).

20. Merchan, A. F., Lee, H. & Maravelias, C. T. Discrete-time mixed-integer programming models and solution methods for production scheduling in multistage facilities. *Comput. Chem. Eng.***94**, 387–410 (2016).

21. Lee, H. & Maravelias, C. T. Discrete-time mixed-integer programming models for short-term scheduling in multipurpose environments. *Comput. Chem. Eng.***107**, 171–183 (2017).

22. Lee, H. & Maravelias, C. T. Mixed-integer programming models for simultaneous batching and scheduling in multipurpose batch plants. *Comput. Chem. Eng.***106**, 621–644 (2017).

23. Schilling, G. & Pantelides, C. C. A simple continuous-time process scheduling formulation and a novel solution algorithm. *Comput. Chem. Eng.***20**, S1221–S1226 (1996).

24. Castro, P. M., Barbosa-Póvoa, A. P., Matos, H. A. & Novais, A. Q. Simple Continuous-Time Formulation for Short-Term Scheduling of Batch and Continuous Processes. *Ind. Eng. Chem. Res.***43**, 105–118 (2004).

25. Maravelias, C. T. & Grossmann, I. E. New General Continuous-Time State–Task Network Formulation for Short-Term Scheduling of Multipurpose Batch Plants. *Ind. Eng. Chem. Res.* **42**, 3056–3074 (2003).

26. Janak, S. L., Floudas, C. A., Kallrath, J. & Vormbrock, N. Production scheduling of a large-scale industrial batch plant. I. Short-term and medium-term scheduling. *Ind. Eng. Chem. Res.* **45**, 8234–8252 (2006).

27. Shaik, M. A. & Floudas, C. A. Unit-specific event-based continuous-time approach for short-term scheduling of batch plants using RTN framework. *Comput. Chem. Eng.* **32**, 260–274 (2008).

28. Mostafaei, H. & Harjunkoski, I. Continuous-time scheduling formulation for multipurpose batch plants. *AIChE J.* **66**, e16804 (2020).

29. Ierapetritou, M. G. & Floudas, C. A. Effective Continuous-Time Formulation for Short-Term Scheduling. 1. Multipurpose Batch Processes. *Ind. Eng. Chem. Res.* **37**, 4341–4359 (1998).

30. Maravelias, C. T. Mixed-Time Representation for State-Task Network Models. *Ind. Eng. Chem. Res.* **44**, 9129–9145 (2005).

31. Westerlund, J., Hästbacka, M., Forssell, S. & Westerlund, T. Mixed-Time Mixed-Integer Linear Programming Scheduling Model. *Ind. Eng. Chem. Res.* **46**, 2781–2796 (2007).

32. Lee, H. & Maravelias, C. T. Combining the advantages of discrete- and continuous-time scheduling models: Part 1. Framework and mathematical formulations. *Comput. Chem. Eng.* **116**, 176–190 (2018).

33. Castro, P. M., Harjunkoski, I. & Grossmann, I. E. Optimal Short-Term Scheduling of Large-Scale Multistage Batch Plants. *Ind. Eng. Chem. Res.* **48**, 11002–11016 (2009).

34. Kopanos, G. M., Méndez, C. A. & Puigjaner, L. MIP-based decomposition strategies for large-scale scheduling problems in multipurpose multistage batch plants: A benchmark scheduling problem of the pharmaceutical industry. *Eur. J. Oper. Res.* **207**, 644–655 (2010).

35. Stefansson, H., Sigmarsdottir, S., Jensson, P. & Shah, N. Discrete and continuous time representations and mathematical models for large production scheduling problems: A case study from the pharmaceutical industry. *Eur. J. Oper. Res.* **215**, 383–392 (2011).

36. Lakhdar, K., Zhou, Y., Savery, J., Titchener-Hooker, N. J. & Papageorgiou, L. G. Medium Term Planning of Biopharmaceutical Manufacture using Mathematical Programming. *Biotechnol. Prog.* **21**, 1478–1489 (2005).

37. Kabra, S., Shaik, M. A. & Rathore, A. S. Multi-period scheduling of a multistage multiproduct bio-pharmaceutical process. *Comput. Chem. Eng.* **57**, 95–103 (2013).

38. Liu, S., Yahia, A. & Papageorgiou, L. G. Optimal Production and Maintenance Planning of Biopharmaceutical Manufacturing under Performance Decay. *Ind. Eng. Chem. Res.* **53**, 17075–17091 (2014).

39. Moniz, S., Barbosa-Póvoa, A. P., de Sousa, J. P. & Duarte, P. Solution Methodology for Scheduling Problems in Batch Plants. *Ind. Eng. Chem. Res.* **53**, 19265–19281 (2014).

40. Eberle, L. *et al.* Rigorous approach to scheduling of sterile drug product manufacturing. *Comput. Chem. Eng.* **94**, 221–234 (2016).

41. Zyngier, D. & Kelly, J. D. Multi-Product Inventory Logistics Modeling in the Process Industries BT - Optimization and Logistics Challenges in the Enterprise. in (eds. Chaovalitwongse, W., Furman, K. C. & Pardalos, P. M.) 61–95 (Springer US, 2009). doi: https://doi.org/10.1007/978-0-387-88617-6_2.

42. Velez, S. & Maravelias, C. T. Advances in Mixed-Integer Programming Methods for Chemical Production Scheduling. *Annu. Rev. Chem. Biomol. Eng.* **5**, 97–121 (2014).

43. Guéret, C., Prins, C., Sevaux, M. & Heipcke, S. *Applications of Optimization with Xpress-MP.* (Dash Optimization Limited, 2002).

Model-Based Risk Assessment of mAb Developability

M. Karlberg, A. Kizhedath, and J. Glassey

Monoclonal antibodies were already one of the fastest growing sectors of bio-pharmaceutical industry [1]. Recent research on the significant benefits of various antibodies in reducing the risks of fatality or reducing the symptoms of COVID-19, e.g., tocilizumab and sarilumab (Cortegiani et al. 2021), inevitably increases the importance of the rapid discovery of mAbs and the development of efficient manufacturing processes. Research reports frequently concentrated on the rapid discovery of new mAbs, but the developability and the manufacturability of mAbs were less explored until recently [1–4]. This chapter adopts the framework of quality by design (QbD), concentrating particularly on the model-based risk assessment of mAb developability. A case study highlights specific areas where advanced modelling approaches can contribute to speeding up the manufacturability and developability of mAbs and demonstrates the benefits and the challenges of this approach.

1 Quality by Design

The QbD paradigm was introduced in 2004 and is a systematic approach that aligns with the Process Analytical Technology (PAT) principles and aims to build quality into the product through product and process understanding (US FDA 2004). The framework is especially useful for the process development of mAbs, which consists of many different steps (unit operations). A typical mAb process can be divided into two parts: the upstream (USP) or the cell culture processing where the mAbs are expressed and the downstream (DSP) or purification where the mAbs are isolated

M. Karlberg · A. Kizhedath · J. Glassey (✉)
School of Engineering, Newcastle University, Newcastle upon Tyne, UK
e-mail: jarka.glassey@ncl.ac.uk

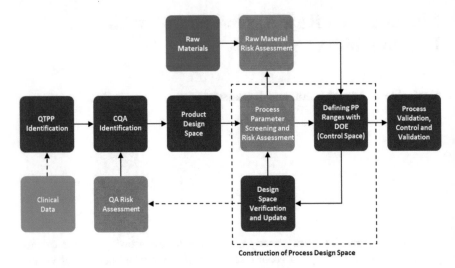

Fig. 1 General outline of the QbD methodology. The process design space is shown as the dashed box where the effects of process parameters and raw material input (*blue box*) on the product quality are characterised. Steps highlighted in *red* indicate risk assessment of either product quality attributes, process parameters or raw materials. The *green box* indicates the availability of clinical data which can be used to better define the QTPP

and contaminants removed. Typically, a mAb process will consist of between 15 and 20 different unit operations which must be individually characterised, e.g. finding the optimal process parameters that deliver consistent drug quality and safety of use [5]. The major steps of a QbD implementation to develop and characterise a product/process are illustrated in Fig. 1. It is important to note that these are a subset of steps involved in the whole QbD process. For more details on QbD, including important aspects such as Critical Material Attributes (CMAs), which will not be discussed in this contribution in detail, please refer to Rathore [6] and Lawrence et al. [7].

1.1 Quality Target Product Profile

The implementation of QbD starts by defining the Quality Target Product Profile (QTPP) which forms the basis of the design for the development and contains information about the drug quality criteria such as delivery mechanisms, intended use and route of administration for the intended product to ensure clinical safety and efficacy. The QTPP is generated from knowledge that is based on literature research, clinical trials and existing experience from industry or academia [8, 9]. For mAbs, the QTPP relates to the product's intended use and properties that can affect patients and needs to be clearly stated to avoid adverse effects in patients.

Issues with the lack of efficacy, adverse effects and/or high manufacturing costs have led to the withdrawal or discontinuation of several mAb products (Kizhedath et al. 2017). It is thus important that QTPPs include antigen binding, pharmacokinetics, effector function, stability and half-life of the mAb [6, 10]. However, much of this information does not become available until later when clinical data has been obtained. Thus, instead, many aspects of the QTPP are based on prior knowledge in early process development of a mAb. Recently, the computational prediction and simulation of the mAb structure have been shown to be a valuable tool for mAb design due to their ability to provide estimates of behaviour and protein stability which can aid in more accurate QTPP specification [11, 12].

1.2 Critical Quality Attributes and Risk Assessment

QTPP provides the basis for the identification of Critical Quality Attributes (CQAs) from a list of Quality Attributes (QAs) using risk-based analysis. This is in accordance with the ICH Q9 guideline to investigate properties that might affect product quality. The CQAs are physical, chemical or biological properties of the drug product that need to be within appropriate ranges to ensure the desired product quality. These ranges, similar to the generation of QTPP, are obtained through literature research, clinical data and previous experience, but they are also updated during process development as new information from characterisation studies becomes available. The most frequently used method for risk assessment in industries is Failure Mode and Effect Analysis (FMEA) where the impact of different unit operations in the process on the QAs is listed. Each effect is ranked according to a Severity rating (S), an Occurrence rating (O) and a Detectability rating (D). A final Risk Priority Number (RPN) is calculated by multiplying the ratings which are then ranked to identify the effects that potentially affect the product quality and efficacy [13, 14]. Tailored risk assessment methods have also been proposed for biopharmaceuticals by Zalai et al. (2013). In their work, the authors argued that traditional methods do not consider the "complexity" of how a process might affect the product or the "uncertainty" which includes the quality of the input material as a possible source of risk and which need to be added as additional factors to the risk assessment.

Once the CQAs have been selected, a process design space is defined by screening process parameters (PPs) for each of the unit operations that have a significant effect on the CQAs. PPs that have a significant impact on the CQAs are called Critical Process Parameters (CPPs) and are identified and controlled using the following steps:

1. Similar to identification of CQAs, risk analysis methods, such as FMEA, are used to reduce the large number of PPs to those that may affect CQAs.

2. Systematic experimental studies using Design of Experiments (DoE) over a range of PP settings are carried out in small scale to obtain experimental data for process characterisation to identify CPPs and their optimal ranges. This is referred to as the control space.

3. Multivariate data analysis (MVDA) is used for the implementation of appropriate real-time monitoring and control strategies needed for the defined CQAs and CPPs to ensure product quality. Movement outside of the defined control space would cause the product quality to drop below that of the desired quality stated in the QTPP.

The use of statistical DoE is preferred over univariate analysis in process development of pharmaceuticals as it can generate qualitative and quantitative information about important process parameters and their impact on the product quality [15]. Response Surface Modelling (RSM) and leverage plots are often used to analyse the DoE data to investigate the significance of PPs on the explored CQAs as well as to define allowed ranges for the identified CPPs [16]. Various experimental designs exist, and selecting an appropriate design is critical in order to maximise the information gained from the experiments. Kumar et al. [17] compared different experimental designs for the DoE of downstream unit operations to demonstrate how these affect the response surface of each unit operation [17]. Tai et al. [18] showed that a well-chosen experimental design can lead to diverse and informative data about the system and when combined with high-throughput experimentation techniques, it can be a powerful tool in defining the process design space.

The fundamental principle of the QbD framework is to increase process understanding in terms of the effect that PPs have on product quality. Zurdo [19] suggested that the QbD framework needed to be extended to incorporate product understanding in terms of the developability of the pharmaceutical which would include manufacturability, safety, pharmacology and biological activity. The author argued that by using in silico risk assessment tools based on structural features of the mAbs and historic development data, predictions concerning manufacturability of an mAb could be made. In a later publication, two case studies were presented where structural properties of mAbs were successfully linked to CQAs related to aggregation and half-life [4]. Such tools can add great value to early process development of mAbs when implementing the QbD framework where little is known about both the process and product. Thus, a more in-depth investigation of Quantitative Structure-Activity Relationship (QSAR) framework and its potential benefits for QbD integration is explored here.

2 Advanced Modelling Approaches in QbD

The QSAR framework relates structural properties and features (also known as descriptors) of a compound to biological or physicochemical activity [20, 21].

This methodology was first introduced by Hammet in the 1930s and was later refined by Hansch and Fujita and has become a standard tool for small-molecule drug discovery [22]. A method derived from QSAR, referred to as Quantitative Sequence-Activity Modelling (QSAM), has been introduced in recent years and focuses on relating structural descriptors of proteins, peptides and nucleic acids to activity [23]. The only difference between QSAR and QSAM is the development of descriptors, whereas the guidelines for the predictive model development remain the same. Given the complex protein structure of mAbs, the QSAM methodology for descriptor generation will be of more relevance, and the workflow described below will therefore focus more on protein-based rather than small molecule-based QSAR.

2.1 Descriptor Generation

One of the most important steps in QSAR is the numerical representation of structures of the pharmaceuticals so that they can be used in correlation studies with prediction outputs of interest. For proteins, such as mAbs, two approaches to generate descriptors are discussed here: (1) descriptors generated from the amino acid primary sequence and (2) descriptors generated from three-dimensional models of the mAbs. It has been shown that a combination of both physicochemical and 3D structure descriptors works best and also ensures that the model is not overly reliant on a single type of a descriptor [24].

2.2 Amino Acid Composition-Based Descriptor Generation

Extensive research has been carried out to develop new informative descriptors for peptides and proteins generated from their primary sequence [25]. This was first introduced by Sneath [26] who derived amino acid descriptors for the 20 naturally occurring amino acids from qualitative data. Later on, Kidera et al. [27] used 188 properties of the 20 naturally occurring amino acids, which were converted into ten orthogonal new descriptors to describe the amino acids. Later, the Z-scale, which consists of three new amino acid descriptors derived by applying PCA to 29 physiochemical properties [28, 29], was introduced. Other amino acid scales, which were also derived through PCA, include the extended Z-scale and T-scale [30, 31]. Other descriptors include the so-called isotropic surface area (ISA) and the electronic charge index (ECI), which are derived from the 3D structures of the amino acids [32]. All these descriptors were tested and performed well in respective studies on small peptides. In a two-part review by van Westen et al. [33, 34], many of the existing amino acid scales were benchmarked and compared. The authors demonstrated that the different scales described different physiochemical and topological properties which is useful when deciding on which scales to use [33, 34]. Doytchinova et al. [35] applied the Z-scale's descriptors to successfully predict ligand binding of peptides, and Obrezanova et al. [3] used several amino acid scales to predict mAb aggregation propensity based on the primary sequence. However, even though amino acid descriptors explain the differences in the primary sequence, they do not take into consideration potential interactions between the amino acids in or between primary chains. It has been argued that this simplification can lead to a loss of information concerning properties of secondary and tertiary structure in larger proteins [25].

Descriptors can also be generated by using empirical equations on the entire primary sequence to infer protein properties such as the isoelectric point, hydrophobicity, molecular weight, physicochemical properties and secondary structure content, to name a few. Many such tools and applications are available on bioinformatics sites, such as Expert Protein Analysis System (ExPASy) [36] and European Bioinformatics Institute at European Molecular Biology Laboratory (EMBL-EBI) [37].

2.3 Homology Modelling and Molecular Dynamics for Descriptor Generation

Descriptors capturing structural and surface properties can be generated by using existing crystal or Nuclear Magnetic Resonance (NMR) structures or by building models using homology modelling. The latter is performed by finding proteins with existing 3D structures that have a high level of similarity to the primary sequence of the protein of interest. These proteins are then used as templates to predict the likely structure of the queried protein [38]. This has been successfully used in many studies where information such as surface areas, angles and surface properties was extracted [39–41]. The method is especially useful when no crystal structure exists. Caution needs to be exercised, however, as the homology models are only predicted structures. Breneman et al. [42] introduced a methodology for generating 2D surface descriptors, also called transferable atom equivalent (TAE) descriptors, by reconstructing the electronic surface properties of the molecular structures from a library of atomic charge density components. This has the advantage of representing surface variations such as hydrophobicity and charge distributions numerically, which is of great importance when studying, for example, protein binding to an anion exchange chromatographic column packing using different salts [43]. Robinson et al. [44] used the TAE descriptors to relate the structural differences between several Fab fragments to predict column performance between different chromatographic systems. It has been argued, however, that caution needs to be exercised when using library-based descriptors as these are usually directly related to a specific state of a compound that was measured in a unique environment. This means that these descriptors should only be applied if experiments were carried out in an identical or in a similar environment. Otherwise, this might cause the descriptors to be biased [24]. Other structural properties, such as molecular angles and solvent accessible surface areas extracted from homology models, were used by Sydow et al. [41] to determine the risk of degradation of asparagine and aspartate in mAbs as PTMs. Similarly, Sharma et al. [40] investigated the risk of oxidation of surface accessible tryptophans.

Due to the flexibility and size of the mAbs, it is very difficult to produce good 3D structures based on X-ray crystallography and NMR. Instead, homology modelling has proven to be a good alternative to circumvent this problem. However, due to the size and the many flexible parts in the mAbs, pure homology models might not give a sufficiently accurate representation of the reality. Molecular dynamics (MD) is a useful tool that can be used to minimise the energy of the entire protein and to simulate the dynamics of the protein of interest in different environments [45]. MD simulations have also shown very high similarities in the internal dynamics of mAbs when comparing the simulated results to those observed in reality [46]. It is therefore recommended to apply MD simulation to all homology models before descriptors are generated in order to mimic the environment of the samples that are used in QSAR studies. However, implementation of MD simulations is still computationally expensive and time-consuming, and its practical use is therefore still limited. Alternatives, such as coarse-grained MD might therefore be preferable where computational power is lacking, but it is computationally cheaper. In coarse-grained MD, groups of atoms, e.g. residue side chains, are simulated as a single static structure or point. This in turn aids in drastically reducing the number of atoms in the system that needs to be simulated [47]. It should be noted that smaller structural fluctuations and dynamics will be lost when using coarse-grained MD, which needs to be considered prior to developing the descriptors.

2.4 QSAR for Protein Behaviour Prediction

The QSAR framework has been applied to a diverse range of challenges where structural properties of pharmaceuticals have been used directly for the prediction of different process-related aspects such as the prediction of isotherm parameters in ion-exchange chromatography [48], ligand-binding in ion-exchange chromatography under high salt concentrations [49], binding of proteins in ion-exchange chromatography under different pH conditions [50], protein surface patch analysis for the choice of purification methods [51], chromatographic separation of target proteins from Host Cell Proteins (HCPs) [39], viscosity, clearance and stability prediction for mAbs [40] and degradation prediction of asparagine and aspartate in mAbs [41], to mention a few. This also showcases one of the main strengths of the QSAR/QSAM framework with its ability to link structural features to many different forms of prediction outputs. It is important to note, however, that identical experiments must have been performed on different mAbs to compare the differences in structure and their effect on the output. Equally important is that sufficient excitation is present in the output data in order for the effects to be linked to the corresponding structural feature [52].

3 Model-Based Prediction of Developability

There have been significant advances in computational prediction methods, and they are starting to become more common in process development [53]. As mentioned by Zurdo et al. [4], the ability to predict product-related characteristics that strongly relate to the QTPP and/or CQAs can greatly simplify process development, especially in the early stages when the product or process knowledge is limited. The implementation of QSAR in process-related areas, such as protein purification, has been researched extensively [2, 44, 48–50, 54–57]. Though not all the mentioned examples concern mAbs specifically, the outlined methodology used in the different research articles is still applicable. Given the significant proportion of mAb develop-ment cost that is incurred during downstream processing, considerable advantages can be gained by being able to predict the performance of chromatographic columns and their effect on product quality early in the process development. In the case of mAbs, much of the cost is incurred during the purification due to the strict regulations surrounding clinical safety of the end product [58, 59]. Examples of regulations for mAbs include the removal of harmful structural variants while retaining the desired structure based on evidence from clinical trials. The removal of contaminants, such as HCPs, DNA and viruses, is also necessary in order to avoid undesired immune responses in patients. Thus, for therapeutic use, a mAb purity of >99% is required in the final formulation [60]. Therefore, the integration of QSAR into QbD is proposed based on the valuable insight that QSAR can provide in early process development and is illustrated in Fig. 2, which also shows how the QbD framework can add to and improve the QSAR modelling with addition of new data.

Two main approaches of integrating the QSAR framework into the QbD paradigm can be considered. The first approach is by only using generated structural descriptors for development of models able to predict protein behaviours [56]. The method is, however, more constrained as it requires data generated from identical experimental setups, and therefore identical PP settings, in order to satisfy the assumption that the observed effect is caused only by the differences in structure between the proteins. Therefore, models developed this way are better for assessing the manufacturing feasibility and/or potential CQAs before starting the process development.

The second approach is to use the PPs of interest, taken from previous mAb processes to use directly in the model development by either (1) adding the PPs together with the generated structural descriptors as inputs [61] or (2) structural descriptors are calculated to be dependent on the PPs, meaning that the values of the descriptors will change with changing values of the PPs [50]. The latter is easiest done by generating descriptors from MD simulations where changes in the soluble environment can be implemented. This, however, requires that data is gathered from similar experimental setups where only the PPs of interest have been varied. This would usually not be a problem when gathering historic data generated from the

QbD (Process Understanding)

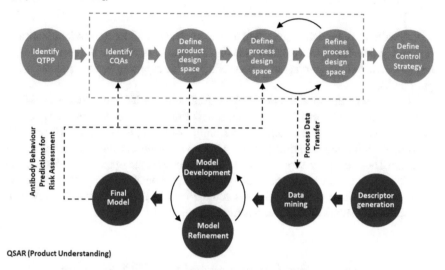

QSAR (Product Understanding)

Fig. 2 Proposed integration of QSAR into QbD where the upper half illustrates the simplified framework of QbD (*red circles*) and the lower half illustrates a simplified version of the QSAR framework (*black circles*). Transfer of characterisation data from previous mAb processes can be used directly for model development using QSAR. Depending on the purpose of the developed QSAR model, it can be used to directly aid in assessing CQAs or provide insight into PPs and ranges

QbD paradigm as it will often conform to experimental designs based on DoEs where the experimental environment is strictly controlled. The added benefit of this approach is that the developed model will be able to account for both the structural differences and the impact from the studied PPs when predicting protein behaviour. This can potentially have great value in process development of new mAbs as PP ranges can be assessed in silico and therefore greatly aid in reducing the number of needed experiments, seen as grey arrows in Fig. 2.

The methods described above provide a reference for further risk assessment and characterisation to be performed in the QbD framework, as they provide information such as the behaviour of the product in different scenarios and increase the product understanding. As additional information from new mAb processes becomes available, models can be improved by expanding the data sets used in the model development. This in turn will aid in providing more accurate predictions due to lowering the sparsity by incorporating more protein structures. Available characterisation research studies can also be used as additional sources of data in order to improve the models by expanding the data set for model development.

4 Case Studies

In line with the approaches described above, we have developed a model identification and parametrisation workflow (see Fig. 3) in order to explore the capabilities of advanced modelling approaches in predicting the behaviour of various mAbs during purification.

The development of a hybrid QSAR-based model with a structured workflow and clear evaluation metrics, with several optimisation steps, was described in detail in Kizhedath et al. [2]. Furthermore, using cross reactivity (from CIC data) or solubility/aggregation (from HIC data) as responses and physicochemical characteristics (primary sequence and 3D structure) of mAbs as descriptors, the QSAR models generated for different applicability domains allow for rapid early-stage screening and developability as summarised in the case studies below and detailed in Kizhedath et al. [2] and Karlberg et al. [56].

4.1 Cross-Interaction Chromatography as CQA Screening Method

As indicated earlier, the success of a new mAb product depends not only on its efficacy and manufacturability but also on the lack of undesirable side effects and interactions. Bailly et al. [1] provide a useful overview of a range of analytical methods that can be used during the sequence selection and product/process development in order to evaluate important CQAs. One such method is the cross-interaction chromatography used in early screening to detect undesirable interactions with other mAbs [62].

Kizhedath et al. [2] detailed the development of a hybrid QSAR-based model with a structured workflow and clear evaluation metrics, with several optimisation steps, that could be beneficial for broader and more generic PLS modelling. Based on the results and observations from this study, a structured selection of data sets and variables demonstrated increased model performance and allowed for further optimisation of these hybrid models. Furthermore, using cross reactivity (from CIC data) as responses and physicochemical characteristics of mAbs as descriptors, the QSAR models generated for different applicability domains allow for rapid early-stage screening and developability [2].

The generated descriptors captured the physicochemical properties of mAbs with varying degrees of resolution (local to global; singular to cluster). These descriptors from different data blocks were subjected to an exploratory analysis to study any separation based on intrinsic properties such as light and heavy chain isotypes as well as species type of mAbs that would then allow for selection of descriptor sets that could be used for QSAR model development. Exploratory analysis of the descriptor data was carried out using unsupervised pattern recognition methods such as principal component analysis (PCA) to visualise any intrinsic property-

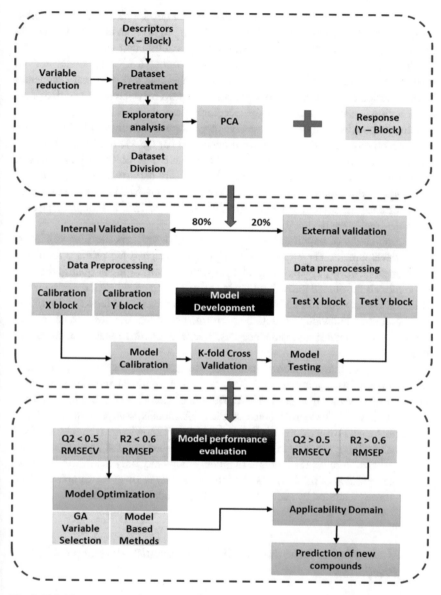

Fig. 3 Hybrid model development workflow outlining the different steps involved in descriptor generation, pre-treatment and variable reduction; model development followed by model evaluation and optimisation. *PCA* principal component analysis, *GA* genetic algorithm, *RMSECV* root mean square error of cross-validation, *RMSEP* RMSE of prediction. (Adapted from Ref. [2])

based separation or clustering. The descriptor sets were assessed for the influence of intrinsic properties that could hamper with predictive model development that facilitates mAb developability. Based on the results, the descriptors of the hypervariable region were chosen for further model development. Furthermore, the samples were divided into appropriate heavy chain, light chain and species type for developing models that have a better-defined applicability domain.

These descriptors were then used for developing a QSAR model for the prediction of cross-interaction chromatographic retention times. Primary sequence-based descriptors do not take into account interactions between amino acid residues or the antibody-antigen and antibody-receptor interaction space. To address this, 3D structures of mAbs were first generated via homology modelling and MD simulation upon which structural descriptors were generated for QSAR model development. Similar to the primary descriptors, resolution and type of descriptors selected were similar, i.e. local and cluster-based substructure data set with electronic and charge-based descriptors were identified to be important. Most of these descriptors of importance arise from the hypervariable regions of mAbs similar to primary sequence-based descriptors [63].

A combination of sequence-based and structural descriptors was also utilised for model development. The structural descriptors outweighed the primary sequence-based ones; however, the overall model performance was of lower quality than that of the models developed individually using primary sequence-based descriptors and structural descriptors, respectively. This implies that careful selection of variables based on expert knowledge should be performed such that the descriptors selected capture both structural and sequence-based aspects of functional characterisation [63].

Modelling techniques, such as those that use categorical responses (partial least squares discriminant analysis, PLS-DA), as well as nonlinear modelling methods, such as support vector machines (SVM), were also briefly investigated in this project (data not shown). The performance of PLS-DA models was poor mainly due to class imbalance. Furthermore, the influence of expert knowledge is greater for these models as defining the classes is arbitrary. With regard to the SVM-based models with non-linear kernels, the increase in model complexity only led to similar model performance as that of the PLS models. Interpretability is lower for complex models such as those generated by such SVM for similar model performance.

4.2 Hydrophobic Interaction Chromatography Retention Time Prediction

Another important experimental assay, highlighted by Bailly et al. [1], is hydrophobic interaction chromatography (HIC), which is used in the assessment of mAb aggregation and solubility. HIC is also a common polishing step in downstream purification of mAbs [62]. Thus, successful prediction of HIC retention times can yield important information for risk assessment of the feasibility of a mAb candidate to be manufactured. It can also provide insight into process characterisation of the HIC polishing step.

In a study of Karlberg et al. [56], a QSAR modelling workflow linking mAb structures to corresponding HIC retention times was implemented where the necessary level of intramolecular interactions for successful prediction was explored. More specifically, descriptors were generated from three potential sources: (1) primary sequence, (2) 3D structure from homology modelling and (3) 3D structure from 50 ns MD simulations. This in order to compare the predictive performance of a model based on descriptors sets that containing residue-to-residue interactions (3D structures) with a model based on descriptor sets without residue-to-residue interactions (primary sequence). As described previously in the CIC case study, the three descriptors sets were subjected to an exploratory data analysis with PCA prior to model development to investigate the presence of intrinsic structural variation originating from the light and heavy chains as well as the species type that could potentially impact model performance.

All QSAR models were fitted according to the workflow outlined in Fig. 3. Here, an SVM algorithm for regression was used with a linear kernel to allow for high model interpretability [64]. The QSAR model developed on primary sequence-based descriptors yielded suboptimal predictions of HIC retention times. This resulted from a high model bias (under-fitting), meaning that critical information was either missing or confounded in the generated descriptors and the resulting model was therefore unable to correlate the mAb structure to the HIC retention time. On the contrary, the QSAR model developed on descriptors generated from 3D homology structures was found to suffer from high variance (over-fitting). This resulted from the fitting of non-informative noise present in the descriptor set which resulted in poor model generalisation when evaluated on an external test set. The main source for this was identified to be biased 3D structures originating from the structure generation step with homology modelling. More specifically, the generated 3D structures were found to be in unfavourable structural conformations which resulted in biased descriptors that were unable to represent the true structural properties of the mAbs. Instead, MD simulations were applied in order to allow residue side chains and domains in the mAb homology structures to relax and attain more energetically favourable conformations as seen in Fig. 4 [56].

The QSAR model developed using the resulting MD descriptors achieved much higher performance in the evaluation of the external test set ($R^2 = 0.63$) compared to the homology model-based descriptors ($R^2 = -0.08$). It was found that descriptors generated from the hypervariable regions, or more specifically the CDR loops column binding where properties such as surface charge and hydrophobicity, were especially important. This is consistent with previous research [65].

5 Conclusions

This chapter reviewed the opportunities and the challenges in model-based risk assessment of mAb developability. A structured workflow was proposed for hybrid

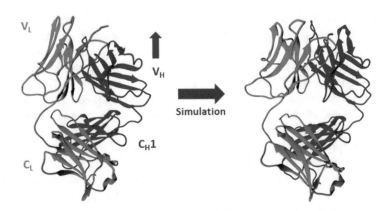

Fig. 4 Displacement of the V_H domain (*blue arrow*) and loops during the MD simulation of eldelumab. The heavy chain and light chain are represented in *blue* and *red*, respectively

QSAR model development to assist in the evaluation of important mAb developability characteristics.

Two case studies highlighted the benefits of such a workflow and the use of PLS and SVM models in predicting Cross Interaction Chromatography (CIC) and Hydrophobic Interaction Chromatography (HIC) retention times as important mAb characteristics related to risks of aggregation and non-specific binding. While some positive observations were reported, further work exploring non-linear modelling techniques, applying the modelling framework on larger and/or more industrial data sets as well as newer types of mAbs such as bispecifics, and developing QSAR models around other substructural and species-related applicability domains of MAbs, including glycoform conformation as a feature for model development, to name a few would provide robust basis for evaluation of this workflow. For example, further investigation to ascertain the applicability of complex modelling techniques such as artificial neural networks, random forests, and Bayesian models for early stage screening of mAb therapeutics would be beneficial. Model predictability and utility can be further improved with the inclusion of better mAb features such as glycoform conformation and distribution, which are linked to mAb efficacy and safety. Increasing the sample sizes within each substructure and specifying applicability domain could expand the applicability of this QSAR modelling framework. Furthermore, this methodology could then extend to different therapeutic types such as fusion proteins, bispecifics, single chain fragment variable and other novel mAb-based therapeutics.

There is a need for carefully designed predictive models to assess the efficacy as well as toxicity of potential drug candidates at an early stage. A more effective, high-throughput rapid screening of candidates based on adverse effects is required at an early stage to filter out the number of candidates proceeding to clinical trials.

From a safety perspective, animal models are not representative of human systems for assessing the efficacy and safety of biopharmaceuticals in specialised therapy areas like oncology and immunology. In this regard, computational toxicology tools like expert/hybrid systems provide a powerful complement during design phases as they will allow for development of automated and reliable models for predicting toxicity or adverse effect of monoclonal antibody therapeutics. To make these predictive platforms more robust, descriptor calculation, feature extraction, inclusion of pharmacokinetics and bioavailability characteristics, mechanistic understanding and multidisciplinary expert knowledge will be of paramount importance. This could aid in reducing the number of lead candidates that could go forward into the bioprocessing /manufacturing pipeline.

Thus, this would tackle two of the main setbacks biopharmaceutical industries face today: manufacturing failure and attrition. This will pave the way for the advancement of rapid bioprocess development strategies for faster development of effective and safe biopharmaceuticals and may in fact change the face of biopharmaceutical manufacturing as we see today.

References

1. Bailly, M., Mieczkowski, C., Juan, V., Metwally, E., Tomazela, D., Baker, J., Uchida, M., Kofman, E., Raoufi, F. & Motlagh, S. Predicting antibody developability profiles through early stage discovery screening. Mabs, 2020. Taylor & Francis, 1743053.
2. Kizhedath, A., Karlberg, M. & Glassey, J. 2019. Cross-interaction chromatography-based Qsar model for early-stage screening to facilitate enhanced developability of monoclonal antibody therapeutics. *Biotechnology Journal,* 14, 1800696.
3. Obrezanova, O., Arnell, A., de la Cuesta, R. G., Berthelot, M. E., Gallagher, T. R. A., Zurdo, J. & Stallwood, Y. 2015. Aggregation risk prediction for antibodies and its application to biotherapeutic development. *mAbs,* 7, 352–363.
4. Zurdo, J., Arnell, A., Obrezanova, O., Smith, N., de la Cuesta, R. G., Gallagher, T. R. A., Michael, R., Stallwood, Y., Ekblad, C., Abrahmsen, L. & Hoiden-Guthenberg, I. 2015. Early Implementation of QbD in Biopharmaceutical Development: A Practical Example. *Biomed Research International.*
5. Rathore, A. S., Singh, S. K., Kumar, J. & Kapoor, G. 2018. Implementation of QbD for Manufacturing of Biologics—Has It Met the Expectations? *Biopharmaceutical Processing.* Elsevier.
6. Rathore, A. S. 2009. Roadmap for implementation of quality by design (QbD) for biotechnology products. *Trends Biotechnol,* 27, 546-53.
7. Lawrence, X. Y., Amidon, G., Khan, M. A., Hoag, S. W., Polli, J., Raju, G. & Woodcock, J. 2014. Understanding pharmaceutical quality by design. *The AAPS Journal,* 16, 771-783.
8. Herwig, C., Garcia-Aponte, O. F., Golabgir, A. & Rathore, A. S. 2015. Knowledge management in the QbD paradigm: manufacturing of biotech therapeutics. *Trends Biotechnol,* 33, 381-7.
9. Rathore, A. S. 2014. QbD/PAT for bioprocessing: moving from theory to implementation. *Current Opinion in Chemical Engineering,* 6, 1-8.
10. Alt, N., Zhang, T. Y., Motchnik, P., Taticek, R., Quarmby, V., Schlothauer, T., Beck, H., Emrich, T. & Harris, R. J. 2016. Determination of critical quality attributes for monoclonal antibodies using quality by design principles. *Biologicals,* 44, 291-305.
11. Tiller, K. E. & Tessier, P. M. 2015. Advances in antibody design. *Annual Review of Biomedical Engineering,* 17, 191-216.

12. Yamashita, T. 2018. Toward rational antibody design: recent advancements in molecular dynamics simulations. *International Immunology,* 30, 133-140.

13. Harms, J., Wang, X., Kim, T., Yang, X. & Rathore, A. S. 2008. Defining process design space for biotech products: case study of Pichia pastoris fermentation. *Biotechnol Prog,* 24, 655-62.

14. Zimmermann, H. F. & Hentschel, N. 2011. Proposal on how to conduct a biopharmaceutical process Failure Mode and Effect Analysis (FMEA) as a Risk Assessment Tool. *PDA J Pharm Sci Technol,* 65, 506-12.

15. Leardi, R. 2009. Experimental design in chemistry: A tutorial. *Anal Chim Acta,* 652, 161-72.

16. Rathore, A. S. 2016. Quality by design (QbD)-based process development for purification of a biotherapeutic. *Trends in biotechnology,* 34, 358-370.

17. Kumar, V., Bhalla, A. & Rathore, A. S. 2014. Design of experiments applications in bioprocessing: concepts and approach. *Biotechnology Progress,* 30, 86-99.

18. Tai, M., Ly, A., Leung, I. & Nayar, G. 2015. Efficient high-throughput biological process characterization: Definitive screening design with the Ambr250 bioreactor system. *Biotechnology Progress,* 31, 1388-1395.

19. Zurdo, J. 2013. Surviving the valley of death. *Eur Biopharmaceutical Rev,* 195, 50-4.

20. Dehmer, M., Varmuza, K., Bonchev, D. & Ebrary Academic Complete International Subscription Collection. 2012. Statistical modelling of molecular descriptors in QSAR/QSPR. *Quantitative and network biology v 2.* Weinheim: Wiley-Blackwell,.

21. Dudek, A. Z., Arodz, T. & Galvez, J. 2006. Computational methods in Developing quantitative structure-activity relationships (QSAR): A review. *Combinatorial Chemistry & High Throughput Screening,* 9, 213-228.

22. Du, Q. S., Huang, R. B. & Chou, K. C. 2008. Recent advances in QSAR and their applications in predicting the activities of chemical molecules, peptides and proteins for drug design. *Current Protein & Peptide Science,* 9, 248-259.

23. Zhou, P., Chen, X., Wu, Y. Q. & Shang, Z. C. 2010. Gaussian process: an alternative approach for QSAM modeling of peptides. *Amino Acids,* 38, 199-212.

24. Hechinger, M., Leonhard, K. & Marquardt, W. 2012. What is Wrong with Quantitative Structure-Property Relations Models Based on Three-Dimensional Descriptors? *Journal of Chemical Information and Modeling,* 52, 1984-1993.

25. Zhou, P., Tian, F. F., Wu, Y. Q., Li, Z. L. & Shang, Z. C. 2008. Quantitative Sequence-Activity Model (QSAM): Applying QSAR Strategy to Model and Predict Bioactivity and Function of Peptides, Proteins and Nucleic Acids. *Current Computer-Aided Drug Design,* 4, 311-321.

26. Sneath, P. H. 1966. Relations between chemical structure and biological activity in peptides. *J Theor Biol,* 12, 157-95.

27. Kidera, A., Konishi, Y., Oka, M., Ooi, T. & Scheraga, H. A. 1985. Statistical-analysis of the physical-properties of the 20 naturally-occurring amino-acids. *Journal of Protein Chemistry,* 4, 23-55.

28. Hellberg, S., Sjostrom, M., Skagerberg, B. & WOLD, S. 1987. Peptide Quantitative Structure-Activity-Relationships, a Multivariate Approach. *Journal of Medicinal Chemistry,* 30, 1126-1135.

29. Hellberg, S., Sjostrom, M. & Wold, S. 1986. The prediction of bradykinin potentiating potency of pentapeptides. An example of a peptide quantitative structure-activity relationship. *Acta Chem Scand B,* 40, 135-40.

30. Sandberg, M., Eriksson, L., Jonsson, J., Sjostrom, M. & Wold, S. 1998. New chemical descriptors relevant for the design of biologically active peptides. A multivariate characterization of 87 amino acids. *Journal of Medicinal Chemistry,* 41, 2481-2491.

31. Tian, F. F., Zhou, P. & Li, Z. L. 2007. T-scale as a novel vector of topological descriptors for amino acids and its application in QSARs of peptides. *Journal of Molecular Structure,* 830, 106-115.

32. Collantes, E. R. & Dunn, W. J. 1995. Amino-Acid Side-Chain Descriptors for Quantitative Structure-Activity Relationship Studies of Peptide Analogs. *Journal of Medicinal Chemistry,* 38, 2705-2713.

33. van Westen, G. J. P., Swier, R. F., Cortes-Ciriano, I., Wegner, J. K., Overington, J. P., Ijzerman, A. P., Van Vlijmen, H. W. T. & Bender, A. 2013b. Benchmarking of protein descriptor sets in

proteochemometric modeling (part 2): modeling performance of 13 amino acid descriptor sets. *Journal of Cheminformatics,* 5.

34. Van Westen, G. J. P., Swier, R. F., Wegner, J. K., Ijzerman, A. P., Van Vlijmen, H. W. T. & Bender, A. 2013a. Benchmarking of protein descriptor sets in proteochemometric modeling (part 1): comparative study of 13 amino acid descriptor sets. *Journal of Cheminformatics,* 5.

35. Doytchinova, I. A., Walshe, V., Borrow, P. & Flower, D. R. 2005. Towards the chemometric dissection of peptide - HLA-A*0201 binding affinity: comparison of local and global QSAR models. *Journal of Computer-Aided Molecular Design,* 19, 203-212.

36. Gasteiger, E., Hoogland, C., Gattiker, A., Duvaud, S. E., Wilkins, M. R., Appel, R. D. & Bairoch, A. 2005. *Protein identification and analysis tools on the ExPASy server,* Springer.

37. Li, W., Cowley, A., Uludag, M., Gur, T., Mcwilliam, H., Squizzato, S., Park, Y. M., Buso, N. & Lopez, R. 2015. The EMBL-EBI bioinformatics web and programmatic tools framework. *Nucleic Acids Research,* 43, W580-W584.

38. Liao, C., Sitzmann, M., Pugliese, A. & Nicklaus, M. C. 2011. Software and resources for computational medicinal chemistry. *Future Med Chem,* 3, 1057-85.

39. Buyel, J. F., Woo, J. A., Cramer, S. M. & Fischer, R. 2013. The use of quantitative structure-activity relationship models to develop optimized processes for the removal of tobacco host cell proteins during biopharmaceutical production. *Journal of Chromatography A,* 1322, 18-28.

40. Sharma, V. K., Patapoff, T. W., Kabakoff, B., Pai, S., Hilario, E., Zhang, B., Li, C., Borisov, O., Kelley, R. F., Chorny, I., Zhou, J. Z., Dill, K. A. & Swartz, T. E. 2014. In silico selection of therapeutic antibodies for development: viscosity, clearance, and chemical stability. *Proc Natl Acad Sci U S A,* 111, 18601-6.

41. Sydow, J. F., Lipsmeier, F., Larraillet, V., Hilger, M., Mautz, B., Molhoj, M., Kuentzer, J., Klostermann, S., Schoch, J., Voelger, H. R., Regula, J. T., Cramer, P., Papadimitriou, A. & Kettenberger, H. 2014. Structure-based prediction of asparagine and aspartate degradation sites in antibody variable regions. *PLoS One,* 9, e100736.

42. Breneman, C. M., Thompson, T. R., Rhem, M. & Dung, M. 1995. Electron-density modeling of large systems using the transferable atom equivalent method. *Computers & Chemistry,* 19, 161.

43. Tugcu, N., Song, M. H., Breneman, C. M., Sukumar, N., Bennett, K. P. & Cramer, S. M. 2003. Prediction of the effect of mobile-phase salt type on protein retention and selectivity in anion exchange systems. *Analytical Chemistry,* 75, 3563-3572.

44. Robinson, J. R., Karkov, H. S., Woo, J. A., Krogh, B. O. & Cramer, S. M. 2017. QSAR models for prediction of chromatographic behavior of homologous Fab variants. *Biotechnology and Bioengineering,* 114, 1231-1240.

45. Brandt, J. P., Patapoff, T. W. & Aragon, S. R. 2010. Construction, MD simulation, and hydrodynamic validation of an all-atom model of a monoclonal IgG antibody. *Biophys J,* 99, 905-13.

46. Kortkhonjia, E., Brandman, R., Zhou, J. Z., VOELZ, V. A., Chorny, I., Kabakoff, B., Patapoff, T. W., Dill, K. A. & Swartz, T. E. 2013. Probing antibody internal dynamics with fluorescence anisotropy and molecular dynamics simulations. *mAbs,* 5, 306-22.

47. Kmiecik, S., Gront, D., Kolinski, M., Wieteska, L., Dawid, A. E. & Kolinski, A. 2016. Coarse-grained protein models and their applications. *Chemical Reviews,* 116, 7898-7936.

48. Ladiwala, A., Rege, K., Breneman, C. M. & Cramer, S. M. 2005. A priori prediction of adsorption isotherm parameters and chromatographic behavior in ion-exchange systems. *Proceedings of the National Academy of Sciences of the United States of America,* 102, 11710-11715.

49. Yang, T., Breneman, C. M. & Cramer, S. M. 2007a. Investigation of multi-modal high-salt binding ion-exchange chromatography using quantitative structure-property relationship modeling. *Journal of Chromatography A,* 1175, 96-105.

50. Yang, T., Sundling, M. C., Freed, A. S., Breneman, C. M. & Cramer, S. M. 2007b. Prediction of pH-dependent chromatographic behavior in ion-exchange systems. *Analytical Chemistry,* 79, 8927-8939.

51. Insaidoo, F. K., Rauscher, M. A., Smithline, S. J., Kaarsholm, N. C., Feuston, B. P., Ortigosa, A. D., Linden, T. O. & Roush, D. J. 2015. Targeted purification development enabled by computational biophysical modeling. *Biotechnology Progress,* 31, 154-164.
52. Bishop, C. M. 2006. Introduction. *Pattern recognition and machine learning.* Springer.
53. Jiang, W. L., KIM, S., Zhang, X. Y., Lionberger, R. A., Davit, B. M., Conner, D. P. & Yu, L. X. 2011. The role of predictive biopharmaceutical modeling and simulation in drug development and regulatory evaluation. *International Journal of Pharmaceutics,* 418, 151-160.
54. Chen, J., Yang, T. & Cramer, S. M. 2008. Prediction of protein retention times in gradient hydrophobic interaction chromatographic systems. *Journal of Chromatography A,* 1177, 207-214.
55. Hou, Y., Jiang, C. P., Shukla, A. A. & Cramer, S. M. 2011. Improved process analytical technology for protein A chromatography using predictive principal component analysis tools. *Biotechnology and Bioengineering,* 108, 59-68.
56. Karlberg, M., De Souza, J. V., Fan, L., Kizhedath, A., Bronowska, A. K. & Glassey, J. 2020. QSAR Implementation for HIC Retention Time Prediction of mAbs Using Fab Structure: A Comparison between Structural Representations. *International Journal of Molecular Sciences,* 21, 8037.
57. Woo, J., Parimal, S., Brown, M. R., Heden, R. & Cramer, S. M. 2015. The effect of geometrical presentation of multimodal cation-exchange ligands on selective recognition of hydrophobic regions on protein surfaces. *Journal of Chromatography A,* 1412, 33-42.
58. Farid, S. S. 2007. Process economics of industrial monoclonal antibody manufacture. *Journal of Chromatography B-Analytical Technologies in the Biomedical and Life Sciences,* 848, 8-18.
59. Hammerschmidt, N., Tscheliessnig, A., Sommer, R., Helk, B. & Jungbauer, A. 2014. Economics of recombinant antibody production processes at various scales: Industry-standard compared to continuous precipitation. *Biotechnology Journal,* 9, 766-775.
60. European Medicines Agency 2016. Guideline on development, production, characterisation and specification for monoclonal antibodies and related products. Committee for medicinal products for human use (CHMP).
61. Rodrigues de Azevedo, C., von Stosch, M., Costa, M. S., Ramos, A. M., Cardoso, M. M., Danhier, F., Preat, V. & Oliveira, R. 2017. Modeling of the burst release from PLGA micro- and nanoparticles as function of physicochemical parameters and formulation characteristics. *Int J Pharm,* 532, 229-240.
62. Jain, T., Sun, T., Durand, S., Hall, A., Houston, N. R., Nett, J. H., Sharkey, B., Bobrowicz, B., Caffry, I., Yu, Y., Cao, Y., Lynaugh, H., Brown, M., Baruah, H., Gray, L. T., Krauland, E. M., XU, Y., Vasquez, M. & Wittrup, K. D. 2017. Biophysical properties of the clinical-stage antibody landscape. *Proc Natl Acad Sci U S A,* 114, 944-949.
63. Kizhedath, A. 2019. *QSAR model development for early stage screening of monoclonal antibody therapeutics to facilitate rapid developability.* (Doctoral Dissertation, Newcastle University).
64. Chang, C.-C. & Lin, C.-J. 2011. LIBSVM: a library for support vector machines. *ACM transactions on intelligent systems and technology (TIST),* 2, 27.
65. Hebditch, M. & Warwicker, J. 2019. Charge and hydrophobicity are key features in sequence-trained machine learning models for predicting the biophysical properties of clinical-stage antibodies. *PeerJ,* 7, e8199.
66. Cortegiani, A., Ippolito, M., Greco, M., Granone, V., Protti, A., Gregoretti, C., Giarratano, A., Einav, S. & Cecconi, M. 2021. Rationale and evidence on the use of tocilizumab in COVID-19: a systematic review, *Pulmonology,* 27, 52–6
67. US Food & Drug Administration. 2004. Guidance for Industry PAT — A Framework for Innovative Pharmaceutical Development, Manufacturing, and Quality Assurance https://www.fda.gov/media/71012/download
68. Kizhedath, A., Wilkinson, S. & Glassey, J. 2017. Applicability of predictive toxicology methods for monoclonal antibody therapeutics: status Quo and scope, Arch Toxicol, 91, 1595–1612

69. Zalai, D., Dietzsch C. & Herwig C. 2013. Risk-based process development of biosimilars as part of the Quality by Design paradigm, *PDA Journal of Pharmaceutical Science and Technology*, 67, 569–580

Design Framework and Tools for Solid Drug Product Manufacturing Processes

Kensaku Matsunami, Sara Badr, and Hirokazu Sugiyama

1 Introduction

Solid drug products, e.g., tablets and capsules, represent a large fraction of drug product sales, with their sales accounting for more than 50% of the Japanese market [1]. Solid drug products are of different types, e.g., generic, orphan, and blockbuster drugs, which differ in physical properties, demand, and price of raw materials. With the rising pressure for cost reduction in the pharmaceutical industry, solid drug product manufacturing has gained increased attention. An example of a solid drug product manufacturing process, which produces tablets from an active pharmaceutical ingredient (API) in a powder state, is given in Fig. 1. This process is one of the typical manufacturing processes, but there are numerous solid drug product manufacturing process alternatives, e.g., wet granulation, dry granulation, and direct compression. Process alternatives are usually selected in conjunction with clinical trials, where many kinds of uncertainty still exist, e.g., undetermined process parameters and success/failure of the clinical development.

Continuous manufacturing has attracted the attention of the pharmaceutical industry, regulatory authorities, and academia in and beyond solid drug product manufacturing. The pharmaceutical industry traditionally uses batchwise operations, where all the materials are processed at once within each individual unit. Continuous technology enables all unit operations to be interconnected and the materials to be processed at a specific flow rate throughout the entire process. Unlike the chemical industry, continuous technology in the pharmaceutical industry normally has a defined running time, which can also be classified as semicontinuous manufacturing [2]. Continuous technology is expected to have merits regarding

K. Matsunami · S. Badr · H. Sugiyama (✉)
Department of Chemical System Engineering, The University of Tokyo, Tokyo, Japan
e-mail: sugiyama@chemsys.t.u-tokyo.ac.jp

© The Author(s), under exclusive license to Springer Nature Switzerland AG 2022   393
A. Fytopoulos et al. (eds.), *Optimization of Pharmaceutical Processes*, Springer
Optimization and Its Applications 189, https://doi.org/10.1007/978-3-030-90924-6_15

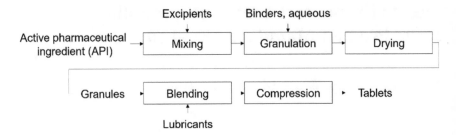

Fig. 1 Typical example of a solid drug product manufacturing process

flexibility to change in demand, reduced efforts for scale-up, and fewer required operators. By contrast, there are concerns such as start-up operations, variability of the inputs, and the necessity of real-time quality control. Although continuous technology has the potential to contribute to cost reduction, the benefits vary depending on the product and process characteristics. Thus, process design should reflect such characteristics to adequately evaluate the choice of continuous technology.

Numerous studies have dealt with further innovations, including implementation of continuous technology, development of process control [3, 4], and physical modeling of unit operations [5, 6]. Regarding comparative studies between batch and continuous technologies, case studies of economic assessment (e.g., [7]) and small-scale experimental investigations [8] have been conducted. However, there is still difficulty in applying these studies to practical decision-making in the pharmaceutical industry because previous studies have focused on specific unit operations, alternatives, and products. A pathway of process design needs to be established that has a broader scope covering newer technologies such as continuous manufacturing.

This chapter presents a design framework for solid drug product manufacturing, considering continuous technology as an alternative. First, the design framework is described in the form of an activity model, which defines two newly developed mechanisms as additional design elements. Next, the details of the introduced mechanisms are presented with applications in various case studies. The chapter combines and partly reproduces previous works from our research group published in collaboration with other industrial partners [9–13] and demonstrates their integration into the proposed design framework.

2 Design Framework

The design framework was described by using the type zero method of integration definition for function modeling (IDEF0). The IDEF0 is a function model systematically representing the functions, activities, or processes [14]. This method has been applied to describe various design frameworks, such as chemical process design

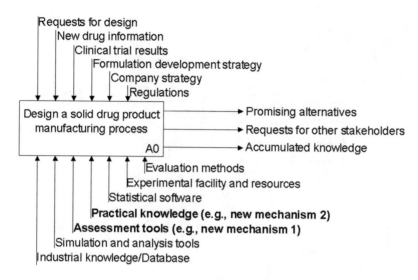

Fig. 2 Top activity A0: Design a solid drug product manufacturing process

[15, 16]. The model consists of boxes and arrows (Fig. 2). Each activity is shown in a box as a verb form, e.g., "design a process." The arrows are classified into four types: input, output (e.g., promising alternatives), control (e.g., regulations), and mechanism (e.g., industrial knowledge) of the activity.

In this study, the IDEF0 viewpoint was set as designers and researchers of formulation and processes. The top activity was defined as "Design a solid drug product manufacturing process" (see Fig. 2). The activity is controlled by the constraints that are characteristic of the pharmaceutical industry, e.g., regulations and clinical trial results. Moreover, the mechanisms of the model define tools and knowledge, which are essential for the process design. Two mechanisms were newly developed by the authors' research group, in collaboration with industrial experts. One is a tool that enables uncertainty-conscious economic assessment with superstructure-based comprehensive alternative generation (new mechanism 1). The other introduces practical knowledge of continuous technology obtained through experimental investigations (new mechanism 2). The top activity, A0, was divided into four sub-activities (Fig. 3). Sub-activities are managed in activity A1, and both simulations (A2) and experiments (A3) are performed interactively before evaluating alternatives (A4).

The developed design framework can be applied at any decision phase. Controls and mechanisms progressively evolve at each phase; for example, the regulatory constraints become more specific and detailed toward the implementation of the process. This chapter focuses on conceptual design in earlier decision phases, where the degree of uncertainty in product, process, and business is high. Thus, the examples given in this chapter will consider the establishment of conceptual process design during the clinical development phase. The controls and mechanisms

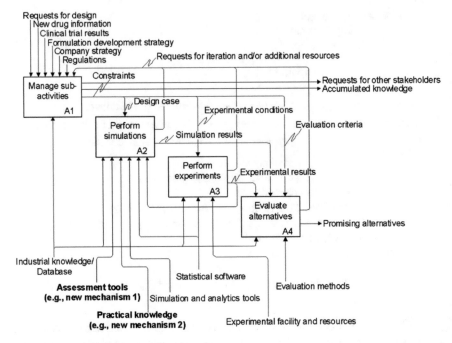

Fig. 3 Sub-activities of the top activity A0 (activities A1 to A4)

will be adjusted for that purpose. The outputs of the framework in this phase are the promising alternatives regarding process and formulation strategy (to be explained in more detail later).

The application of the framework can be described as follows. After receiving a design request, a design case is defined in A1, which includes the API properties, e.g., solubility, and design phase, e.g., clinical phase. The candidate dosage forms, e.g., tablets or capsules, and types of potential excipients, e.g., mannitol or lactose, are also specified in the design case. The uncertainty regarding the new drug, e.g., expected market size, and the clinical trial results, e.g., drug efficacy, are also considered. Activity A1 manages the conducting and iteration of activities A2 to A4. The simulation (A2) can be further divided into three sub-activities: "generate alternatives" (A21), "analyze processes" (A22), and "assess processes" (A23). Alternatives regarding process and formulation strategy are generated in A21 based on the design case. For each alternative, the process is analyzed to clarify the process characteristics (A22), e.g., start-up time, product loss, required resources (person hours), and the impacts of process parameters on product quality. In activity A23, the economic performance of the alternative is assessed, where the results reflect the uncertainty in the phase concerned, e.g., undetermined process parameters, potential change of the market demand, and success or failure of the clinical development. The two new developed mechanisms are introduced for use in activity A2. New mechanism 1 (assessment tool) is for the systematic generation, analysis, and assessment of alternatives, the application of which can be assisted by new mechanism 2 (practical knowledge of continuous technology). The details are discussed in the later sections. These simulation activities are conducted concurrently with experiments (A3). Experiments can provide missing but critical information in simulation (represented by the path from activity A3 to A2 through A4 and A1), and simulation can help conduct designed experiments (the path from activity A2 to A3 through A4 and A1). Finally, in activity A4, promising alternatives for processes and the formulation strategy are determined as an output based on the assessment results. During the process design activities, requests for other stakeholders, e.g., clinical developers and API designers, are produced in A1. New findings from the process and product design are integrated with the existing know-how, which is indicated as accumulated knowledge for new drug products in the output.

In the existing framework for bulk chemical process design [15, 16], nonexperimental activities, such as flowsheeting and steady-state simulation, were considered as the core of the process design. Because of the nature of the product and the process, our proposed framework highlights the collaboration between the experimental and simulation investigations. Heterogeneous characteristics of powder materials are, by their nature, difficult to simulate. Repetition of the start-up and shutdown operations for lot-based manufacturing (even for continuous manufacturing) could cause unforeseen phenomena such as clogging of powder materials or machine deterioration/malfunctions. Thus, the effective use of simulation techniques, in particular new mechanism 1 (the economic assessment tool), requires interaction with experiments. In our framework, this point is reflected in the presence of A3 as the main activity and as new mechanism 2 (practical knowledge obtained from experimental analyses) for activity A2.

3 New Mechanism 1: Superstructure-Based Economic Assessment Tool

In activity A2, alternatives are generated, analyzed, and assessed according to the specifications in the design case, e.g., the potential dosage form or type of excipients. The choice of the processing technologies (wet and dry granulation, or continuous and batch) and formulation strategy (common and proportional, explained later) can be considered. The economic assessment is performed considering the uncertainty in clinical development. New mechanism 1 (Fig. 3) was developed to support these activities and was implemented as an original software "SoliDecision" (the name is a combination of the words "solid" and "decision"). This section introduces this software, together with the implemented algorithm. The full details of the mechanism are presented elsewhere [9].

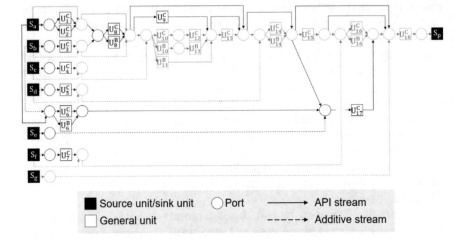

Fig. 4 Developed superstructure for solid drug product manufacturing processes [9]

3.1 Generation of Alternatives

Process Alternatives Represented as a Superstructure

The superstructure of the solid drug product manufacturing processes was defined to comprehensively generate possible process alternatives. Figure 4 presents the superstructure, covering various units such as size reduction, spray drying, mixing, granulation, drying, tableting, coating, and encapsulation, from units 1 to 18. Superscripts B and C represent batch and continuous operation in the unit. To describe the superstructure, the unit, port, conditioning stream (UPCS) representation [17] was adopted. Units are categorized as sources representing the provision of raw materials, sinks for the collection of final products, and general unit operations. Ports represent interfaces between units, e.g., materials transferred such as granules and tablets. The presence of the API in a stream is represented by a solid arrow, while streams with no API are represented as dotted arrows. One process alternative is defined as the connected options of streams, ports, and units starting from source to sink units, which represent the combination of raw materials, processing technologies, and dosage forms.

The superstructure in Fig. 4 was developed after conducting a thorough literature survey and consulting the expert knowledge of the industrial collaborators [9]. In total, 9452 process alternatives were specified, some of which are well-known alternatives, e.g., wet granulation, dry granulation, and direct compression methods. Among these 9452 alternatives, process alternatives were counted under "continuous technology" if all interconnected unit operations were run in continuous operation mode with a single manufacturing rate for the entire process. If any of the units was operated in batch mode, then the alternative is counted under "batch technology" with stepwise implementation of the process units. New units or combinations thereof could be added as needed to update the superstructure.

Formulation Strategy

In addition to process alternatives, the formulation concept for doses is another important decision point. Two options are available: "proportional dosage" where all doses have the same composition ratios but different product weights and "common dosage" where all doses have the same weights but different composition ratios. In clinical development, at least two doses are generally produced in either of the formulation options or in combinations thereof. The choice greatly impacts the amounts of processed materials for products and placebos and consequently impacts the economic assessment.

An alternative that is an output of activity A2 was defined as a combination of the process alternative and formulation strategy; that is, a maximum of 18,904 alternatives can be generated within the superstructure as the product of 9,452 processes and two formulation strategies. Each alternative is assessed individually. The number of practical alternatives can be obtained by applying case-specific constraints such as resource availability for development and production, the characteristics of the powder materials, and past production experience or market characteristics affecting company preferences. For example, six alternatives, consisting of three process alternatives and two formulation strategies, can be considered if a drug product of interest is suitable for wet granulation.

3.2 Stochastic Economic Assessment

Overview of Economic Assessment

A stochastic economic assessment tool was developed, where the probability density functions (PDFs) of the net present value (NPV) can be calculated. In the present and the next sections, figures and equations are presented by assuming the beginning of phase II (clinical development) as the decision stage. The cash flow in the drug life cycle can be illustrated as in Fig. 5. The design problem was defined as finding the best combination of process alternatives (dosage forms, processing technologies, and raw materials) and formulation strategy (proportional or common dosage) to maximize the economic objective function, denoted by $NPV(l)$ [USD], for a given product formulation. Equation 1 defines the NPV for alternative l as

$$NPV(l) = -\sum_{\tau=0}^{\tau_3} \frac{C_{dev}(\tau)}{(1+r)^{\tau}}\bigg|_l - \sum_{\tau=0}^{\tau_{prod}} \frac{C_{invest}(\tau)}{(1+r)^{\tau}}\bigg|_l + \sum_{\tau=\tau_{lau}}^{\tau_{prod}} \frac{C_{sales}(\tau) - C_{op}(\tau)}{(1+r)^{\tau}}\bigg|_l,$$

$$(1)$$

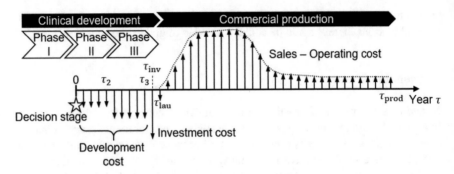

Fig. 5 Overview of cash flow in the drug life cycle with an indication of the decision stage [9]

where $C_{dev}(\tau)$ [USD yr^{-1}], $C_{invest}(\tau)$ [USD yr^{-1}], $C_{sales}(\tau)$ [USD yr^{-1}], and $C_{op}(\tau)$ [USD yr^{-1}] represent the development cost, investment cost, sales, and operating cost, respectively, when the time between the decision stage and target phases is τ years. The dimensionless parameter r represents the interest rate. The parameters τ_3 [yr], τ_{inv} [yr], τ_{lau} [yr], and τ_{prod} [yr] represent the periods from the decision stage to the clinical trials in phase III, the investment in production facilities (e.g., the continuous manufacturing machine), the product launch, and the end of the commercial production, respectively. For more details regarding the economic assessment, refer to [9].

The design problem can be expressed, as shown in Eq. (2).

$$
\begin{aligned}
&\max E_\theta \left(NPV(l)\right) \\
&\text{s.t.} \\
&E_\theta \left(NPV(l)\right) > 0 \\
&\text{(Mass balance constraints)} \\
&\text{(Processing time constraints)} \\
&\text{(Pharma-specific constraints)} ,
\end{aligned}
\tag{2}
$$

where the objective function is the expected value (E) of NPV, the design variable is alternative l, and the parameter θ represents the vector of uncertainty parameters. The first constraint serves as the rejection criterion for an alternative. Mass balance constraints consider the mass balance of raw materials and products/losses. The examples of process time and pharma-specific constraints are the validated runtime for continuous technology and safety stock, respectively. The following three pharma-specific constraints were considered as worth incorporating in the model [18]. At product launch, the production of a specific number of lots, typically three in the pharmaceutical industry, is required for process validation. The number of lots becomes flexible later in commercial production. Another important constraint is avoiding drug shortages and therefore determining the required production volume to provide sufficient inventory levels. The third constraint is expiration dates, which also determines the shipping deadline.

Equation 3 describes the difference in *NPV* between two alternatives l_1 and l_2 denoted as $\Delta NPV_{l_1,l_2}$ [USD].

$$\Delta NPV_{l_1,l_2} = NPV\,(l_1) - NPV\,(l_2) \tag{3}$$

The area of the positive region where $\Delta NPV_{l_1,l_2} > 0$ gives the probability of alternative l_1 being preferable to l_2. This can be thus used as an additional mechanism for comparison of alternatives.

Monte Carlo Simulation (MCS)

Uncertainty is the highest at earlier stages, such as during clinical development, with variables becoming better defined at later stages. Process variables such as continuous manufacturing rates are classified as internal variables, while others such as demand volume and success/failure of clinical development are defined as external variables. Defining PDF of input parameters is used to quantify uncertainty in clinical development and commercial production through MCS.

A triangular distribution was used to describe the PDF for parameters with potential ranges/multiple values. Triangular distributions specify minimum, maximum, and peak parameter values. Such distributions are more convenient to use at early design stages, e.g., phase II, since the required information of upper and lower ends can be available then. Furthermore, the distribution can be asymmetric, adding flexibility to the analysis. Equation 4 describes the PDF $f(x)$ of continuous variables such as the manufacturing rate.

$$f(x) = \begin{cases} \frac{2(x-x_{min})}{(x_{max}-x_{min})(x_{std}-x_{min})} & |x_{min} \leq x \leq x_{std} \\[2mm] \frac{2(x_{max}-x)}{(x_{max}-x_{min})(x_{max}-x_{std})} & |x_{std} \leq x \leq x_{max}, \\[2mm] 0 & |x < x_{min}, x > x_{max} \end{cases} \tag{4}$$

where x_{min}, x_{max}, and x_{std} represent the minimum, maximum, and standard (i.e., peak) values of an input parameter, respectively.

After calculating the PDFs of $\Delta NPV_{l_1,l_2}$, a global sensitivity analysis (GSA) can be performed to identify critical parameters for decision-making. The Spearman rank correlation coefficient (RCC), ρ_x [–] [19], was used as an indicator, as shown in Eq. 5:

$$\rho_x = 1 - \frac{6 \sum d^2}{N\,(N^2-1)}, \tag{5}$$

where N [–] and d [–] represent the iteration number and the difference between the ranks of the parameters x and $\Delta NPV_{l_1,l_2}$, respectively.

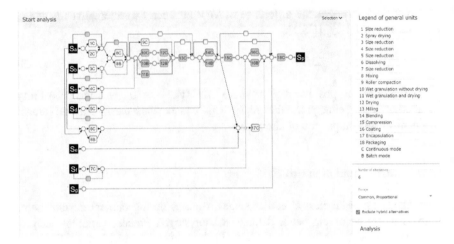

Fig. 6 Screenshot of the superstructure section in the "SoliDecision" software (a prototype version)

3.3   Implementation of "SoliDecision"

The developed mechanism was implemented as an original software called "SoliDecision." The software consists of three sections: superstructure, data input, and result. The following describes the workflow when using the software.

Superstructure Section

A screenshot of the superstructure section in SoliDecision (a prototype version) is presented in Fig. 6. As a first step of the economic assessment, alternatives for the target product are generated (a maximum of 9452 process alternatives and two formulation strategies). By activating or deactivating the boxes, the number of alternatives is calculated and displayed.

Input Data Section

The input parameters are categorized according to the relevant stages (phase II, phase III, and commercial production). The default values of all parameters that are set in the software can be altered according to the product characteristics and the company standards. The uncertainty of the input parameters can be specified by setting the minimum, maximum, and standard values of each parameter. Triangular or uniform distributions are available, besides simply using the deterministic value.

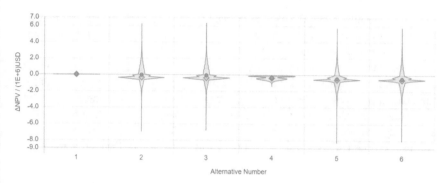

Fig. 7 An example of the produced violin plots for PDFs of ΔNPV by SoliDecision (a prototype version)

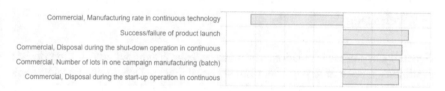

Fig. 8 The results of SoliDecision (a prototype) for the sensitivity analysis in the demonstration

Results Section

The results section provides the ranking of alternatives in terms of $E_\theta(NPV(l))$, PDFs of NPV and ΔNPV, and the sensitivity analysis results. The alternative of interest is highlighted in the superstructure with the results of $E_\theta(\Delta NPV)$. PDFs of NPV and ΔNPV are presented by box plots and violin plots (Fig. 7); the Spearman RCCs of critical parameters are shown by a bar chart (Fig. 8).

The practical use of the software was demonstrated for a case study involving six alternatives: a combination of three process alternatives (continuous high shear, batch high shear, and batch fluidized bed wet granulation methods) and two formulation strategies (proportional and common). As a result, alternative number 1, consisting of the continuous high shear wet granulation method and proportional dosage, showed the highest $E_\theta(NPV(l))$. The violin plots of ΔNPV are shown in Fig. 7. Alternative 1 (continuous) was the best in terms of $E_\theta(NPV(l))$, but the possibility that alternative 2 (batch) became better than alternative 1 was 32%, which could be too high to exclude alternative 2.

A sensitivity analysis was performed for $\Delta NPV_{1,2}$ to find the relevant parameters to maintain the superiority of alternative 1. The results are shown in Fig. 8, where the manufacturing rate in continuous technology was shown to be the most influential parameter among the process-related parameters (i.e., the higher the rate is, the more preferable continuous technology becomes). Because the manufacturing rate affects both loss amounts and production time, the impact was higher than other parameters. By redefining a PDF of the manufacturing rate, a what-if analysis can be performed to understand how much the change in manufacturing rate would affect the results (see Ref. [9] for an example). Overall, alternative 1 can be chosen if the feasibility of a high manufacturing rate is verified.

In the context of the process design framework shown in Figs. 2 and 3, "SoliDecision" as new mechanism 1 can help specify key parameters (e.g., manufacturing rate) that need to be clarified in the earlier stage, as well as the economically optimal alternative (e.g., alternative 1 in the case above). Based on these simulation results as an output of activity A2, the promising alternatives can be determined in activity A4, or a further experiment in activity A3 can be triggered (through activities A4 and A1).

4 New Mechanism 2: Practical Knowledge of Continuous Technology

Generally, in process simulation, a priori knowledge is required to set up appropriate conditions and to interpret the results appropriately. Due to its novelty, such knowledge is yet to be established for continuous technology. New mechanism 2 aims to cover this gap. Three types of experiments were performed for continuous technology: large-scale performance comparison with batch technology [10], key parameter determination regarding product quality and productivity [11], and the analysis of the start-up operation [12, 13].

4.1 Large-Scale Comparison

Material and Methods

The wet granulation process was investigated with small- (5–10 kg) and large-scale (100 kg) experiments. In these experiments, batch fluidized bed granulation, batch high shear granulation, and continuous high shear granulation were tested and compared. In all experiments, 29.4 wt%-ethenzamide was used as the API and mixed with mannitol, microcrystalline cellulose, hydroxypropyl cellulose, and magnesium stearate.

Granules and tablets were sampled and tested to assess the yield and relevant quality attributes. Tablet quality targets were set as (a) tablet hardness $\geq$40 N, (b) 95% $\leq$API content $\leq$105% of the target composition (i.e., 29.4 wt%), and (c) dissolution rate $\geq$80% of the API dissolved within 30 min. The impact of scale-up was analyzed by comparing the results of small- and large-scale experiments. For the comparison of different dissolution behaviors, a similarity factor f_2 [–] was used as shown in Eq. 6.

$$f_2 = 50 \cdot \log \left\{ \left[1 + \frac{1}{n} \sum_{t=1}^{n} (R_t - T_t)^2 \right]^{-0.5} \times 100 \right\} \tag{6}$$

where n [–], R_t [%], and T_t [%] represent the number of time points, the dissolution of the reference product, and the dissolution of the test product at time t, respectively [20]. Two dissolution profiles are considered similar if the value of f_2 is larger than 50.

For process performance, product losses and their sources, for example, powders sticking to the granulator surface, have been analyzed to determine the process yield in addition to quantifying the amounts of the final product. For the large-scale experiments, the yield was calculated as the ratio of the mass of the final product and input raw materials. In the case of continuous technologies, the final product was defined as that obtained after steady-state operation has been reached with a stable output. Tablets produced during start-up operations and during the initial condition setting of the compression were written off as losses.

Results

All tablets in the large-scale experiment achieved the targets mentioned above of tablet hardness, API content, and dissolution. Comparison of the three tested technologies showed that the tablet hardness in batch high shear granulation was the lowest, while API content was lowest with the batch fluidized bed granulation. The latter result is assumed to be due to higher losses of API as higher concentration powders escape the bag filter in fluidized bed granulation. Figure 9a shows the different dissolution profiles in the large-scale experiments, where three profiles were judged as equivalent because all values of f_2 were larger than 60. These results confirmed that all tested manufacturing technologies, including continuous technologies, could achieve the tested tablet quality targets at an industrial scale.

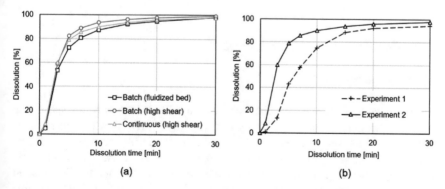

Fig. 9 Comparison of dissolution profiles (**a**) between technologies and (**b**) between small- and large-scale experiments in continuous technology [10]

Further findings were obtained regarding scale-up. The dissolution profiles of each technology were compared between the small- and large-scale experiments. As presented in Fig. 9b, the dissolution profiles changed significantly in continuous technology from small- to large-scale experiments, where f_2 was lower than 50. Both profiles fulfilled the product quality targets in the experiments, but the scale-dependent change in dissolution profiles highlights scale-up is a key factor that could affect the final product quality. In continuous operations, scale-up through runtime extension was found to be not straightforward when using the same core granulation and drying units in both the small- and large-scale experiments. When the large-scale experiment was conducted under the same conditions as the small-scale experiment, the run failed due to equipment clogging and subsequent malfunction. Additional adjustments were required in the large-scale experiments to complete the required 4-h operation needed for a 100-kg production scale. First, the ratio of binder–water (liquid–solid ratio) was reduced from 22 wt% to 18 wt%. Second, the blade rotation speed was reduced from 6000 to 5000 rpm. Lastly, the screw type in the kneading part of the granulator was changed to reduce the equipment's pressure. These changes affected the dissolution profiles. This experiment was an actual case where unexpected complications could arise with scale-up.

From the results of process performance, continuous technology showed the lowest yield. The yield was more than 93% in batch technologies with both fluidized bed and high shear granulation, whereas the yield in continuous technology was 90.6%. Critical causes of loss in continuous technology were determined to be residues remaining in the feeder and losses during the start-up process, which accounted for 4.95% of input materials. The inline monitoring results revealed that the median granule diameter was higher at the first 4.5 min and stabilized afterward.

To summarize the results, the experimental results provided a feasibility analysis of new continuous technology. The product quality equivalence was confirmed, but critical technical challenges were also found, i.e., scale-up issues and start-up operation. The key factors for solving the scale-up issues in the experiments were the liquid–solid ratio and the screw specification.

4.2   Key Parameter Determination

Material and Methods

The same equipment and raw materials were used as in the previous subsection with ethenzamide as the API. Design of experiment (DoE) was applied. Five input parameters were selected as factors and changed during the experiments: two material parameters (API content and the molecular weight of the binder) and three process parameters (manufacturing rate, blade rotation speed, and the liquid–solid ratio). As intermediate parameters, granule properties were measured, e.g., granule size distribution and circularity distribution. As output parameters, tablet quality, e.g., dissolution, and productivity, e.g., drying time, were measured.

Based on fractional factorial designs, 22 experimental runs were planned and performed. The experimental results were analyzed using a five-way analysis of variance (ANOVA) and the partial least squares (PLS) method. ANOVA was used to analyze the effects of input parameters, whereas PLS was used to observe the impacts of intermediate parameters.

Results

The effects of input parameters on granule and product quality were judged by p-values of ANOVA. The null hypothesis was "there is no difference in the mean of each property when varying the factors." Two material parameters showed high impacts on tablet properties, but the effects were not observed on measured granule properties. The effects of process parameters on granule properties were confirmed in the experiments, and the liquid–solid ratio further affected tablet properties such as dissolution.

The PLS regression coefficients of raw material and granule properties were calculated for each item of tablet quality. The coefficients for the % of API dissolved at 3 min, which represented tablet dissolution, are summarized in Fig. 10. Besides raw material properties (granule properties 1 and 2 in Fig. 10), 10-percentile circularity was the most relevant parameter; the high impacts of circularity were also observed for other tablet properties such as disintegration time. This PLS analysis showed that circularity is a new key parameter that can be monitored to predict tablet quality. A possible explanation for the correlation between circularity and dissolution is that high circularity is the result of high levels of agglomeration during granulation. This would result in a higher granule true density and a delay in dissolution.

For the drying time as a measure of productivity, ANOVA determined that the manufacturing rate and the liquid–solid ratio were the most relevant parameters. The

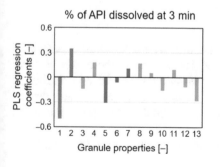

Granule properties [–]
1. API content
2. Molecular weight of binder
3. Median diameter
4. Geometric standard deviation of granule size
5. 10-percentile circularity
6. Median circularity
7. 90-percentile circularity
8. Loose bulk density
9. Tapped density
10. Compressibility index
11. Repose angle
12. Flowability
13. Water content

Fig. 10 PLS regression coefficients of granule properties for % of API dissolved at 3 min [11]

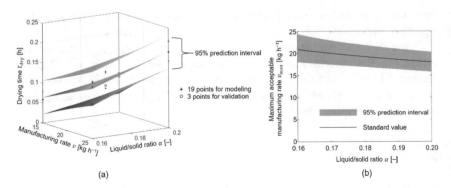

Fig. 11 Results generated from the effects on drying time: (**a**) regression model of drying time and (**b**) the relationship between liquid–solid ratio and maximum acceptable manufacturing rate [11]

regression model of drying time was then developed with a 95% prediction interval (Fig. 11a). Because the acceptable drying time is governed by the manufacturing rate, an inequality equation of the manufacturing rate and the liquid–solid ratio was derived (see Ref. [11] for details) and applied (Fig. 11b). The results thus show that low liquid–solid ratios are preferable in high-speed continuous manufacturing. This could be further used in product development, e.g., for the selection and development of excipients for continuous processing.

Through the experiments, the liquid–solid ratio and granule circularity were determined as the key parameters of continuous wet granulation in terms of tablet quality and productivity. More specifically, the following practical findings were obtained: (1) lower liquid–solid ratios are preferred for high-speed manufacturing and (2) the impact of high circularity on slowing down tablet disintegration and dissolution.

4.3 Start-Up Operation

Material and Methods

Premixed powders containing 5.0 wt% theophylline were used for the experiments. A full factorial experimental design was performed to assess the effects of screw speed, manufacturing rate, and the liquid–solid ratio on the start-up operation in continuous wet granulation. The torque profiles in the twin-screw granulator and the particle size distribution of granules were measured during each 1-h production run.

The torque y at time t was fitted by the first-order system, as shown in Eq. (7).

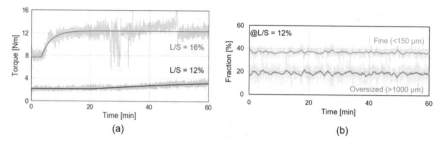

Fig. 12 Experimental results of the start-up operation: (**a**) torque profiles at different liquid–solid ratios and (**b**) profiles of fractions of fine and oversized granules [12]

$$y = a - b \exp\left(-\frac{t-d}{c}\right), t \ge d,$$ (7)

where a, b, c, and d are the fitting parameters. The effects of process parameters on the values of the fitting parameters were assessed by ANOVA. The particle size distributions were monitored inline and were measured by an offline measurement. Several indicators were used to find the appropriate indicator for the judgment of start-up, e.g., median size, fractions of fine or oversized granules, and the principal components of size distributions.

Results

The torque profiles of the two runs are summarized in Fig. 12a, where raw and fitted data are shown as light and dark color, respectively. In all runs, the effects of the start-up operation were observed through profiles dependent on runs. The liquid–solid ratio was the most influential parameter on the torque profiles; significant differences were measured in the value of a. The increase in torque was larger for the high liquid–solid ratio, but the torque was slightly increased for the low liquid–solid ratio. These differences were thought to be due to the differences in the agglomeration rate and sticking.

A profile of fractions of fine and oversized granules is shown in Fig. 12b, where a run of the low liquid–solid ratio was measured using an inline measurement. The dark lines are the moving averages of the raw data, which are shown as the light lines. Unlike the results of the torque profiles, the start-up effects were not obvious in the results of particle size distributions. The principal component analysis also showed that the effects of the start-up were small compared to the deviations of particle size through the operation. While torques and particle sizes have correlations in general, it was not observed in the investigated start-up.

4.4 Summary of Three Experiments

The large-scale experimental comparison specified two critical aspects of continuous technology, namely, scale-up issues and start-up operation. DoE-based experiments determined key parameters for both product quality and productivity, i.e., the liquid–solid ratio and circularity. Moreover, the definition of the start-up operation was found to be different depending on torque and granule size. In the context of the design framework in Figs. 2 and 3, these findings, despite being limited to specific materials and processes, could still help specify appropriate input parameters in activity A2. For example, when applying a high manufacturing rate in continuous technology, the value of the liquid–solid ratio needs to be checked to ascertain whether it is too high (see Fig. 11). In specifying the liquid–solid ratio, the time required for the start-up operation could also be scrutinized, considering the influence of the parameter on process behavior (see Fig. 12). If further experimental support is needed to validate the simulation results, activity A3 could be activated.

5 Conclusion

This chapter presented a design framework and the associated new tools for solid drug product manufacturing processes. IDEF0 activity modeling was applied to define a process design pathway. To deal with the difficulty of the powder processes, the developed activity model highlighted the interactions between simulation and experimental investigation. Two newly developed mechanisms were introduced for conducting simulation-oriented analysis. One was the superstructure-based economic assessment tool for the comprehensive generation, analysis, and assessment of process alternatives. Stochastic simulation was integrated to propagate the uncertainty of the input parameters into the NPV assessment result. The algorithm was implemented as an original software called "SoliDecision." The other mechanism was the practical knowledge of continuous technology obtained through experiments. Although the experiment was limited to specific raw materials and process conditions, investigation of the scale-up and start-up operations and key process parameters provided useful insights for process simulation. These new mechanisms in the framework can effectively assist simulation-based, and more rational and efficient, design of solid drug product manufacturing processes.

The proposed framework can serve as a "hub" for various other mechanisms to be developed in the future. For example, population balance models can be integrated with our economic assessment tool to incorporate material and process characteristics in the calculation. Further experiments with different raw materials, processes, and equipment setups could provide more general insights, which could be also useful for the simulation-oriented design activities. To this end, more collaborative efforts between simulation and experiment are desired.

Acknowledgments The authors acknowledge Dr. Hiroshi Nakagawa, Dr. Shuichi Tanabe, and Mr. Keita Yaginuma from Daiichi Sankyo Co., Ltd.; Mr. Koji Hasegawa and Mr. Takuya Nagato from Powrex Corporation; Prof. Thomas De Beer, Prof. Ingmar Nopens, Dr. Alexander Ryckaert, and Mr. Michiel Peeters at Ghent University; and Mr. Fabian Sternal at Friedrich-Alexander University Erlangen-Nürnberg for useful discussions. H.S. is thankful for the financial support by a Grant-in-Aid for Young Scientists (A) [Grant number 17H04964] and a Grant-in-Aid for Scientific Research (B) [Grant number 21H01704] from the Japan Society for the Promotion of Science (JSPS) in conducting part of this research. K. M. used the financial support of a Grant-in-Aid for JSPS Research Fellows [Grant number 18 J22793] for conducting part of this research.

References

1. Ministry of Helath, Labour and Welfare, 2019. Statistics of production by pharmaceutical industry, URL https://www.mhlw.go.jp/toukei/list/105-1.html (Accessed March 27, 2021)
2. Khinast, J., Bresciani, M., 2017. Continuous manufacturing: definitions and engineering principles, in: Continuous Manufacturing of Pharmaceuticals. John Wiley & Sons Ltd, Chichester, UK, pp. 1–31. doi: https://doi.org/10.1002/9781119001348.ch1
3. Pereira, G.C., Muddu, S.V., Román-Ospino, A.D., Clancy, D., Igne, B., Airiau, C., Muzzio, F.J., Ierapetritou, M., Ramachandran, R., Singh, R., 2019. Combined feedforward/feedback control of an integrated continuous granulation process. J. Pharm. Innov. 14, 259–285. doi: https://doi.org/10.1007/s12247-018-9347-8
4. Nicolaï, N., De Leersnyder, F., Copot D., Stock M., Ionescu C.M., Gernaey K.V., Nopens I., De Beer, T., 2018. Liquid-to-solid ratio control as an advanced process control solution for continuous twin-screw wet granulation. AIChE J. 64, 2500–2514. https://doi.org/10.1002/aic.16161
5. Van Hauwermeiren, D., Verstraeten, M., Doshi, P., Am Ende, M.T., Turnbull, N., Lee, K., De Beer, T., Nopens, I., 2019. On the modelling of granule size distributions in twin-screw wet granulation: Calibration of a novel compartmental population balance model. Powder Technol 341, 116–125. https://doi.org/10.1016/j.powtec.2018.05.025
6. Toson, P., Lopes, D.G., Paus, R., Kumar, A., Geens, J., Stibale, S., Quodbach, J., Kleinebudde, P., Hsiao, W.-K., Khinast, J., 2019. Model-based approach to the design of pharmaceutical roller-compaction processes. Int. J. Pharm. X 1, 100005. https://doi.org/10.1016/j.ijpx.2019.100005
7. Schaber, S.D., Gerogiorgis, D.I., Ramachandran, R., Evans, J.M.B., Barton, P.I., Trout, B.L., 2011. Economic analysis of integrated continuous and batch pharmaceutical manufacturing: A case study. Ind. Eng. Chem. Res. 50, 10083–10092. https://doi.org/10.1021/ie2006752
8. Järvinen, M.A., Paavola, M., Poutiainen, S., Itkonen, P., Pasanen, V., Uljas, K., Leiviskä, K., Juuti, M., Ketolainen, J., Järvinen, K., 2015. Comparison of a continuous ring layer wet granulation process with batch high shear and fluidized bed granulation processes. Powder Technol 275, 113–120. https://doi.org/10.1016/j.powtec.2015.01.071
9. Matsunami, K., Sternal, F., Yaginuma, K., Tanabe, S., Nakagawa, H., Sugiyama, H., 2020. Superstructure-based process synthesis and economic assessment under uncertainty for solid drug product manufacturing. BMC Chem. Eng. 2, 6. https://doi.org/10.1186/s42480-020-0028-2
10. Matsunami, K., Nagato, T., Hasegawa, K., Sugiyama, H., 2019. A large-scale experimental comparison of batch and continuous technologies in pharmaceutical tablet manufacturing using ethenzamide. Int. J. Pharm. 559, 210–219. https://doi.org/10.1016/j.ijpharm.2019.01.028
11. Matsunami, K., Nagato, T., Hasegawa, K., Sugiyama, H., 2020. Determining key parameters of continuous wet granulation for tablet quality and productivity. Int. J. Pharm. 579, 119160. https://doi.org/10.1016/j.ijpharm.2020.119160

12. Matsunami, K., Nopens, I., Sugiyama, H., De Beer, T., 2020. Abstract of The Society of Chemical Engineer, Japan 51st Autumn Meeting, T216.
13. Matsunami, K., Ryckaert, A., Peeters, M., Badr, S., Sugiyama, H., Nopens, I., De Beer, T., 2021. Analysis of the effects of process parameters on start-up operation in continuous wet granulation. Processes 9(9), 1502. https://doi.org/10.3390/pr9091502
14. National Institute of Standards and Technology (NIST) 1993. Integration Definition for Function Modeling (IDEF0), Federal Information Processing Standards Publication NO. 183, Department of Commerce, Gaithersburg, U.S.A.
15. Sugiyama, H., Hirao, M., Mendivil, R., Fischer, U., Hungerbühler, K., 2006. A hierarchical activity model of chemical process design based on life cycle assessment. Process Saf. Environ. Prot. 84, 63–74. https://doi.org/10.1205/psep.04142
16. Sugiyama, H., Hirao, M., Fischer, U., Hungerbühler, K., 2008. Activity modeling for integrating Environmental, Health and Safety (EHS) consideration as a new element in industrial chemical process design. J. Chem. Eng. Japan 41, 884–897. https://doi.org/10.1252/jcej.07we263
17. Wu, W., Henao, C.A., Maravelias, C.T., 2016. A superstructure representation, generation, and modeling framework for chemical process synthesis. AIChE J. 62, 3199–3214. https://doi.org/10.1002/aic.15300
18. Matsunami, K., Miyano, T., Arai, H., Nakagawa, H., Hirao, M., Sugiyama, H., 2018. Decision support method for the choice between batch and continuous technologies in solid drug product manufacturing. Ind. Eng. Chem. Res. 57(30), 9798–9809. https://doi.org/10.1021/acs.iecr.7b05230
19. Zar, J.H., 1972. Significance testing of the Spearman rank correlation coefficient. J. Am. Stat. Assoc. 67, 578–580. https://doi.org/10.1080/01621459.1972.10481251
20. US FDA, 1997. Guidance for Industry Dissolution Testing of Immediate Release Solid Oral Dosage Forms [WWW Document]. URL https://www.fda.gov/downloads/drugs/guidances/ucm070237.pdf (Accessed May 3, 2021).

Challenges and Solutions in Drug Product Process Development from a Material Science Perspective

Fanny Stauffer, Pierre-François Chavez, Julie Fahier, Corentin Larcy, Mehrdad Pasha, and Gabrielle Pilcer

1 Introduction

Pharmaceutical process development is a delicate balance between scientific process understanding, resource, and time constraints. While drug product (DP) development teams aim at designing optimal processes, the development time is usually limited to accelerate the time to market [1]. In addition, the DP development is usually performed in parallel to the chemical process development, limiting the quantity of active pharmaceutical ingredient (API) available for the formulation and DP process development.

The current regulatory environment clearly highlights the prerequisite of a thorough process understanding. The critical material attributes and process parameters must be identified. In addition, the demonstration of an "enhanced knowledge of product performance over a wide range of material attributes, processing options and process parameters" is encouraged for the filing [2]. On the one hand, the identification of critical process parameters and their impact on product and process performance is well understood and is commonly done during process development. On the other hand, the critical material attributes are more difficult to assess and are less often considered. The considered physiochemical and biological properties of the API are often limited to the parameters that are impacting the biopharmaceutical activity of the product but rarely include considerations regarding the manufacturability of the compound and the interactions between process parameters and material attributes.

The identification of the material attributes impacting the product and process performance is nonetheless a critical aspect of the drug product development, and

F. Stauffer (✉) · P.-F. Chavez · J. Fahier · C. Larcy · M. Pasha · G. Pilcer
UCB Pharma, Braine l'Alleud, Belgium
e-mail: fanny.stauffer@ucb.com

© The Author(s), under exclusive license to Springer Nature Switzerland AG 2022   413
A. Fytopoulos et al. (eds.), *Optimization of Pharmaceutical Processes*, Springer
Optimization and Its Applications 189, https://doi.org/10.1007/978-3-030-90924-6_16

appropriate studies are required to address this challenge. Due to the discrete nature of particulate systems, it is important to understand single-particle properties, inter-particle and particle-boundary interactions, and bulk powder responses. Characterization of single-particle properties is favorable due to limited availability of APIs at early stages of drug product and process development. Although several attempts have been made in the literature to link single-particle properties to the bulk powder behavior either experimentally or via modelling approaches, carrying such characterization is often challenging, time-consuming, and expensive [3–5]. Moreover, the properties at this length scale have variable distributions, which questions the representability and relevance of single-particle measurements. For instance, atomic force microscopy measurements of particles with complex surface morphology and shape yield extremely variable values of adhesion force between two particles [6].

Considering the representativeness and interpretation challenges associated with single-particle measurements, characterizations are often performed at the bulk level. It is hence crucial to account for the relevance and representability of the characterization methods and properties at the bulk level. In bulk powder characterization, it is also most crucial that the samples selected for the measurements should be physically and chemically representative of the bulk [7]. Moreover, bulk powder properties are sensitive to the stress level of particles, dynamics and strain rates of the process, and environmental conditions such as relative humidity and temperature. Examples are as follows: (a) flow properties of cohesive powders deteriorate under stress due to the increased number of contacts and contact area [8], (b) compressibility response is very sensitive to the compaction rate [9], and (c) the presence of moisture and prolonged storage time lead to caking phenomena and deterioration of powder flow properties [10]. As a result, multiplying characterization tests often results in contradictory findings that are then difficult to interpret if the property measured by the selected characterization technique cannot immediately be linked to the process of interest. Unlike liquid and gas systems, fundamental scale-up rules are not established for particle systems and processes [11]. In the absence of representative characterization technique, the best solution can then be the miniaturization and pilot testing in addition to sample characterization.

In this chapter, we identified specific challenges associated with material attributes and solutions that can be applied to overcome them using industrial case studies. In the first case study, quality-by-design (QbD) principles will be used to identify critical material attributes (CMAs) with a limited number of API batches for a product under development. In the second case study, miniaturization will be applied to develop a new process with reduced material consumption. In the third case study, the knowledge acquired on a marketed product will be transposed for the development of a new process. In the fourth case study, targeted characterizations will be applied to new API sources to mitigate troubleshooting for commercial products.

2   Case 1: Identifying CMAs with a Limited Number of API Batches

This first case study describes the development of a new drug product. During development phases, the amount of API batches is limited, and the batch-to-batch variability is unknown. It is therefore difficult to identify relevant CMAs at this stage. Applying an enhanced QbD approach could nonetheless guide early identification of the CMAs.

In the last decade, the pharmaceutical industry was encouraged by authorities to enhance knowledge and understanding of products and manufacturing processes. In order to help industries in this task, the International Conference on Harmonization (ICH) has published several guidelines such as the ICH Q8 guideline on pharmaceutical development. This guideline mainly covers the concept of quality by design (QbD) described as a science- and risk-based approach for which the quality should not be tested into products but should be built in by design. Furthermore, this QbD approach contributes to a continuous improvement of the product quality by a systematic assessment and understanding and refining of the formulation and processes throughout the product life cycle [2, 12].

ICH Q8 focuses on the pharmaceutical development that aims at designing products and manufacturing processes to provide the intended performance of the products and to meet the needs of patients. Therefore, pharmaceutical industries should demonstrate that the proposed manufacturing processes and formulations are suitable for the intended purpose. It can be eased by the achievement of development studies that allow to acquire an enhanced understanding of product performance over a wide range of material attributes and process parameters. This understanding can be earned by preliminary knowledge, design of experiments, and implementation of process analytical technology and can lead to the definition of a design space.

According to ICH Q8(R2), all pharmaceutical development should include, at a minimum, the following deliverables:

- Define the Quality Target Product Profile (QTPP)
- Identify potential Critical Quality Attributes (CQAs)
- Determine the CQAs
- Select an appropriate manufacturing process
- Define a control strategy.

In this case study, the QTPP was first defined, and then, from this QTPP, CQAs that are "physical, chemical, biological or microbiological properties or characteristics that should be within an appropriate limit, range, or distribution to ensure the desired product quality" (ICH Q8) were identified. The DP process was based on continuous twin-screw wet granulation. Wet granulation technology was selected because of the API properties (i.e., poorly flowable, highly cohesive) and relatively high drug load. The continuous manufacturing technology was selected as it allowed reducing API consumption during development and enabled faster development time as no scale-up is necessary [13].

It was moreover decided to apply an enhanced QbD approach that also includes the following deliverables:

- Identify the material attributes and process parameters that can have an effect on product CQAs
- Determine the functional relationship that links material attributes and process parameters to product CQAs
- Use the enhanced product and process understanding in combination with Quality Risk Management (QRM) to establish an appropriate control strategy.

In consequence, knowledge collected during the pharmaceutical development studies supplies an essential scientific understanding for the implementation of design space, specifications, manufacturing controls, and quality risk management.

Quality risk management described in ICH Q9 document is useful to prioritize the list of potential CQAs and to identify the relevant ones [14]. Risk assessment, used in quality risk management, is also helpful to identify material attributes and process parameters that have an impact on product CQAs based on preliminary knowledge and experimental data (screening experiments). In the present case study, a Potential Risk Identification using Severity Matrix (PRISM) analysis was performed to guide the development. A priori risks related to raw material attributes and process parameters were listed and prioritized to design development studies. The API under development was a BCS class II compound. The modeling of the dissolution highlighted the API particle size as a potential CMA for the dissolution rate of the final DP. In the absence of ICH definition, a CMA can be described as a measurable characteristic of a starting material or raw material, whose variability has an impact on a CQA and therefore should be monitored or controlled to ensure the process produces the desired quality. Yu et al. especially mentioned that "drug substance, excipients, and in-process materials may have many CMAs" [15]. Other potential CMAs were indeed identified by the risk analysis such as the API flowability, which could impact feeding stability and therefore final product content uniformity.

Extensive material characterization was performed on each API batch in order to characterize the variability of the API physical attributes. However, as the drug substance (DS) manufacturing process was still under development, a limited variability had been observed between the API batches. The observed variability was moreover not necessarily representative of the future commercial process due to the diversification of API sources. In order to evaluate the impact of API variability on the CQAs and manufacturability, API batches having extreme properties based on the predicted biological activity were manufactured. These extreme batches were then used for process development. The impact of potential CMAs on the CQAs were studied together with the potential CPPs using design of experiments (DoEs). The API particle size being confirmed as a CMA, this material attribute, and the identified CPPs were included in the full line optimization DoE. The design space is defined in ICH Q8 as "the multidimensional combination and interaction

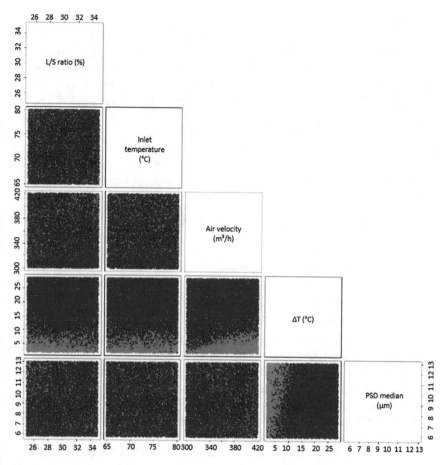

Fig. 1 Map of the probability of success over the experimental space for tablet assay. *Blue*: probability of success ≥0.95, *red*: probability of success <0.95

of input variables (e.g., material attributes) and process parameters that have been demonstrated to provide assurance of quality." Design space is commonly calculated based on process optimization results [16, 17]. The full line design space was defined based on DoE results as illustrated in Fig. 1. In this figure, each combination of process parameters is colored based on their probability of success. The design space corresponds to the blue areas. As seen in the picture, the product temperature (ΔT) is the main driver for the product assay, a low value resulting in a high risk of failure.

The generation of a design space as a sound development practice does not preclude or determine if a design space is included in the registration file. In this case, proven acceptance ranges (PAR) were extracted from the design space study for the registration file. As seen in the design space, the API particle size (PSD median), though being varied only within an acceptable range to ensure adequate biological activity, impacted the tablet assay to an extent that could lead to out-of-specification assay results. It is, however, not advantageous to reduce API specification for commercial manufacturing. The PAR was therefore defined to accommodate for all API batches by restricting the accepted process range. In this case, the design space contained but was not limited to the PAR [18].

In addition to the enhanced scientific understanding and PAR definition, the development of a design space was also used for control strategy with a real-time monitoring of impacting CPPs allowing to decrease end-product testing. A control strategy is defined in ICH Q10 guideline as "a planned set of controls, derived from current product and process understanding, that ensures process performance and product quality" ([12], p. 10). The controls included parameters and attributes related to drug substance and drug product:

- Control of the CMAs including API particle size
- Control of the CPPs
- Product specifications
- Control of critical manufacturing steps
- In-process analysis and control of the CQAs instead of end-product testing
- A planned maintenance to check the multivariate prediction models as the design space was considered for predicting some CQAs

As seen in this case study, applying an enhanced QbD approach during process development allowed identifying API CMAs with limited amount of materials and batches. The risk analysis combined with extensive material characterization identified the potential CMAs and their correlation. The inclusion of API batches manufactured to map the expected future variability in the DoEs then allowed to confirm the CMAs and to design a robust process that can accommodate for this variability. This is only the first step as the knowledge on the raw material CMAs should be continuously built during life cycle management as will be demonstrated in the fourth case study.

This first case study described the development of a new drug product. During development phases, the amount of API batches is limited and the batch-to-batch variability unknown. It is therefore difficult to identify relevant CMAs at this stage. Applying an enhanced QbD approach could nonetheless guide in an early identification of the CMAs.

3   Case 2: Accelerating Process Development Using Miniaturized Equipment

The previous case study used continuous manufacturing to reduce development time and material consumption. Process miniaturization can offer a valuable alternative to full-scale development to characterize raw materials, develop formulation, and run feasibility studies with reduced amount of materials. In the context of development acceleration and reduction of material consumption, a methodology using only 10 g of material has been developed to assess the suitability of a given formulation for roller compaction.

Roller compaction is a dry granulation process in which a blend containing active ingredients and excipients are agglomerated together, thanks to the mechanical stress applied by two rollers of a compactor and directly milled into granules afterward. The resulting granules can then be blended with an external phase prior to compression into tablets or prior to capsule filling. The aim of roller compaction is to increase powder flowability, prevent active ingredient segregation, and improve product stability while decreasing bulk volume.

The development of roller compaction processes is currently performed on pilot scale equipment. Despite best efforts in developing small-scale roller compactors, this approach still requires few kilograms of blend and therefore a corresponding amount of active ingredients that are not always available at the early development stage of a new drug product compound. The amount of materials required is even more significant when different blend compositions are investigated. Moreover, material conveying and powder adhesion to rollers' surface are additional challenges that need to be addressed before evaluating the compaction itself.

According to literature, in order to ensure complete granulation and therefore ensure suitable cohesiveness of the granules, roller compaction development should target [19] (a) a solid fraction of around 0.7 and (b) a tensile strength – defined by a three-point bending flexural test – of at least 1 MPa [20, 21]. Process parameters allowing to obtain these attributes can be generated by roller compaction studies. However, compaction simulators can also be used. In a first step, a compaction simulator equipped with force and displacement sensors on each punch is used, with a set of round flat punches, together with a semiautomatic tablet testing system to characterize the manufactured tablets. Therefore, two tablet attributes can easily and rapidly be evaluated:

1. The compressibility: the ability of a powder to decrease in volume under pressure – expressed as the solid fraction of the tablets as a function of the tableting compression.
2. The tabletability: the ability to form tablets of certain properties under pressure – expressed as the tensile strength of the tablets in function of the tableting compression.

A recent update of the Styl'One Evolution allows to mimic the roller compaction process parameters with uniaxial compaction of the powder to ribbon-like tablets – called ribblets – with a set of rectangular flat punches. This module, called RoCo Pack, uses a model based on the thin layer model described by Peter et al., as seen in Fig. 2 [23]. The model explains that in a roller compactor, the powder between the rolls is divided into thin layers that consist of a mass which remains constant during the process. The layers have a width determined by the roll width and a constant height. Only the length differs, depending on the position between the rolls, which decreases from the nip angle to the gap size. Considering this evolution of the layer length, the density of each layer evolves as well.

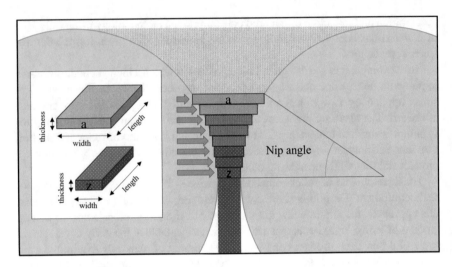

Fig. 2 Thin-layer model [23]

The evolution of the in-die density according to the applied compression along with the characteristics of the formulation allows to convert a hydraulic pressure (expressed in MPa) into a roll force per unit (expressed in kN/cm or MPa) and vice versa. That learning phase of the module allows then to manufacture ribblets corresponding to specific roller compaction process parameters.

The compaction assessment therefore uses the round flat punches to establish the compressibility and tabletability profiles, identifying the hydraulic compression force to apply on the blend to obtain (a) the suitable solid fraction and (b) the aimed diametrical-compression tensile strength. As said before, it is usually advised to target ribbons with a solid fraction of 0.7 and a three-point bending tensile strength of at least 1 MPa. Hilden et al. [24] showed a correspondence 1:2 between the diametrical compression tensile strength and the three-point bending tensile strength. Therefore the target of at least 0.5 MPa of diametrical tensile strength should be aimed. Finally, the RoCo Pack module is used with the rectangular flat punches to determine the hydraulic compression force corresponding to the roller compaction parameters (such as compaction force or gap size) on the equipment of interest.

In this study, the downscaling was performed from a roller compactor to the RoCo Pack for two in-house products and afterward with the 11.28-mm round flat punch in order to verify the miniaturization approach. This would indicate the targets in solid fraction and diametrical-compression tensile strength to aim for a new product using the tablet press simulator. If the approach if verified, the amount of material to be used for roller compaction feasibility and formulation development studies could be reduced from a few kilograms per blend to about 10 g.

Two in-house validated products have been used to develop this methodology: Product A, for which an external phase is added prior to tableting, and Product B, for which the granules are directly tableted. Three batches from those two products have been used, and homogenized blends have been sampled in the commercial facilities. Blends were characterized by true density using helium pycnometry.

For the RoCo Pack learning phase, blends were manually filled into the die cavity. This learning phase allowed to obtain the correspondence between hydraulic force and roll compaction process parameters. Ribblets were characterized in terms of mass and thickness. Once the learning phase was performed and the commercial process parameters (i.e., gap size and compaction force) were entered into the recipe, hydraulic pressures of 140 MPa and 42 MPa appeared to correspond for all batches of Product A and Product B, respectively.

For each blend, the compaction behavior was then characterized using the 1-compression mode provided as a default by manufacturer. At each compaction, 300 mg of powder was accurately weighed and was manually poured into the die cavity. Then, the powder was compacted with the pressure applied from the punch-die set. To correspond to the stress applied during roller compaction, a range of hydraulic pressure from 20 to 200 MPa has been investigated. At least three tablets per compression force have been manufactured. Tablets were characterized in terms of mass, hardness, and thickness. The envelop density (Eq. 1) and the tensile strength (Eq. 2) have been calculated for each tablet. Using the blend true density, the out-of-die solid fraction (Eq. 3) has been determined.

$$\text{Envelop density } \left(\frac{g}{mL}\right) = \frac{4 \times \text{Tablet masse (mg)}}{\pi \times \text{Diameter}^2 \text{ (mm)} \times \text{Thickness (mm)}} \tag{1}$$

$$\text{Solid fraction} = \frac{\text{Envelop density } \left(\frac{g}{mL}\right)}{\text{Preblend true density } \left(\frac{g}{mL}\right)} \tag{2}$$

$$\text{Tensile strength (MPa)} = \frac{2 \times \text{Tablet Hardness (N)}}{\pi \times \text{Tablet diameter (mm)} \times \text{Tablet thickness (mm)}} \tag{3}$$

Therefore, two tablet attributes can be evaluated: (a) the compressibility of the material, by plotting the solid fraction as a function of the compression applied, and (b) the tabletability of the material, by plotting the tensile strength in function of the compression applied.

The compressibility profiles of each batch of Product A and Product B are displayed in Fig. 3 by plotting the obtained round flat tablet solid fraction according to the compression applied. The compressibility profiles were fitted with a logarithmic trendline leading to a fitted $R^2 > 0.98$. This fitting was used to interpolate the solid fraction obtained at the hydraulic pressures estimated for both products. Solid fractions of 0.85 and 0.81 were obtained for Product A and Product B, respectively.

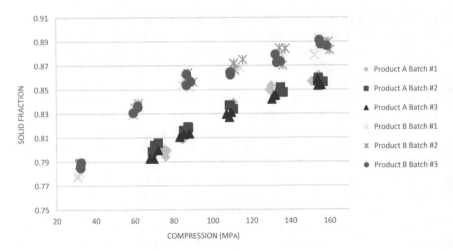

Fig. 3 Compressibility profiles of Product A and Product B

Compared to the reference value of 0.7 found in the literature, it was seen that higher solid fractions were needed to obtain appropriate cohesiveness for the products under investigation.

The tabletability profiles of each batch of Product A and Product B are displayed in Fig. 4 by plotting the obtained round flat tablet tensile strength according to the compression applied. The compressibility profiles were fitted with a linear trendline leading to a fitted $R^2 > 0.98$. This fitting was used to interpolate the tensile strength obtained at the hydraulic pressures estimated for both products. Diametrical compression tensile strengths of 0.52 MPa and 0.41 MPa were obtained for Product A and Product B, respectively. These values are aligned with the one mentioned in the introduction, taking into consideration that 0.5 MPa of diametrical compression tensile strength corresponds to 1 MPa of three-point bending tensile strength.

Through the characterization of the two in-house products via the Styl'One Evolution mounted with round flat tablets manufactured mimicking the commercial process, a solid fraction up to 0.85 and a diametrical-compression tensile strength around 0.5 MPa should be targeted to achieve cohesive ribblets. By miniaturizing the roller compaction process, it was possible to perform the early assessment of this process with only 10 g of blend per tested batch. This methodology could also be used to run feasibility studies for new chemical entities or formulation development rapidly and with minimum amount of materials. Also, the low amount of material required allows to assess different qualitative and quantitative compositions of blends before applying the optimal parameter conditions to a pilot-scale roller compactor. It is therefore well suited to evaluate the impact of various material attributes. It has nonetheless to be noticed that this miniaturization approach cannot anticipate feeding performance and potential powder adhesion to the roller's surface.

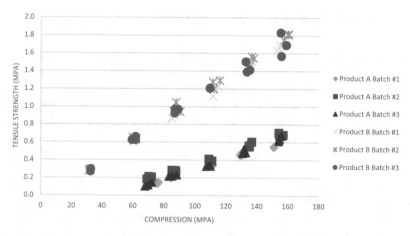

Fig. 4 Tabletability of Product A and Product B

4 Case 3: Coping with Batch-to-Batch Variability in Drug Product Process Improvement

This third case study describes the development of a new process for a commercial product. Process improvement and product extension are common during product life cycle. Existing processes might benefit from process improvement to reduce the cost of good and environmental footprint during product life cycle. Product extension can be considered to develop modified release forms to reduce pill burden. In both cases, the knowledge acquired during initial process development can be utilized to develop a robust improved process or a new formulation.

In the present case, the aim of the process change was to improve the drug product manufacturing process in order to reduce the cost of good. The original process was based on batch high shear wet granulation. Continuous twin-screw wet granulation was considered as an alternative to the batch process. Continuous manufacturing is indeed renowned for being more efficient, more flexible, and greener [13, 25–28]. The main challenges associated with the change of process from batch to continuous were the poor flowability of the API, its high drug load in the formulation, and its batch-to-batch variability which impact on the process was not fully understood. The aim was therefore to design a continuous process, keeping the same formulation and mitigating the impact of the API batch-to-batch variability on processability while ensuring consistent product quality attributes between the batch and the continuous process.

4.1 Identification of the API Variability

The first step toward designing a new and more robust drug product process was to better understand the API batch-to-batch variability. Raw materials indeed present slight variations of physical properties not only from manufacturer to manufacturer but also from batch to batch. In order to capture this variability and to then account for it during process development, a thorough material characterization should be performed on each batch of raw materials. The API was manufactured at different manufacturing sites and using different synthetic routes, crystallization, drying and delumping processes, and manufacturing equipment. The API manufacturing could be grouped into four processes called Processes 1, 2, 3, and 4 in this section. From the experience acquired on the batch drug product process, the API variability existed not only between but also within drug substance processes. The link between API characteristics and drug product manufacturability was, however, missing, leading to drug product process adjustments.

In recent years, scientific researches investigating the link between material attributes and process performance increased dramatically. Standardized approaches involving material science, particle engineering, and process development are indeed being developed to rationalize product development [1, 29] or guide process selection [20].

While historical studies usually based their conclusions on a few selected materials to investigate the impact of specific material attributes [30, 31], the current standard relies on the use of broad material databases and extensive material characterization [32–34]. These databases are then exploited using multivariate statistical analysis to select relevant materials and to link material attributes and process performance. This was especially done for twin-screw feeding [35–38], dry granulation [39], or compression processes [40] for instance. The end use is to predict the behavior of a new compound based on its characteristics or to guide the process selection.

This type of studies has demonstrated their relevance when comparing materials with large differences in terms of material attributes (e.g., cohesive APIs versus free-flowing excipients). It is, however, not suited to address the challenges related to batch-to-batch variability and to identify critical material attributes for a given compound. The methodology is nonetheless transferable, the material database being dedicated to a specific compound and no longer to multiple ones. It was successfully applied to excipients [41–43] but also API [44].

In this project, API batches were systematically characterized in terms of PSD, density, and agglomeration profile. Based on this initial database, eight API batches were selected for process screening, and four more were selected for process optimization. Three batches were selected from drug substance process 1 (P1/1-3), three from process 2 (P2/1-3), two from process 3 (P3/1-2), and three from process 4 (P4/1-3). All batches were within specifications in terms of purity, residual solvents, crystallinity, and polymorphism.

For all batches, the physical characterization was extended to better identify what characteristics are changing between batches and what variability is impacting the drug product process. The selected API batches were therefore characterized for PSD, density, compressibility, agglomeration profile, specific surface area, surface energy, electrostatic charging, angle of avalanche, and rheology. In total, 17 properties were measured for each API batch. Principal component analysis (PCA) was used to extract relevant information from this API database. The methodology is further detailed in a dedicated article [22]. The PCA consisted of three principal components (PCs) and explained 92.9% of the API variability. Figure 5 presents the PC1/PC2 and PC2/PC3 loading scatter plots. The first PC was related to crystal length, agglomerates, flowability, and electrostatic charging. The second PC was related to the span of the PSD and the agglomerate strength. Finally, the third PC was related to surface energy of the API.

The API batches could then be clustered using the corresponding score plots as seen in Fig. 6. It was, for instance, observed that the selected API batches from process 2 were characterized by larger particles and better flowability in opposition to the selected API batches from process 4.

4.2 Process Development

Thanks to the PCA, the API variability was quantified. The next step consisted of including this variability in the process development to ensure the development of a drug process that accounts for the API variability. The drug product consisted of an intra-granular phase and an extra-granular phase. The API represented 64% of the intra-granular phase explaining its prominent impact on processability. For each process step (i.e., feeding [45], granulation [46], drying, milling, final blending, and tableting), both the potential material attributes and the process parameters were included in the design of experiments. In order to quantify the impact of the API variability on process performance, the three PC scores associated to each API were used as quantitative factors to design and interpret process development trials. This allowed including the evaluated variability of the API properties with a limited number of uncorrelated factors.

During granulation screening for instance, the impact of the API variability was studied together with the screw speed and the liquid-to-solid (L/S) ratio. Thanks to this approach, the two first PCs were identified as potential CMA and the L/S ratio as a potential CPP. This information was then used to optimize the full manufacturing process (from pre-blend to tablet) applying the same approach [47]. As a result, a multistep design space including both the API CMAs and the CPPs was defined. The design space (in green in Fig. 7) demonstrated the ability to define process settings leading to conforming product CQAs regardless of the API characteristics. The design space was finally verified with external API batches.

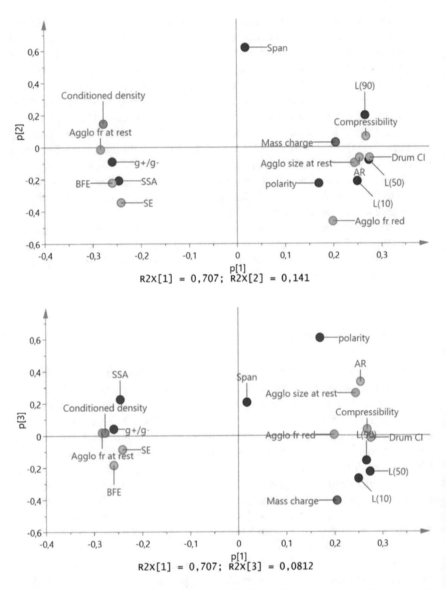

Fig. 5 PC1/PC2 and PC2/PC3 loading plots – colored according to properties characterized. In *blue*: PSD parameter, in *light blue*: agglomerate parameters, in orange: flowability parameters, in *purple*: surface parameters, in *red*: electrostatic charges, in *green*: density [22]

In this case study, the prior knowledge on API batch-to-batch variability was used to design a new process for an existing product. The existing characterization data were complemented for a selected number of API batches in order to identify potential CMAs. API batches were then enrolled in the process development studies

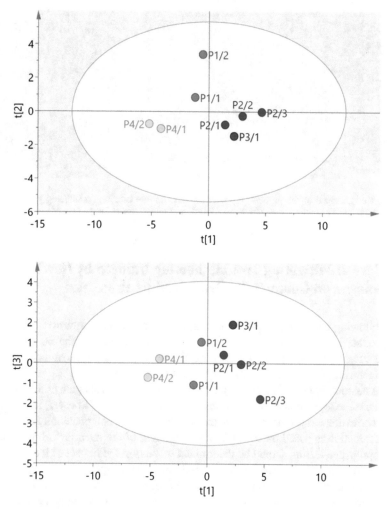

Fig. 6 PC1/PC2 and PC1/PC3 score plot – colored according to the drug substance process. In *green*: process 1, in *blue*: process 2, in *red*: process 3, in *yellow*: process 4 [22]

to link API properties to process and product performance. This approach allowed to design a robust DP process able to cope with the previously identified API batch-to-batch variability.

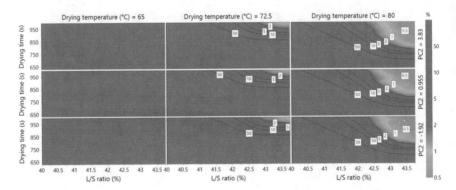

Fig. 7 Design space of the process line with a risk of failure of 1% guaranteeing granule LOD below 3.0%, dryer air flow deviation below 5.0%, and tablet press punch displacement deviation below 0.5% [47]

5   Case 4: Mitigating Troubleshooting Induced by New API Sources on Commercial Drug Product Processes

The following case study focuses on examples of a continual improvement across the product life cycle of a commercial drug product, namely, the new sourcing of the drug substance (DS). Indeed, the development and improvement of API manufacturing process usually continue over its life cycle.

The outsourcing of API manufacturing has several objectives such as the capacity and market extension and the reduction of the cost of good. However, any change should be evaluated for the impact on the quality of the DS and potentially on the DP. This evaluation is based on scientific understanding of the manufacturing process, and appropriate testing should be determined to analyze the impact of the proposed change. Studies should therefore be carried out to demonstrate the equivalence of the sources, usually by comparing the new API source to a reference material. Thus, no influence on DP process and quality should be expected. While this comparison should at least be based on specifications, including relevant material properties that affect the DP process is key to mitigate future troubleshooting. This type of evaluation is even more complex as processability differences often result from a combination of multiple API properties (e.g., granulometry, surface properties, etc.) as highlighted in the previous case study. In extreme cases, DP process adjustment is performed to cope with the new properties of the new API source.

5.1   Impact of Storage Conditions and Shipment

The first example concerns a drug substance A in the form of powder. The drug product process was a dry granulation followed by tableting leading to coated tablets. The drug product contained 90% of DS. The DS properties are then critical and drive the drug product quality. DS A has involved multiple external partners worldwide since the launch of the medicine and has been supplied using different chemical synthetic pathways. One source in particular led to difficulties during the DP process compared to the others. Even though studies demonstrate the equivalence in terms of chemical properties and impurity profile and meet the specification, some observations were reported on the physical behavior of the powder. The manufacturing team especially reported difficulties to load the mixer (5 h loading time instead of 1 h30) because of the tendency of the DS to agglomerate. For this reason, a crushing step was added to the process. Then, the compression step required more adjustments (distributor speed, pre-compression force, compression speed) than usual because of a variability of the tablet mass and a nonconforming friability of the tablets. These adjustments depended on the DS batch due to batch-to-batch variability.

Studies were performed to better understand the behavior of the DS powder. Many factors can be involved: the synthesis pathway, the packaging quality, the type of shipment (i.e., boat, plane), the time of storage (i.e., at supplier site, during transition, at manufacturing site), and the condition of storage (i.e., temperature and relative humidity). During the investigation, the physical properties – PSD, densities, compressibility profile, and mechanical properties – were assessed to identify the physical characteristics varying between batches and sources. The hardness of the DS powder was identified as the main difference between DS batches. The hardness was measured on tablets manufactured with the pure DS by using a tablet tester.

Figure 8 illustrates the compressibility profiles of 12 DS A batches coming from the same supplier. It was seen that the hardness of the DS can vary from 28 to 65 N in the compression range (i.e., 2500–3100 daN).

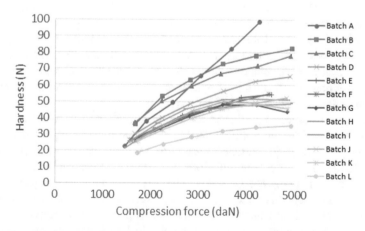

Fig. 8 Compressibility profiles of several DS A batches from the same supplier colored by DS batch

As dry granulation precedes the tableting, it mitigates the difference in terms of tabletability and standardizes the final blend. However, when the hardness of the DS was too low, significant differences in terms of tabletability persisted (tablet hardness and friability typically).

Though the impact of storage conditions is mostly reported for deliquescent drugs [48] or amorphous solid dispersion [49], crystal defects can also induce water sorption of crystalline powders [50] with a direct impact on their physical behavior. To better understand potential causes of the variations between the DS batches, the impact of shipment and storage was then investigated. Storage conditions (temperature and humidity) were found to be highly variable in the warehouse and intermediate storage locations. The variations were even more impacted by the type of shipment (boat or plane). Storage tests were performed by exposing the DS powder in open dish to a variation of temperature and humidity. As expected, variation in storage conditions was found to impact the PSD, particle shape, and hardness. After prolonged storage at 40 °C and 75% RH, the particle size had increased; the powder particles presented smoother edges and looked transparent. Finally, the hardness decreased after exposure to stress conditions.

This case study highlighted that even if the equivalence between the different sources is demonstrated, the impact of storage conditions on DS physical properties is key for the drug product performance.

5.2 Apparition of a New Polymorphic Form

The second example concerns drug substance B, which is also a powder. The drug product was a coated tablet manufactured via direct compression. The drug load was 90%; the DS physical properties were therefore again critical for the DP process. Deviations in tablet thickness and hardness were reported by the manufacturing team leading to out-of-specifications. An investigation was triggered to understand and resolve the issue and implement preventive actions. In view of the high drug load, DS batches were withdrawn and analyzed for PSD, densities, microscopy, X-ray powder diffraction, compressibility behavior, and mechanical properties.

Figure 9 presents the results of optical microscopy for a reference batch (left) and one of the batches under investigation (right).

The optical microscopy allowed to observe a difference in terms of particle opacity. The particles from the reference batch were transparent, whereas a mix of transparent and opaque particles was observed for the batch under investigation.

In addition, another polymorphic form was detected in the batches under investigation, and so not only one form was present but also a mix of two polymorphic forms in the powder. This change of polymorphism means a difference in molecular rearrangements and consequently a modification of particulate properties.

The next step was then to study the mechanical properties and especially the consolidation behavior of the DS (Fig. 10).

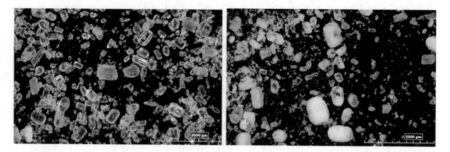

Fig. 9 Optical microscopy of a reference batch (left) versus a batch under investigation (right)

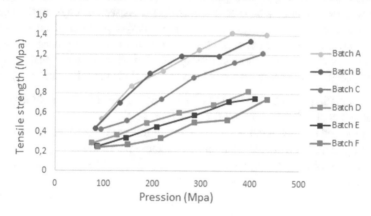

Fig. 10 Tabletability of various DS batches. In orange and red: DS batches under investigation. In green: reference DS batches

Figure 10 represents the tensile strength according to the compression pressure. The DS batches under investigation (in *orange/red*) presented a higher tensile strength at a given compression pressure compared to the reference batches (in *green*) and were therefore more cohesive. Moreover, the brittleness of the particles was estimated using Heckel equation [51, 52] showing lower brittleness of the batches under investigation.

As a conclusion, the investigation allowed to highlight a new polymorphic form that impacted the physical properties of the DS and therefore the manufacturability of the DP. Identifying the source of the apparition of this new polymorphic form will be critical to solve the issue on tableting.

6 Conclusions

This chapter addressed the challenges associated with material attributes during drug product process development and life cycle. As seen in the first case study, material availability and variability are very limited during process development. It is, however, possible to start developing the knowledge around material attributes by applying an enhanced quality-by-design approach. In the second case study, process miniaturization was applied to a roller compaction process, allowing the determination of relevant material attributes for process development and enabling process acceleration and reduction of API consumption. In the third case study, the knowledge acquired about an API variability was utilized to develop a more robust drug product process that is able to cope for this variability. The last case study showed challenges related to life cycle management of a drug product. Batch-to-batch variability indeed evolves by the introduction of new sources that can have a dramatic impact on drug product performance. A targeted material characterization shows to be key to anticipate process adjustments. As seen throughout the chapter, material science should not only be considered at development level but also should play an active role during the entire life of a product to ensure process robustness and therefore an improved product quality and undisturbed supply chains to meet patients' needs. Good practices should therefore include the following:

- A systematic identification of API CMAs, not only in regard to product specifications but also CMAs relevant for the DP process.
- Harmonized characterization guidance for all raw materials since the start of the development, allowing the creation of a database per product.
- Targeted studies allowing to understand the interplay between drug substance properties and drug product process.

References

1. Beg S, Robaian MA, Rahman M, et al (2020) Pharmaceutical drug product development and process optimization: effective use of quality by design. CRC Press
2. International Conference on Harmonisation of Technical Requirements for Registration of Pharmaceuticals for Human Use, Requirements for Registration of Pharmaceuticals for Human Use (2009) Q8(R2): Pharmaceutical Development
3. Capece M, Ho R, Strong J, Gao P (2015) Prediction of powder flow performance using a multi-component granular Bond number. Powder Technol 286:561–571. doi: https://doi.org/10.1016/j.powtec.2015.08.031
4. Pasha M, Hekiem NL, Jia X, Ghadiri M (2020) Prediction of flowability of cohesive powder mixtures at high strain rate conditions by discrete element method. Powder Technol 372:59–67. doi: https://doi.org/10.1016/j.powtec.2020.05.110
5. Williams DR (2015) Particle engineering in pharmaceutical solids processing: surface energy considerations. Curr Pharm Des 21:2677–2694. doi: https://doi.org/10.2174/1381612821666150416100319
6. Hodges CS, Looi L, Cleaver JAS, Ghadiri M (2004) Use of the JKR model for calculating adhesion between rough surfaces. Langmuir 20:9571–9576. doi: https://doi.org/10.1021/la035790f
7. Allen T (2003) Powder Sampling and Particle Size Determination 1st Edition. Elsevier
8. Ogata K (2019) A review: recent progress on evaluation of flowability and floodability of powder. KONA Powder and Particle Journal 36:33–49

9. Jain S (1999) Mechanical properties of powders for compaction and tableting: an overview. Pharm Sci Technol Today 2:20–31. doi: https://doi.org/10.1016/S1461-5347(98)00111-4
10. Zafar U, Vivacqua V, Calvert G, et al (2017) A review of bulk powder caking. Powder Technol 313:389–401. doi: https://doi.org/10.1016/j.powtec.2017.02.024
11. Bell TA (2005) Challenges in the scale-up of particulate processes—an industrial perspective. Powder Technol 150:60–71. doi: https://doi.org/10.1016/j.powtec.2004.11.023
12. International Conference on Harmonisation of Technical Requirements for Registration of Pharmaceuticals for Human Use (2008) Guidance for Industry Q10: Pharmaceutical Quality System
13. Vervaet C, Vercruysse J, Remon JP, Beer TD (2013) Continuous Processing of Pharmaceuticals. In: Encyclopedia of Pharmaceutical Science and Technology, Fourth Edition. Taylor & Francis, pp 644–655
14. International Conference on Harmonisation of Technical Requirements for Registration of Pharmaceuticals for Human Use (2006) Guidance for Industry Q9 Quality Risk Management
15. Yu LX, Amidon G, Khan MA, et al (2014) Understanding pharmaceutical quality by design. AAPS J 16:771–783. doi: https://doi.org/10.1208/s12248-014-9598-3
16. Chavez P-F, Lebrun P, Sacré P-Y, et al (2015) Optimization of a pharmaceutical tablet formulation based on a design space approach and using vibrational spectroscopy as PAT tool. Int J Pharm 486:13–20. doi: https://doi.org/10.1016/j.ijpharm.2015.03.025
17. Lebrun P, Krier F, Mantanus J, et al (2012) Design space approach in the optimization of the spray-drying process. Eur J Pharm Biopharm 80:226–234. doi: https://doi.org/10.1016/j.ejpb.2011.09.014
18. Garcia T, Cook G, Nosal R (2008) PQLI key topics - criticality, design space, and control strategy. J Pharm Innov 3:60–68. doi: https://doi.org/10.1007/s12247-008-9032-4
19. Qiu Y, Chen Y, Zhang GGZ, et al (2016) Developing solid oral dosage forms: pharmaceutical theory and practice. Academic Press
20. Leane M, Pitt K, Reynolds G, Group TMCS (MCS) W (2015) A proposal for a drug product Manufacturing Classification System (MCS) for oral solid dosage forms. Pharm Dev Technol 20:12–21. doi: https://doi.org/10.3109/10837450.2014.954728
21. Leane M, Pitt K, Reynolds GK, et al (2018) Manufacturing classification system in the real world: factors influencing manufacturing process choices for filed commercial oral solid dosage formulations, case studies from industry and considerations for continuous processing. Pharm Dev Technol 23:964–977. doi: https://doi.org/10.1080/10837450.2018.1534863
22. Stauffer F, Vanhoorne V, Pilcer G, et al (2018) Raw material variability of an active pharmaceutical ingredient and its relevance for processability in secondary continuous pharmaceutical manufacturing. Eur J Pharm Biopharm 127:92–103. doi: https://doi.org/10.1016/j.ejpb.2018.02.017
23. Peter S, Lammens RF, Steffens K-J (2010) Roller compaction/Dry granulation: Use of the thin layer model for predicting densities and forces during roller compaction. Powder Technol 199:165–175. doi: https://doi.org/10.1016/j.powtec.2010.01.002
24. Hilden J, Polizzi M, Zettler A (2017) Note on the use of diametrical compression to determine tablet tensile strength. J Pharm Sci 106:418–421. doi: https://doi.org/10.1016/j.xphs.2016.08.004
25. Betz G, Junker-Bürgin P, Leuenberger H (2003) Batch and continuous processing in the production of pharmaceutical granules. Pharm Dev Technol 8:289–297. doi: https://doi.org/10.1081/PDT-120022157
26. Leuenberger H (2001) New trends in the production of pharmaceutical granules: batch versus continuous processing. Eur J Pharm Biopharm 52:289–296. doi: https://doi.org/10.1016/S0939-6411(01)00199-0
27. Matsunami K, Miyano T, Arai H, et al (2018) Decision support method for the choice between batch and continuous technologies in solid drug product manufacturing. Ind Eng Chem Res 57:9798–9809. doi: https://doi.org/10.1021/acs.iecr.7b05230
28. Vanhoorne V, Vervaet C (2020) Recent progress in continuous manufacturing of oral solid dosage forms. Int J Pharm 579:119194. doi: https://doi.org/10.1016/j.ijpharm.2020.119194

29. Hsiao W-K, Hörmann TR, Toson P, et al (2020) Feeding of particle-based materials in continuous solid dosage manufacturing: a material science perspective. Drug Discov Today 25:800–806. doi: https://doi.org/10.1016/j.drudis.2020.01.013

30. Herting MG, Kleinebudde P (2007) Roll compaction/dry granulation: Effect of raw material particle size on granule and tablet properties. Int J Pharm 338:110–118. doi: https://doi.org/10.1016/j.ijpharm.2007.01.035

31. Ohta M, Buckton G (2004) Determination of the changes in surface energetics of cefditoren pivoxil as a consequence of processing induced disorder and equilibration to different relative humidities. Int J Pharm 269:81–88. doi: https://doi.org/10.1016/j.ijpharm.2003.08.015

32. Benedetti A, Khoo J, Sharma S, et al (2019) Data analytics on raw material properties to accelerate pharmaceutical drug development. Int J Pharm 563:122–134. doi: https://doi.org/10.1016/j.ijpharm.2019.04.002

33. Escotet-Espinoza MS, Moghtadernejad S, Scicolone J, et al (2018) Using a material property library to find surrogate materials for pharmaceutical process development. Powder Technol 339:659–676. doi: https://doi.org/10.1016/j.powtec.2018.08.042

34. Van Snick B, Dhondt J, Pandelaere K, et al (2018a) A multivariate raw material property database to facilitate drug product development and enable in-silico design of pharmaceutical dry powder processes. Int J Pharm 549:415–435. doi: https://doi.org/10.1016/j.ijpharm.2018.08.014

35. Beretta M, Hörmann TR, Hainz P, et al (2020) Investigation into powder tribo-charging of pharmaceuticals. Part I: Process-induced charge via twin-screw feeding. Int J Pharm 591:120014. doi: https://doi.org/10.1016/j.ijpharm.2020.120014

36. Bostijn N, Dhondt J, Ryckaert A, et al (2019) A multivariate approach to predict the volumetric and gravimetric feeding behavior of a low feed rate feeder based on raw material properties. Int J Pharm 557:342–353. doi: https://doi.org/10.1016/j.ijpharm.2018.12.066

37. El Kassem B, Heider Y, Brinz T, Markert B (2020) A multivariate statistical approach to analyze the impact of material attributes and process parameters on the quality performance of an auger dosing process. J Drug Deliv Sci Technol 60:101950. doi: https://doi.org/10.1016/j.jddst.2020.101950

38. Van Snick B, Kumar A, Verstraeten M, et al (2018c) Impact of material properties and process variables on the residence time distribution in twin screw feeding equipment. Int J Pharm. doi: https://doi.org/10.1016/j.ijpharm.2018.11.076

39. Yu J, Xu B, Zhang K, et al (2019) Using a material library to understand the impacts of raw material properties on ribbon quality in roll compaction. Pharmaceutics 11:662. doi: https://doi.org/10.3390/pharmaceutics11120662

40. Van Snick B, Grymonpré W, Dhondt J, et al (2018b) Impact of blend properties on die filling during tableting. Int J Pharm 549:476–488. doi: https://doi.org/10.1016/j.ijpharm.2018.08.015

41. Albers J, Knop K, Kleinebudde P (2006) Brand-to-brand and batch-to-batch uniformity of microcrystalline cellulose in direct tableting with a pneumohydraulic tablet press. Pharm Ind 68:1420–1428

42. Fonteyne M, Correia A, De Plecker S, et al (2015) Impact of microcrystalline cellulose material attributes: A case study on continuous twin screw granulation. Int J Pharm 478:705–717. doi: https://doi.org/10.1016/j.ijpharm.2014.11.070

43. Thoorens G, Krier F, Rozet E, et al (2015) Understanding the impact of microcrystalline cellulose physicochemical properties on tabletability. Int J Pharm 490:47–54. doi: https://doi.org/10.1016/j.ijpharm.2015.05.026

44. Vippagunta RR, LoBrutto R, Pan C, Lakshman JP (2010) Investigation of Metformin HCl Lot-to-Lot Variation on Flowability Differences Exhibited during Drug Product Processing. J Pharm Sci 99:5030–5039. doi: https://doi.org/10.1002/jps.22207

45. Stauffer F, Vanhoorne V, Pilcer G, et al (2019a) Managing active pharmaceutical ingredient raw material variability during twin-screw blend feeding. Eur J Pharm Biopharm 135:49–60. doi: https://doi.org/10.1016/j.ejpb.2018.12.012

46. Stauffer F, Vanhoorne V, Pilcer G, et al (2019b) Managing API raw material variability during continuous twin-screw wet granulation. Int J Pharm 561:265–273. doi: https://doi.org/10.1016/j.ijpharm.2019.03.012

47. Stauffer F, Vanhoorne V, Pilcer G, et al (2019c) Managing API raw material variability in a continuous manufacturing line – Prediction of process robustness. Int J Pharm 569:118525. doi: https://doi.org/10.1016/j.ijpharm.2019.118525

48. Stoklosa AM, Lipasek RA, Taylor LS, Mauer LJ (2012) Effects of storage conditions, formulation, and particle size on moisture sorption and flowability of powders: A study of deliquescent ingredient blends. Food Res Int 49:783–791. doi: https://doi.org/10.1016/j.foodres.2012.09.034

49. Shishir MRI, Taip FS, Saifullah MD, et al (2017) Effect of packaging materials and storage temperature on the retention of physicochemical properties of vacuum packed pink guava powder. Food Packag Shelf Life 12:83–90. doi: https://doi.org/10.1016/j.fpsl.2017.04.003

50. Ward GH, Schultz RK (1995) Process-induced crystallinity changes in albuterol sulfate and its effect on powder physical stability. Pharm Res 12:773–779. doi: https://doi.org/10.1023/A:1016232230638

51. Heckel R. W. (1961a) An analysis of powder compaction phenomena. Trans Metall Soc AIME 1001–1008

52. Heckel R. W. (1961b) Density-pressure relationships in powder compaction. Trans Metall Soc AIME 671–675

Printed in the United States
by Baker & Taylor Publisher Services